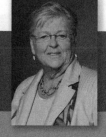

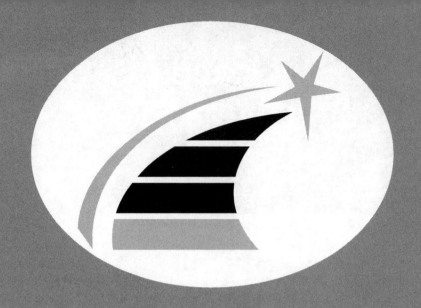

Step 1: Learn

"A journey of a thousand miles begins with a single step."

— Lao-tzu

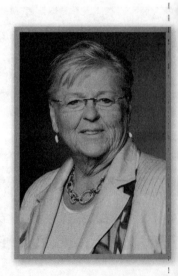

Congratulations! You are embarking on an exciting and rewarding career, and you have taken a great first step. Coding is a career that gives you a chance to pursue excellence at a variety of levels, and I am happy that you have chosen to start with my *Step* line of products. As a lifelong coder and educator, I am dedicated to giving you the tools you need to succeed. ***So, get out there and code!***

— Carol J. Buck, MS, CPC, CPC-H, CCS-P

Track your progress!

**See the checklist in the back of this book
to learn more about your next step toward coding success!**

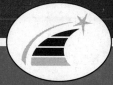
2014
STEP-BY-STEP
MEDICAL CODING

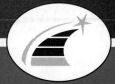

2014

STEP-BY-STEP

MEDICAL CODING

Carol J. Buck
MS, CPC, CPC-H, CCS-P

Former Program Director
Medical Secretary Programs
Northwest Technical College
East Grand Forks, Minnesota

ELSEVIER

3251 Riverport Lane
St. Louis, Missouri 63043

WORKBOOK FOR STEP-BY-STEP MEDICAL CODING,   ISBN: 978-1-4557-4630-9
2014 EDITION

ISBN: 978-1-4557-4630-9

Content Strategy Director: Jeanne R. Olson
Senior Content Development Specialist: Joshua S. Rapplean
Publishing Services Manager: Pat Joiner
Project Manager: Lisa A. P. Bushey
Senior Designer: Amy Buxton

Printed in the United States of America

Last digit is the print number: 9   8   7   6   5   4   3   2   1

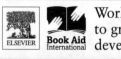

Development of This Edition

LEAD TECHNICAL COLLABORATOR

Jacqueline Klitz Grass, MA, CPC
Coding and Reimbursement Specialist
Grand Forks, North Dakota

QUERY MANAGER

Patricia Cordy Henricksen, MS, CHCA, CPC-I, CPC, CCP-P, ASC-PCS
Auditing and Coding Educator
Soterian Medical Services
Lexington, Kentucky

SENIOR COLLABORATOR AND ICD-10-CM CONSULTANT

Nancy Maguire, ACS, CRT, PCS, FCS, HCS-D, APC, AFC
Physician Consultant for Auditing and Education
Winchester, Virginia

ICD-10-CM CONSULTANT

Kathy Buchda, CPC, CPMA
Revenue Recognition
New Richmond, Wisconsin

EDITORIAL REVIEW BOARD

Monique Andrews-Ferguson, CPC
Associate Director, Revenue Cycle Operations
University of Chicago Physicians Group
Chicago, Illinois

Deborah Bennett, CCS-P, AA, BS
Medical Coder
Cleveland, Ohio

**Diane Roche Benson, CMA (AAMA), BSHCA, MSA, CFP, CPC,
CMRS, NSC-SCFAT, ASE, CDE, AHA BCLS/First Aid-Instructor,
PALS, ACLS, CCT, NCI-I**
Professor
Wake Technical Community College
Raleigh, North Carolina
Johnston Community College
Smithfield, North Carolina
University of Phoenix
Phoenix, Arizona

Patricia A. Cox, CPC, CPC-H, CPMA, CPC-I, CEMC, CCS-P
Director of Coding, Compliance and Credentialing
Riverside Medical Group
Owner
Pat Cox Professional Medical Education
Gloucester, Virginia

Diane S. Friedman, RHIA
Retired Educator
Tamarac, Florida

Donna Fuchs, CPC, RMA
Medical Instructor
Arnold, Missouri

Mary Lou Hilbert, MBA, RHIT, LHRM
Program Manager
Medical Coding and Billing and Health Information Technology
Seminole State College of Florida
Altamonte Springs, Florida

Janice Manning, MBA, CPC, CMRS
Program Chair, Medical Insurance Specialist
Baker College of Michigan, Jackson Campus
Jackson, Michigan

Genieve Nottage, MBA, BSHA, CPC-I, CPMA, CMRS, CMBS
CEO/Owner
Chronicles Billing Inc.
Stockbridge, Georgia

Kathy O'Brien, MBA-HM, CPC, CPC-H
Allied Health Instructor
Brown Mackie College
Fenton, Missouri

Sharon J. Oliver, CPC, CPC-I, CPMA
Senior Inpatient Coder
East Tennessee State University Physicians & Associates
Johnson City, Tennessee

Letitia Patterson, MPA, CPC, CCS-P
Consultant
A Coder's Resource
Chicago, Illinois

Terri Pizzano, MBA Mkt, CHTS-IM & TR
Owner
Pizzano Consulting, LLC
Clinical Applications Project Manager
Educator and Instructional Designer
Indianapolis, Indiana

Mary Lynn Taylor, MA-HIM, CMS, CPC, CPC-I
CEO
Professional Coding Services
Fairbanks, Alaska

LET THIS BE YOUR GOAL:

People who have accomplished worthwhile [goals] have had a very high sense of the way to do things. They have not been content with mediocrity. They have not confined themselves to the beaten tracks; they have never been satisfied to do things just as others do them, but always a little better. They always pushed things that came to their hands a little higher up, a little farther on. It is this little higher up, this little farther on, that counts in the quality of life's work. It is the constant effort to be first class in everything one attempts that conquers the heights of excellence.

Orison Swett Marden

This *Workbook* has been developed to assist you in the application of the theoretical and practical coding knowledge presented in the textbook *Step-by-Step Medical Coding*. The *Workbook* parallels the textbook with presentation of Chapters 1 through 31 and includes ample opportunity to practice the skill of medical coding. The *Workbook* contains three levels of questions—theory, abbreviated patient service and diagnosis descriptions, and original reports. The first level of question is the theory question; these questions are fill-in-the-blanks, multiple choice, true or false, and matching and often include medical terminology based on the specific area of coding presented in the coding manuals. The theory information serves as the foundational knowledge necessary to correctly code services and diagnoses. The second level of question is the abbreviated patient service and diagnosis descriptions; these questions begin the practical application of coding. The descriptions are condensed statements that provide broad-based coding experience. The final level is presented at the end of each *Workbook* chapter and contains reports that represent more complex services and diagnosis descriptions, such as operative, pathology, radiology, and emergency services.

The format for the answers has been developed to guide you in the development of your coding ability by using a format that includes four response variations:

- **One answer blank** for coding questions that require one code for the answer
- **Multiple answer blanks** for coding questions that require more than one code for the answer
- Key terms next to the blank(s) to guide you through the most difficult coding scenarios
- **Answer blanks with ☺ preceding the blank to indicate that you must decide the number of codes necessary to correctly answer the question**

Appendix B of the *Workbook* contains the answers to the odd-numbered questions, and the full answer key is available only in the TEACH Instructor Resources on Evolve. It is very important that you first complete the questions and then check your answers. The skill of medical coding can be acquired only through practice and by learning from mistakes that we all make along the way. It is from the understanding of why a service or diagnosis is coded in a certain way that you will develop a strong foundation that will serve you well throughout your coding career. Always take the time to read each code description fully, all notes connected with the code, and any applicable guidelines.

It is my sincere hope that you find the material presented in the *Workbook* challenging, enlightening, and worth your time and effort. Do your very best, and it will show in the quality of your work.

Carol J. Buck, MS, CPC, CPC-H, CCS-P

Some of the CPT code descriptions for physician services include physician extender services. Physician extenders, such as nurse practitioners, physician assistants, and nurse anesthetists, etc., provide medical services typically performed by a physician. Within this educational material the term "physician" may include "and other qualified health care professionals" depending on the code. Refer to the official CPT® code descriptions and guidelines to determine codes that are appropriate to report services provided by non-physician practitioners.

Contents

Some of the CPT code descriptions for physician services include physician extender services. Physician extenders, such as nurse practitioners, physician assistants, and nurse anesthetists, etc., provide medical services typically performed by a physician. Within this educational material the term "physician" may include "and other qualified health care professionals" depending on the code. Refer to the official CPT® code descriptions and guidelines to determine codes that are appropriate to report services provided by non-physician practitioners.

CHAPTER 1

Reimbursement, HIPAA, and Compliance

THEORY

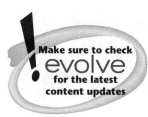

Without the use of reference material, answer the following:

1. What two groups of persons were added to those eligible for Medicare benefits after the initial establishment of the Medicare program?

   a. _persons eligible for disability benefits from social security_

   b. _permanent kidney failure_

2. To what government organization did the Secretary of the Department of Health and Human Services delegate the responsibility for administering the Medicare program?

   CMS

3. What government organization handles the funds for the Medicare program?

   Social security administration

4. There are three items that Medicare beneficiaries are responsible for paying before Medicare will begin to pay for services. What are these three items? _deductible_ , _premiums_ , and _coinsurance_

5. Medicare publishes the Medicare fee schedule and usually pays what percentage of the amounts indicated for services? _80%_

6. The three components of work, overhead (practice expense), and malpractice are part of an RVU. What do the initials RVU stand for?

   relative value unit

Odd-numbered answers are located in Appendix B, while the full answer key is only available in the TEACH Instructor Resources on Evolve.

7. According to the filing guidelines, providers must file claims for their

   Medicare patients within ____12____ months of the date of service.

8. What editions of the *Federal Register* would the outpatient facilities be interested in?

   ____November____ and ____december____

9. Under what act was a major change in Medicare in 1989 made possible?

   ____OBRA____

10. Can a physician charge a patient to complete a Medicare form?

    ____No____

11. Individuals covered under Medicare are termed ____beneficiaries____.

12. The ____MAC____ _____ _____
    do the paperwork for Medicare and are usually insurance companies
    that have bid for a contract with CMS to handle the Medicare program
    for a specific area.

13. Medicare Part C is also known as ____medicare advantage____.

14. HIPAA stands for ____health insurance____
    ____portability and accountability act____

15. The most major change to the health care industry as a result of HIPAA

    was as a result of what portion of the act? ____administrative____
    ____simplification____

16. The transfer of electronic documentation is accomplished through the

    use of ____electronic____ ____data____ Interchange technology.

17. The number that is assigned to all providers as a result of HIPAA:

    ____National____ ____provider____ Identification

18. Under the Relative Value Unit system, ____unit____ values are
    assigned to each service and are determined on the basis of the
    resources necessary to the physician's performance of the service.

19. The ____limiting____ charge historically was specific for each
    physician, but in 1993, the charge for a service was the same for all
    physicians within a locality, regardless of the specialty.

Odd-numbered answers are located in Appendix B, while the full answer key is only available in the TEACH Instructor Resources on Evolve.

20. For co-surgeons, Medicare pays the lesser of the actual charge or

    _____125_____% of the global fee, dividing the payment equally between the two surgeons.

21. Specific regulations for Medicare are contained in the

    _____Internet_____ _____only_____ Manual.

22. Within an HMO, there is usually an individual who has been assigned to monitor the services provided to the patient both inside the facility and outside the facility. This person is known as the

    _____gatekeeper_____.

23. In this model of HMO, the HMO directly employs the physicians.

    _____Staff_____ Model

24. In this model of HMO, the HMO contracts with the physician to provide the service at a set fee. This organization is known as

    _____Individual_____ _____practice_____ Associations.

25. An all-inclusive care program for the elderly that provides a comprehensive package of services that permits the client to continue

    to live at home is known as _____Program_____ for

    _____all_____-_____inclusive_____ Care for the Elderly (PACE).

Odd-numbered answers are located in Appendix B, while the full answer key is only available in the TEACH Instructor Resources on Evolve.

An Overview of ICD-10-CM

THEORY

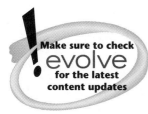

Make sure to check evolve for the latest content updates

Answer the following questions about the Overview of ICD-10-CM:

1. I-10 replaces I-9 Volumes 1 and 2.

   True   False

2. Mapping is a type of crosswalk to find corresponding diagnosis codes between I-9 and I-10.

   True   False

3. ICD-10 is widely used in Europe.

   True   False

4. The National Center for Health Statistics is responsible for the disease classification system (Volumes 1 and 2) in the United States.

   True   False

5. The 10th revision of the International Classification of Diseases (ICD-10) was issued in 1989 by the World Health Organization.

   True   False

6. The latest update for ICD-10-CM was in 2009.

   True   False

7. The implementation date for ICD-10-CM is October 1, 2014.

   True   False

8. The ICD-10-CM contains 20 chapters.

   True   False

Odd-numbered answers are located in Appendix B, while the full answer key is only available in the TEACH Instructor Resources on Evolve.

9. All I-10 codes start with a letter sand can have as many as 7 characters.

    True   False

10. GEMs refers to mapping files that crosswalk ICD-9-CM to ICD-10-CM and ICD-10-CM to ICD-9-CM.

    True   False

CHAPTER 2 ■ An Overview of ICD-10-CM

PRACTICAL

Using the I-9 to I-10 GEMs file, map the following codes:

11. 401.9 _____

12. V30.00 _____

13. 787.01 _____

14. 174.9 _____

15. E875.1 _____

16. 789.02 _____

    a. C50.919

    b. R11.2

    c. Y64.1

    d. Z38.00

    e. R10.12

    f. I10

Using the I-10 to I-9 GEMs file, map the following codes:

17. A07.3 _____

18. N13.721 _____

19. Z98.810 _____

20. M25.841 _____

21. H81.8x9 _____

22. E13.610 _____

    a. 593.71

    b. 719.84

    c. 250.60

    d. 007.2

    e. 386.8

    f. V49.82

Odd-numbered answers are located in Appendix B, while the full answer key is only available in the TEACH Instructor Resources on Evolve.

Copyright © 2014 by Saunders, an imprint of Elsevier Inc. All rights reserved.

CHAPTER 3

ICD-10-CM Outpatient Coding and Reporting Guidelines

THEORY

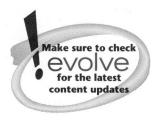

Using a current copy of the ICD-10-CM Guidelines for Coding and Reporting for Outpatient Services, *answer the following questions:*

1. Section IV Diagnostic Coding and Reporting Guidelines for Outpatient Services take precedence over the general and disease specific guidelines.

   True   False

2. Always begin the search for the correct code assignment in the Alphabetic Index.

   True   False

3. When a patient presents for outpatient surgery and the surgery is canceled, report the reason why the surgery was canceled as the first-listed diagnosis.

   True   False

4. The codes from A00 through Z99 are always reported as first-listed diagnoses.

   True   False

5. When a final diagnosis has not been established by the provider, it is acceptable to report codes for the presenting signs and symptoms.

   True   False

6. External Cause codes are located in the Alphabetical Index for Diseases under External Causes.

   True   False

Odd-numbered answers are located in Appendix B, while the full answer key is only available in the TEACH Instructor Resources on Evolve.

7. Report all conditions that coexist, even if they are not addressed or do not affect management/treatment during that encounter.

   True   False

8. For patients receiving diagnostic services only during an encounter/ visit, sequence first the reason for the encounter/visit indicated in the medical record.

   True   False

9. A patient with primary lung cancer with metastasis to the spine presents for radiation treatment of the spine. The first-listed diagnosis reported is the primary lung cancer.

   True   False

10. For patients receiving preoperative evaluations, sequence first a code from the subcategory Z01.81, Encounter for preprocedural examinations, followed by findings related to the preoperative evaluation.

    True   False

11. Routine prenatal outpatient visits for high-risk patients are reported with a first-listed diagnosis from category O09, Supervision of high-risk pregnancy.

    True   False

12. Z codes may be reported as a principal diagnosis in the hospital setting.

    True   False

13. Heart transplant status code Z94.1 should not be reported with a code from subcategory T86.2, Complications of heart transplant.

    True   False

14. The External Cause codes can be reported as a first-listed diagnosis.

    True   False

15. When a patient is admitted to observation for a complication following outpatient surgery, report the complication as the first-listed diagnosis.

    True   False

Odd-numbered answers are located in Appendix B, while the full answer key is only available in the TEACH Instructor Resources on Evolve.

PRACTICAL

Assign ICD-10-CM first-listed diagnosis followed by additional diagnoses if appropriate:

16. Established 50-year-old patient with end-stage renal disease, currently receiving dialysis, is seen for acute left upper quadrant pain.

    First-listed Diagnosis: _____

    Code: _____

    Other Diagnosis: _____

    Code: _____

    Other Diagnosis: _____

    Code: _____

17. Established patient with complaints of shortness of breath. Upon examination, the physician determined she needed more aggressive treatment for her current congestive heart failure.

    First-listed Diagnosis: _____

    Code: _____

18. Patient is seen for unstable angina. He has a history of arteriosclerotic coronary artery disease.

    First-listed Diagnosis: _____

    Code: _____

19. Patient is seen for follow-up for hypertension. He has end-stage renal disease.

    First-listed Diagnosis: _____

    Code: _____

    Other Diagnosis: _____

    Code: _____

Odd-numbered answers are located in Appendix B, while the full answer key is only available in the TEACH Instructor Resources on Evolve.

20. Encounter for chemotherapy for prostate cancer.

    First-listed Diagnosis: _____

    Code: _____

    Other Diagnosis: _____

    Code: _____

21. Patient with chronic obstructive pulmonary disease (COPD) is seen for an acute lower respiratory tract infection.

    First-listed Diagnosis: _____

    Code: _____

22. Patient was scheduled for outpatient surgery for right inguinal hernia repair; however, he has a fever and a URI and the procedure is canceled.

    First-listed Diagnosis: _____

    Code: _____

    Other Diagnosis: _____

    Code: _____

    Other Diagnosis: _____

    Code: _____

23. An otherwise healthy patient is seen in the clinic for exposure to tuberculosis.

    First-listed Diagnosis: _____

    Code: _____

24. Patient presents for an outpatient chest x-ray, due to chest pain with breathing. Finding later indicated: normal x-ray.

    First-listed Diagnosis: _____

    Code: _____

Odd-numbered answers are located in Appendix B, while the full answer key is only available in the TEACH Instructor Resources on Evolve.

25. Patient, with known cardiovascular disease, is seen for a follow-up visit to discuss results of a cardiac perfusion study (cardiovascular function study), which was abnormal.

First-listed Diagnosis: _____

Code: _____

Other Diagnosis: _____

Code: _____

26. Following outpatient surgery for a right bunionectomy for hallux valgus, the patient was admitted to observation due to an exacerbation of her asthma post procedure.

First-listed Diagnosis: _____

Code: _____

Other Diagnosis: _____

Code: _____

27. A patient presents with a contusion to the left cheek that resulted from a fist fight, initial encounter.

First-listed Diagnosis: _____

Code: _____

Other Diagnosis: _____

Code: _____

28. Patient presents with a fracture of the right femur shaft due to a fall from her horse while riding, initial encounter.

First-listed Diagnosis: _____

Code: _____

Other Diagnosis: _____

Code: _____

Other Diagnosis: _____

Code: _____

Odd-numbered answers are located in Appendix B, while the full answer key is only available in the TEACH Instructor Resources on Evolve.

29. Encounter for insulin pump titration.

   First-listed Diagnosis: _____

   Code: _____

30. Patient in her second trimester is seen for a regular prenatal visit. She has a history of ectopic pregnancy.

   First-listed Diagnosis: _____

   Code: _____

31. Twin born via vaginal delivery, liveborn in the hospital.

   First-listed Diagnosis: _____

   Code: _____

32. Encounter for change of nephrostomy tube.

   First-listed Diagnosis: _____

   Code: _____

33. A patient was seen for an abrasion of the left upper arm, initial encounter.

   First-listed Diagnosis: _____

   Code: _____

34. Established patient is seen for hypertension and a prescription is refilled for psoriasis.

   First-listed Diagnosis: _____

   Code: _____

   Other Diagnosis: _____

   Code: _____

35. A patient who smokes 2 packs of cigarettes per day and suffers with chronic pulmonary disease is seen in follow-up for acute bronchitis.

   First-listed Diagnosis: _____

   Code: _____

   Other Diagnoses: _____, _____

   Code: _____, _____

Odd-numbered answers are located in Appendix B, while the full answer key is only available in the TEACH Instructor Resources on Evolve.

CHAPTER 4

Using ICD-10-CM

THEORY

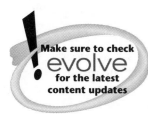

Make sure to check
evolve
for the latest
content updates

Without the use of reference material, answer the following:

1. An example of a late effect is hemorrhage after a surgery requiring a return to the operating room.

   True   False

2. You may report a code from the Index, without verifying in the Tabular when there is no indication that the code requires additional characters.

   True   False

3. If a patient has a confirmed diagnosis, the signs and symptoms related to that condition should also be reported.

   True   False

4. If the same condition is described as both acute and chronic, and separate subentries exist in the Alphabetic Index at the same indentation level, report both codes and sequence the acute code first.

   True   False

5. A dash (-) at the end of an Index entry indicates that an additional character or characters is/are required.

   True   False

6. Cholelithiasis with chronic cholecystitis without obstruction (K80.10) is an example of a dual code.

   True   False

7. A code is invalid if it has not been reported to the full number of characters available, including the 7th character, if applicable.

   True   False

Odd-numbered answers are located in Appendix B, while the full answer key is only available in the TEACH Instructor Resources on Evolve.

8. In most cases the manifestation codes will have in the code title, "in diseases classified elsewhere."

    True   False

9. A late effect usually occurs within 1 month of the illness or injury.

    True   False

10. In diabetic retinopathy, the retinopathy is the etiology and the diabetes is the manifestation.

    True   False

11. In the outpatient setting, it is correct to report a "probable" condition as if it exists, such as probable appendicitis as appendicitis.

    True   False

12. When sequencing codes for residuals and late effects, the late effect code is sequenced first followed by a code describing the residual condition.

    True   False

13. Section II of the *ICD-10-CM Official Guidelines for Coding and Reporting* includes instructions on outpatient coding and reporting.

    True   False

14. Diagnosis codes are always reported to the highest number of characters available.

    True   False

15. The cooperating parties for the development and approval of the *Official Guidelines for Coding and Reporting* are CMS, AMA, and NCHS.

    True   False

16. List two common symptoms associated with acute myocardial infarction.

    _____   _____

17. List two common symptoms associated with gastroesophageal reflux.

    _____   _____

18. List two common symptoms associated with seasonal allergies.

    _____   _____

Odd-numbered answers are located in Appendix B, while the full answer key is only available in the TEACH Instructor Resources on Evolve.

19. List two symptoms of a broken nose.

    _____ _____

Identify the Residual and Cause of the following diagnoses:

20. Acute renal failure due to previous viral encephalitis.

    Residual: _____

    Cause: _____

21. Constrictive pericarditis due to old tuberculosis infection.

    Residual: _____

    Cause: _____

22. Hemiplegia/hemiparesis affecting right dominant side due to cerebrovascular accident 4 months ago.

    Residual: _____

    Cause: _____

Odd-numbered answers are located in Appendix B, while the full answer key is only available in the TEACH Instructor Resources on Evolve.

PRACTICAL

Using the ICD-10-CM, code the following:

23. Acute and chronic sinusitis.

    ICD-10-CM Codes: _____, _____

24. Acute and chronic tonsillitis.

    ICD-10-CM Codes: _____, _____

25. Pneumoconiosis due to lime dust.

    ICD-10-CM Code: _____

26. Neuritis due to herniation of nucleus pulposus.

    ICD-10-CM Codes: _____, _____

27. Pneumonitis due to *Hemophilus influenzae*.

    ICD-10-CM Code: _____

28. Patient has unstable angina.

    ICD-10-CM Code: _____

29. Threatened shock, patient is hypotensive.

    ICD-10-CM Code: _____

30. Adult osteomalacia due to malnutrition.

    ICD-10-CM Code: _____

31. Pancreatitis, acute and chronic.

    ICD-10-CM Codes: _____, _____

32. Systemic lupus erythematosus causing endocarditis.

    ICD-10-CM Code: _____

33. Vitamin D-resistant rickets.

    ICD-10-CM Codes: _____, _____

34. Febrile complex convulsions with status epilepticus.

    ICD-10-CM Code: _____

35. Ascites in alcoholic hepatitis, alcohol use unspecified.

    ICD-10-CM Codes: _____, _____

Odd-numbered answers are located in Appendix B, while the full answer key is only available in the TEACH Instructor Resources on Evolve.

Chapter-Specific Guidelines (ICD-10-CM Chapters 1-10)

THEORY

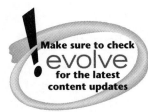

Answer the following questions about the overview of ICD-10-CM:

1. Combination coding is when one code fully describes the conditions and/or manifestations.

   True   False

2. For hemiplegia and hemiparesis and other paralytic syndromes, report the right side as dominant if the documentation does not specify which side is dominant.

   True   False

3. When reporting an infection other than *Staphylococcus aureus*, that is antibiotic resistant, report the infection first followed by a code from category Z16, Infection with drug resistant microorganisms.

   True   False

4. Diabetes mellitus codes are combination codes that include the type of diabetes as well as the body system involved and complications affecting the body system.

   True   False

5. Methicillin-resistant *Streptococcus aureus* is also referred to as MRSA.

   True   False

6. For reporting purposes, urosepsis is not considered sepsis.

   True   False

7. If the medical documentation indicates the patient has two conditions that are both included in one diagnosis code, report that diagnosis code only once.

   True   False

Odd-numbered answers are located in Appendix B, while the full answer key is only available in the TEACH Instructor Resources on Evolve.

8. Multiple coding is when it takes more than one code to fully describe the condition, circumstance, or manifestation.

   True   False

9. When the histological type of neoplasm is documented, reference the Alphabetical Index first rather than going immediately to the Neoplasm Table.

   True   False

10. SIRS is the diagnosis when all of the following are diagnosed: hypothermia or fever, tachycardia, tachypnea, increased or decreased white blood count.

    True   False

11. Viral hepatitis codes are divided based on the type of hepatitis and if the condition is with or without hepatic coma.

    True   False

12. If a patient is admitted with pneumonia and while hospitalized develops severe sepsis, you would report the pneumonia first, followed by the severe sepsis.

    True   False

13. When an encounter is for treatment of anemia due to a malignancy, the first-listed diagnosis would be the malignancy, followed by the anemia.

    True   False

14. An "Uncertain" neoplasm is one that is not clearly benign or malignant.

    True   False

15. Septic shock is considered organ failure.

    True   False

16. Hepatitis A was formerly known as infectious or epidemic hepatitis.

    True   False

17. Epiphora is a blockage of the lacrimal passage.

    True   False

Odd-numbered answers are located in Appendix B, while the full answer key is only available in the TEACH Instructor Resources on Evolve.

18. When reporting hypertensive chronic kidney disease, an additional code to report the type of chronic kidney disease is not required.

    True   False

19. A Q-wave or transmural myocardial infarction, also known as STEMI, is the most severe type of infarction.

    True   False

20. Sepsis is classified as severe sepsis when it causes organ dysfunction.

    True   False

Odd-numbered answers are located in Appendix B, while the full answer key is only available in the TEACH Instructor Resources on Evolve.

PRACTICAL

Using the ICD-10-CM, code the following:

21. Acute renal failure and acute respiratory failure due to sepsis.

    ICD-10-CM Codes: _____, _____,

    _____, _____

22. A patient with early onset Alzheimer's progresses to combative behavior.

    ICD-10-CM Codes: _____, _____

23. Patient with known Hepatitis B seen in the clinic complaining of joint pain, loss of appetite, nausea and vomiting, and weakness and fatigue. He is admitted to the hospital for severe dehydration.

    ICD-10-CM Codes: _____, _____

24. An obstetric patient in her third trimester of pregnancy is admitted for *Pneumocystis carinii* pneumonia due to AIDS.

    ICD-10-CM Codes: _____, _____, _____

25. Lung abscess due to MRSA (Methicillin resistant *Staphylococcus aureus*).

    ICD-10-CM Codes: _____, _____, _____

26. Patient in a homosexual relationship presents for HIV screening; patient is asymptomatic.

    ICD-10-CM Code: _____

27. Patient presents for follow-up exam following reconstructive surgery to repair hypospadias.

    ICD-10-CM Codes: _____, _____

28. Initial encounter for a 45-year-old woman receiving her first cycle of chemotherapy for pancreatic cancer is seen in the emergency room for severe nausea and vomiting due to the chemotherapy. She is admitted for dehydration.

    ICD-10-CM Codes: _____, _____, _____

29. Patient seen in an outpatient clinic with ascites due to disseminated malignant neoplasm.

    ICD-10-CM Codes: _____, _____

Odd-numbered answers are located in Appendix B, while the full answer key is only available in the TEACH Instructor Resources on Evolve.

30. Hypertensive heart disease, with congestive heart failure.

    ICD-10-CM Codes: _____, _____

31. Patient seen for cellulitis of left lower leg. He is a type 2 diabetic controlled with oral medications. The cellulitis has elevated his blood glucose and the physician elects to treat with sliding scale insulin regime.

    ICD-10-CM Codes: _____, _____

32. A 62-year-old man admitted to the hospital from the emergency room diagnosed with a transmural Q wave infarction. He has ASHD and had a pacemaker placed 5 years ago.

    ICD-10-CM Codes: _____, _____, _____

33. Patient seen in consult by a high-risk obstetrician. She is two months pregnant and was diagnosed with a malignant neoplasm of the left breast.

    ICD-10-CM Codes: _____, _____

34. Initial encounter for a patient with sepsis due to a blood transfusion. He has hemophilia.

    ICD-10-CM Codes: _____, _____, _____

35. Patient with anemia due to prostate cancer.

    ICD-10-CM Codes: _____, _____

36. Patient is admitted for chemotherapy for primary liver cancer.

    ICD-10-CM Codes: _____, _____

37. Patient admitted to hospital for bowel obstruction. This patient is also hypertensive with chronic kidney disease, stage 5.

    ICD-10-CM Codes: _____, _____, _____

38. Patient is following up at her oncologist's office for treatment options of metastatic cancer to right axillary lymph nodes. She has a history of right upper-outer quadrant breast cancer, still receiving treatment.

    ICD-10-CM Codes: _____, _____

39. Patient underwent a biopsy of the brain. The pathology report indicates secondary cancer from the primary site of the breast. The patient had a left mastectomy 5 years ago and currently receives no treatment for breast cancer.

    ICD-10-CM Codes: _____, _____, _____

Odd-numbered answers are located in Appendix B, while the full answer key is only available in the TEACH Instructor Resources on Evolve.

40. Patient underwent fulguration of malignant bladder tumors.

    ICD-10-CM Code: _____

41. Patient with polycythemia vera presented to an outpatient clinic for a phlebotomy.

    ICD-10-CM Code: _____

42. A 45-year-old man seen in the office is diagnosed with right carpal tunnel syndrome.

    ICD-10-CM Code: _____

43. Initial encounter for failure of insulin pump causing an overdose of insulin and hypoglycemic coma. The patient is a type 1 diabetic.

    ICD-10-CM Codes: _____, _____, _____

44. Patient diagnosed with dementia with Lewy bodies.

    ICD-10-CM Codes: _____, _____

45. Patient admitted to the hospital for resection of a malignant lung tumor from the right upper lobe.

    ICD-10-CM Code: _____

46. A man arrested for disorderly conduct is brought to the emergency room. He is a known alcoholic-dependent patient. Alcohol blood level indicates intoxication.

    ICD-10-CM Code: _____

47. Patient with chest pain is admitted to the hospital. He is diagnosed with acute Q wave myocardial infarction.

    ICD-10-CM Code: _____

48. Initial encounter for cardiac arrest due to cocaine dependence.

    ICD-10-CM Codes: _____, _____, _____

49. Schizophrenic with disorderly conduct noncompliance with his medications.

    ICD-10-CM Codes: _____, _____, _____

50. Delirium tremors due to withdrawal from cocaine dependence.

    ICD-10-CM Code: _____

Odd-numbered answers are located in Appendix B, while the full answer key is only available in the TEACH Instructor Resources on Evolve.

51. Meningitis caused by measles.

    ICD-10-CM Code: _____

52. Mononeuropathy of right lower limb due to diabetes, type 2.

    ICD-10-CM Code: _____

53. Polyneuropathy and arthritis due to syphilis.

    ICD-10-CM Codes: _____, _____

54. Streptococcal arthritis.

    ICD-10-CM Codes: _____, _____

55. Patient admitted with left hemiplegia and cerebral palsy for evaluation for possible Baclofen pump to treat spasticity.

    ICD-10-CM Code: _____

User to decide number of codes necessary to correctly answer the question.

56. Bilateral sensorineural deafness following bacterial meningitis.

    ICD-10-CM Code(s): _____

57. Ménière's disease.

    ICD-10-CM Code(s): _____

58. Right carotid stenosis causing a cerebral infarct.

    ICD-10-CM Code(s): _____

59. Acute pulmonary edema due to left heart failure. Patient now intubated and on a respirator.

    ICD-10-CM Code(s): _____

Odd-numbered answers are located in Appendix B, while the full answer key is only available in the TEACH Instructor Resources on Evolve. codes necessary to correctly answer the question.

REPORTS

Toward the end of this textbook, you will find a section titled Reports, which contains original reports. Read the report indicated below and supply the appropriate ICD-10-CM codes on the following lines:

60. Report 90

ICD-10-CM Code(s): _____

CHAPTER 6

Chapter-Specific Guidelines (ICD-10-CM Chapters 11-14)

THEORY

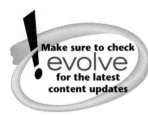

Answer the following questions about the ICD-10-CM Guidelines for Coding and Reporting *for Outpatient Services:*

1. Includes and Excludes notes are only listed in the Tabular of the ICD-10-CM.

   True   False

2. Chapter 12, Diseases of the Skin and Subcutaneous Tissue, describes diseases or conditions of the integumentary and musculoskeletal systems.

   True   False

3. In the ICD-10-CM, pressure ulcers are graded and reported based on the depth of the ulcer.

   True   False

4. Code range M00-M02 reports infectious arthropathies due to infections that are direct or indirect.

   True   False

5. Chapter 13 of the *ICD-10-CM Guidelines for Coding and Reporting* indicates the 7th character D is assigned as long as the patient is receiving active treatment for a fracture.

   True   False

6. The two types of indirect infections are reactive and postinfective arthropathy.

   True   False

7. To report a hemorrhage, active bleeding must be present.

   True   False

Odd-numbered answers are located in Appendix B, while the full answer key is only available in the TEACH Instructor Resources on Evolve.

8. The categories in Chapter 11, Diseases of the Digestive System, begin when food enters the mouth and continue to when it leaves the body through the anus.

   True   False

9. Conditions affecting the nails, sweat glands, and hair are located in Chapter 12.

   True   False

10. The "Code first" note directs the coder to report first the underlying disease.

    True   False

PRACTICAL

Using the ICD-10-CM, code the following:

11. Patient is seen for erosion of the teeth due to diet.

    ICD-10-CM Code: _____

12. Abscess of the salivary glands.

    ICD-10-CM Code: _____

13. Hemorrhage of the fallopian tube.

    ICD-10-CM Code: _____

14. Chronic prostatitis with hematuria.

    ICD-10-CM Codes: _____, _____

15. Cellulitis of female external genital organs.

    ICD-10-CM Code: _____

16. Stiffness of the right wrist.

    ICD-10-CM Code: _____

17. Congenital paraphimosis.

    ICD-10-CM Code: _____

18. Submandibular abscess.

    ICD-10-CM Code: _____

19. Secondary amenorrhea.

    ICD-10-CM Code: _____

20. Ligament disorder of the right foot joint.

    ICD-10-CM Code: _____

21. Patient suffers a nontraumatic hematoma of the soft tissue.

    ICD-10-CM Code: _____

22. Old sacroiliac joint lesion.

    ICD-10-CM Code: _____

Odd-numbered answers are located in Appendix B, while the full answer key is only available in the TEACH Instructor Resources on Evolve.

23. Inflammatory polyps of colon with intestinal obstruction.

   ICD-10-CM Code: _____

24. Hypertrophic scar.

   ICD-10-CM Code: _____

25. Chronic ulcer of the right thigh, non-pressure, with exposure of fat layer.

   ICD-10-CM Code: _____

26. Acute recurrent sialoadenitis.

   ICD-10-CM Code: _____

27. Unilateral internal inguinal hernia with gangrene, recurrent.

   ICD-10-CM Code: _____

28. Acute osteomyelitis of the right radius and ulna.

   ICD-10-CM Code: _____

29. Chronic nephritic syndrome with focal glomerulonephritis.

   ICD-10-CM Code: _____

30. Patient with end-stage renal disease, currently on hemodialysis.

   ICD-10-CM Codes: _____, _____

31. Infected pilonidal fistula with abscess.

   ICD-10-CM Code: _____

32. Cradle cap.

   ICD-10-CM Code: _____

33. Interstitial myositis of the left lower leg.

   ICD-10-CM Code: _____

34. Abnormal uterine bleeding, unrelated to menstrual cycle.

   ICD-10-CM Code: _____

35. Systemic lupus erythematosus with lung involvement.

   ICD-10-CM Code: _____

Odd-numbered answers are located in Appendix B, while the full answer key is only available in the TEACH Instructor Resources on Evolve.

36. *Staphylococcus aureus* arthritis of right carpal bones.

    ICD-10-CM Codes: _____, _____

37. Streptococcal group B arthritis of the metacarpus and phalanges, left hand.

    ICD-10-CM Codes: _____, _____

38. Endometriosis of the left ovary and fallopian tube.

    ICD-10-CM Codes: _____, _____

39. Patient is seen for a foreign body granuloma of the soft tissue, right upper arm.

    ICD-10-CM Code: _____

User to decide number of codes necessary to correctly answer the question.

40. Acute appendicitis with peritonitis with perforation of appendix.

    🔮 ICD-10-CM Code(s): _____

41. Chronic abscess of the areola of the right breast, unrelated to the puerperium.

    🔮 ICD-10-CM Code(s): _____

42. Cyst of the Bartholin's gland.

    🔮 ICD-10-CM Code(s): _____

🔮 **User to decide number of codes necessary to correctly answer the question.**
Odd-numbered answers are located in Appendix B, while the full answer key is only available in the TEACH Instructor Resources on Evolve.

REPORTS

Toward the end of this textbook, you will find a section titled Reports, which contains original reports. Read the reports indicated below and supply the appropriate ICD-10-CM codes on the following lines:

43. Report 91

   🔗 ICD-10-CM Code(s): _____

44. Report 92

   🔗 ICD-10-CM Code(s): _____

45. Report 93

   🔗 ICD-10-CM Code(s): _____

🔗 **User to decide number of codes necessary to correctly answer the question.**
Odd-numbered answers are located in Appendix B, while the full answer key is only available in the TEACH Instructor Resources on Evolve.

Chapter-Specific Guidelines (ICD-10-CM Chapters 15-21)

THEORY

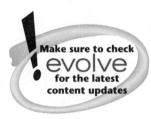

Make sure to check **evolve** for the latest content updates

Answer the following questions about the ICD-10-CM Guidelines for Coding and Reporting *for Outpatient Services:*

1. Chapter 17, Congenital Anomalies, can be reported any time during a person's life, as appropriate.

   True   False

2. Chapter 15 codes are never reported on the mother's record.

   True   False

3. The first-listed diagnosis for a routine outpatient prenatal visit is a code from category Z34, Encounter for supervision of normal pregnancy.

   True   False

4. The outcome of delivery is reported only on the newborn's record.

   True   False

5. The third trimester is considered 28 weeks 0 days from the first day of LMP until delivery occurs.

   True   False

6. A hydatidiform mole is a tumor that only forms in the uterus.

   True   False

7. When there is an encounter for a complication and no delivery occurred, report the complication as the first-listed condition.

   True   False

Odd-numbered answers are located in Appendix B, while the full answer key is only available in the TEACH Instructor Resources on Evolve.

8. When coding the birth episode in a newborn record, assign a code from Category Z38, Liveborn infants, according to place of birth and type of delivery, as the first-listed diagnosis.

   True   False

9. ICD-10-CM contains combination codes that identify only definitive diagnoses.

   True   False

10. The aftercare Z codes should not be reported for aftercare of injuries.

    True   False

11. Multiple fractures are sequenced in accordance to the location of the fracture.

    True   False

12. Corrosions are a result of a chemical contact and are classified by the depth, extent, and corrosive agent.

    True   False

13. You would assign an adverse effect code when a drug that was correctly prescribed and administered resulted in an adverse effect.

    True   False

14. When reporting multiple burns, sequence first the code that reports the highest degree of burn.

    True   False

15. Functional quadriplegia is the lack of ability to use one's limbs and is not associated with neurologic deficit or injury.

    True   False

With the use of reference material, answer the following:

16. When assigning one of the O10 codes that include hypertensive heart disease or hypertensive chronic kidney disease, it is necessary to add a

    _____ code from the appropriate hypertension category to specify the type of heart failure or chronic kidney disease.

17. A(n) _____ is an abnormality of a structure or organ.

Odd-numbered answers are located in Appendix B, while the full answer key is only available in the TEACH Instructor Resources on Evolve.

18. A _____ is defined as objective evidence of a disease that can be observed by the physician. A _____ is a subjective observation reported by the patient.

19. One method to locate abnormal findings in the Index of the I-10 is to reference the main term _____ and subterm by specific test.

20. Most categories in Chapter 19 of the ICD-10 have 7th character extensions. Most categories in this chapter have three extensions (with the exception of fractures): A, initial encounter, D, subsequent encounter, and _____, sequela.

21. A patient presents with second- and third-degree burns of the arm. What is the only degree of burn reported?

    _____

22. According to the guidelines on poisoning, _____ refers to taking less of a medication than is prescribed by a provider.

23. Codes from Chapter _____ of the Tabular of the I-10 report symptoms, signs, and abnormal clinical and laboratory findings.

24. Chapter _____ of the Tabular of the I-10 is probably the most difficult chapter from which to report diagnoses due to the complexity of coding.

25. According to the guidelines, when sequencing multiple fractures, sequence in accordance with the _____ of the fracture.

Odd-numbered answers are located in Appendix B, while the full answer key is only available in the TEACH Instructor Resources on Evolve.

PRACTICAL

Using the ICD-10-CM, code the following:

26. Induced abortion complicated by endometritis.

    ICD-10-CM Code: _____

27. Abrasion of the left upper arm, initial encounter.

    ICD-10-CM Code: _____

28. Hepatomegaly.

    ICD-10-CM Code: _____

29. Anaphylactic shock, initial encounter.

    ICD-10-CM Code: _____

30. Failure to gain weight, child.

    ICD-10-CM Code: _____

31. Pelvic peritonitis following ectopic pregnancy.

    ICD-10-CM Codes: _____, _____

32. Initial encounter of a patient transported to emergency department. Patient died from cardiac arrest due to an accidental overdose from heroin abuse.

    ICD-10-CM Codes: _____, _____, _____

33. Concealed penis.

    ICD-10-CM Code: _____

34. Crush syndrome, subsequent encounter.

    ICD-10-CM Code: _____

35. A 24-year-old woman at 32 weeks' gestation has hypotension.

    ICD-10-CM Code: _____

36. Newborn with cellulitis of the navel with mild hemorrhage.

    ICD-10-CM Code: _____

37. Inability to swallow.

    ICD-10-CM Code: _____

Odd-numbered answers are located in Appendix B, while the full answer key is only available in the TEACH Instructor Resources on Evolve.

38. Absence of bowel sounds.

    ICD-10-CM Code: _____

39. Sprain, left ankle, initial encounter.

    ICD-10-CM Code: _____

40. Newborn with obstructive sleep apnea.

    ICD-10-CM Code: _____

41. First- and second-degree burn, right hand, subsequent encounter.

    ICD-10-CM Code: _____

42. Partial traumatic amputation of the left index finger, initial encounter.

    ICD-10-CM Code: _____

43. Patient with persistent proteinuria.

    ICD-10-CM Code: _____

44. Accidental overdose of ibuprofen [NSAID], initial encounter.

    ICD-10-CM Code: _____

45. Hematoma of the nose, subsequent encounter.

    ICD-10-CM Code: _____

46. Newborn female delivered in the hospital by cesarean delivery.

    ICD-10-CM Code: _____

47. Fragile X syndrome.

    ICD-10-CM Code: _____

48. Anemia due to prematurity of infant.

    ICD-10-CM Code: _____

49. A 26-year-old woman at 30 weeks' gestation with quadruplets.

    ICD-10-CM Code: _____

Odd-numbered answers are located in Appendix B, while the full answer key is only available in the TEACH Instructor Resources on Evolve.

User to decide number of codes necessary to correctly answer the question.

50. Unexplained death, prior to entering health care facility.

    🌐 ICD-10-CM Code(s): _____

51. Tremors due to accidental overdose of monoamine oxidase, initial encounter.

    🌐 ICD-10-CM Code(s): _____

52. Nausea and vomiting.

    🌐 ICD-10-CM Code(s): _____

53. Blister of the right wrist, initial encounter.

    🌐 ICD-10-CM Code(s): _____

54. Acute gastritis with bleeding due to adverse effect of omeprazole, initial encounter.

    🌐 ICD-10-CM Code(s): _____

55. Subsequent encounter for fracture, right clavicle, with delayed healing.

    🌐 ICD-10-CM Code(s): _____

56. Positive occult blood in stools.

    🌐 ICD-10-CM Code(s): _____

57. Adult with respiratory distress and extreme fatigue.

    🌐 ICD-10-CM Code(s): _____

58. Vaginal pain.

    🌐 ICD-10-CM Code(s): _____

🌐 **User to decide number of codes necessary to correctly answer the question.**
Odd-numbered answers are located in Appendix B, while the full answer key is only available in the TEACH Instructor Resources on Evolve.

REPORTS

Toward the end of this textbook, you will find a section titled Reports, which contains original reports. Read the reports indicated below and supply the appropriate ICD-10-CM codes on the following lines:

59. Report 94

    🌐 ICD-10-CM Code(s): _____

60. Report 95

    🌐 ICD-10-CM Code(s): _____

🌐 **User to decide number of codes necessary to correctly answer the question.**
Odd-numbered answers are located in Appendix B, while the full answer key is only available in the TEACH Instructor Resources on Evolve.

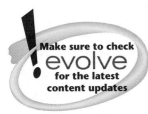

CHAPTER 8

An Overview of ICD-9-CM

THEORY

Make sure to check **evolve** for the latest content updates

Match the abbreviations, punctuation, symbols, words, or typeface to the correct descriptions:

1. __F__ [ ]

2. __G__ NOS

3. __A__ :

4. __I__ Subterms

5. __H__ Italics

6. __L__ Excludes

7. __J__ Includes

8. __L__ }

9. __D__ NEC

10. __E__ ( )

11. __B__ [ ]

12. __C__ Bold type

a. Incomplete term that needs one of the modifiers to make a code assignable

b. Used in Volume 2 to enclose the disease codes that are recorded with the code they are listed with

c. Typeface used for all codes and titles in Volume 1

d. Information is not available to code to a more specific category

e. Encloses a series of terms that are modified by the statement to the right

f. Encloses synonyms, alternative words, or explanatory phrases

g. Equals unspecified

h. Typeface used for all exclusion notes and codes that are never listed first

i. Located under the main terms and indented to the right

j. Appears under a three-digit code title to further define or explain category content

k. Encloses supplementary words and does not affect the code

l. Indicates terms that are to be coded elsewhere

Odd-numbered answers are located in Appendix B, while the full answer key is only available in the TEACH Instructor Resources on Evolve.

Without the use of reference material, answer the following:

13. E codes are located in Volume 2, Section:
    a. 3
    b. 2
    c. 1
    d. 0

14. Synchronous means:
    a. location of an opening
    b. occurring at the same time
    c. creation of an opening
    d. none of the above

Match the convention to the definition:

15. __F__ See category

16. __B__ Modifiers

17. __C__ See

18. __D__ Notes

19. __A__ Subterms

20. __E__ See also

21. __G__ Eponym

a. Indented under main term and are essential to code selection

b. Terms in parentheses that are nonessential

c. Explicit direction to look elsewhere

d. Follows terms to define and give instructions

e. Directs coder to look under another term since all information is not under the first term

f. Directs coder to Volume 1 for important information

g. Disease/syndrome named for a person

Circle the correct answer for each of the following:

22. Volume 3 is primarily used by which of the following?
    a. clinics
    b. ambulatory centers
    c. hospitals
    d. nursing homes

23. Volume 3 is used to code what type of procedures?
    a. surgical
    b. therapeutic
    c. diagnostic
    d. all of the above

Odd-numbered answers are located in Appendix B, while the full answer key is only available in the TEACH Instructor Resources on Evolve.

Identify if the following statements are True or False:

24. The location of the Includes and Excludes notes has no bearing on the code selection.

    (True)   False

25. Use of fourth and fifth digits, if available, is mandatory.

    (True)   False

26. Appendix D—Classification of Industrial Accidents According to Agency—was deleted October 1, 2004.

    True   (False)

27. Four-digit codes are referred to as subcategory codes in Volume 1.

    (True)   False

28. In Volume 2, Alphabetic Index, when the main term is modified by terms listed in parentheses following the main term, these modifiers are considered essential for code selection.

    True   (False)

Underline the main term in the following:

29. Grief reaction

30. Fracture radius and ulna

31. Bowel obstruction

32. Erb's palsy

33. Supervision of high-risk pregnancy

34. Aortic stenosis

35. Rapid respiration

36. Actinomycosis meningitis

Identify as category, subcategory, or subclassification:

37. 066.1 Subcategory

38. 070.43 subclassification

39. 220 category

40. 274.11 subclass

Odd-numbered answers are located in Appendix B, while the full answer key is only available in the TEACH Instructor Resources on Evolve.

41. 284.9 _subcategory_

42. 337.21 _subclass_

Are the following codes procedure codes or diagnosis codes?

43. 214.0 _diagnosis code_

44. 251.0 _diagnosis code_

45. 31.41 _procedure code_

46. 37.96 _procedure code_

47. 663.61 _diagnosis code_

Odd-numbered answers are located in Appendix B, while the full answer key is only available in the TEACH Instructor Resources on Evolve.

PRACTICAL

Using ICD-9-CM, Volume 1, Tabular List, locate the first page of Chapter 10 and answer the following questions about the chapter:

48. The name of the chapter: Diseases of the Genitourinary System (580-629)

49. The name of the first section: Nephritis, nephrotic syndrome and nephrosis (580-589)

50. The description of the first category: 580 acute glomerulonephritis

51. The description of the first subcategory: 580.0 with lesion of proliferative glomerulonephritis

52. The description of the first subclassification: acute glomerulonephritis in diseases classified elsewhere

Using ICD-9-CM, Volume 2, Alphabetic Index, locate the following main terms and identify if the bolded subterm is an essential or nonessential modifier:

53. **Alcoholic** gastritis   (Essential)   Nonessential

54. **Hemorrhagic** gastroenteritis   Essential   (Nonessential)

55. **Salmonella** gastroenteritis   (Essential)   Nonessential

56. **Obstructive** cardiomyopathy   Essential   (Nonessential)

57. **Ischemic** cardiomyopathy   (Essential)   Nonessential

Using the Tabular List, answer the following questions:

58. Is septicemia due to anthrax assigned code 038.8? NO

    If not, what code is assigned? 022.3

59. Is congenital pneumonia assigned code 771.2? NO

    If not, what code is assigned? 770.0

60. Is acute mesenteric lymphadenitis assigned code 683? Yes

    If not, what code is assigned? _____

Using the Tabular and instructional notes, assign and sequence the following code(s):

61. See category 484.8; assign code(s) for patient with pneumonia due to typhoid fever. 002.0, 484.8

62. See category 713.1; assign a code for patient with arthropathy due to ulcerative colitis. 556.9, 713.1

63. See category 573.1; assign a code for patient with hepatitis due to infectious mononucleosis. 075, 573.1

Odd-numbered answers are located in Appendix B, while the full answer key is only available in the TEACH Instructor Resources on Evolve.

CHAPTER 9

ICD-9-CM Outpatient Coding and Reporting Guidelines

THEORY

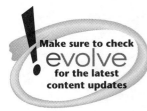

Answer the following questions about the ICD-9-CM Guidelines for Coding and Reporting *for Outpatient Services:*

1. It is not acceptable to code a symptom when a definitive diagnosis has been confirmed.

   (True)   False

2. Codes from Chapter 11 should not be reported in conjunction with V22.0 and V22.1.

   (True)   False

3. It is acceptable to code suspected pneumonia to the pneumonia code 486.

   True   (False)

4. In the physician office, V codes should only be assigned as secondary codes.

   True   (False)

5. When a patient is to have outpatient surgery and the surgery is canceled, the V code to indicate the reason for the cancellation is the first-listed diagnosis.

   True   (False)

6. When coding an encounter for a preoperative evaluation, the appropriate V code that indicates the type of preoperative evaluation is the first-listed diagnosis.

   (True)   False

7. The guidelines for coding and reporting are the same for inpatient and outpatient services.

   True   (False)

Odd-numbered answers are located in Appendix B, while the full answer key is only available in the TEACH Instructor Resources on Evolve.

8. The definition for principal diagnosis applies only to inpatient in acute, short-term, long-term care, and psychiatric hospitals.

 True   False

9. The first-listed ICD-9-CM code is usually the diagnosis, condition, problem, or other reason for the encounter shown in the medical record to be chiefly responsible for the services provided.

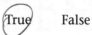 True   False

10. History V codes should be assigned if the historical condition or family history has an impact on current care or influences treatment.

 True   False

PRACTICAL

Assign ICD-9-CM codes to the following:

11. Family history of gout.

    ICD-9-CM Code: V18·19

12. Encounter for plaster cast removal.

    ICD-9-CM Code: V54.89

13. Encounter for vision examination.

    ICD-9-CM Code: V72.0

14. Status post cardiac pacemaker placement.

    ICD-9-CM Code: V45.01

15. Screening for yellow fever.

    ICD-9-CM Code: V73.4

16. Screening for malignant neoplasm of the colon.

    ICD-9-CM Code: V76.51

17. Observation for an alleged suicide attempt.

    ICD-9-CM Code: V71.89

18. Personal history of an allergy to latex.

    ICD-9-CM Code: V15.07

19. Vaccination for smallpox.

    ICD-9-CM Code: V04.1

20. Adjustment of a colostomy tube for fitting. *reaction, adjustment*

    ICD-9-CM Code: V55.3

21. Screening for cystic fibrosis.

    ICD-9-CM Code: V77.6

22. Screening for unspecified immunity disorder.

    ICD-9-CM Code: V77.99

Odd-numbered answers are located in Appendix B, while the full answer key is only available in the TEACH Instructor Resources on Evolve.

23. MMR immunization.

    ICD-9-CM Code: _V06.4_

24. Suspected carrier of diphtheria.

    ICD-9-CM Code: _V02.4_

25. Patient admitted to donate bone marrow for brother with aplastic anemia (used by facility coder only).

    ICD-9-CM Code: _V59.3_

26. Exposure to rabies.

    ICD-9-CM Code: _V01.5_

27. Closure of colostomy (used by facility coder only).

    ICD-9-CM Code: _V55.3_

28. Reprogramming of cardiac pacemaker.

    ICD-9-CM Code: _V53.31_

Odd-numbered answers are located in Appendix B, while the full answer key is only available in the TEACH Instructor Resources on Evolve.

CHAPTER 10

Using ICD-9-CM

THEORY

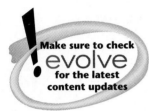

Make sure to check evolve for the latest content updates

Without the use of reference material, answer the following:

1. The *ICD-9-CM Guidelines for Coding and Reporting* are updated every other year.

   True   ~~False~~ (circled)

2. If there are separate codes for both the acute and chronic forms of a condition, the code for the acute condition is sequenced first.

   ~~True~~ (circled)   False

3. If a patient has a certain disease or condition, the routine signs and symptoms that the patient has should also be coded.

   True   ~~False~~ (circled)

4. The term "use additional code" indicates that a secondary code should be added if supported by documentation in the medical record.

   ~~True~~ (circled)   False

5. A late effect is the residual effect after the acute phase of an illness or injury has terminated.

   ~~True~~ (circled)   False

6. A late effect usually occurs within 6 months of the illness or injury.

   True   ~~False~~ (circled)

7. In the outpatient setting, it is acceptable to code a "threatened" condition as if it exists.

   True   ~~False~~ (circled)

Odd-numbered answers are located in Appendix B, while the full answer key is only available in the TEACH Instructor Resources on Evolve.

8. When sequencing codes for residuals and late effects, the late effect code is generally sequenced first followed by a code describing the residual.

   True   **False**

9. It is acceptable to assign codes directly from the Alphabetic Index.

   True   **False**

10. Codes must be assigned to the highest level of specificity to be valid codes.

    True   False

PRACTICAL

11. List two common symptoms associated with a urinary tract infection.

   urgency, burning pain

12. List two common symptoms associated with gastroenteritis.

   nausea, vomiting

13. Severe intellectual disabilities due to previous viral encephalitis.

   Residual: _mental retardation_ ICD-9-CM Code: _318.1_

   Cause: _viral encephalitis_ ICD-9-CM Code: _139.0_

14. Nonunion of left tibia fracture (closed).

   Residual: nonunion fracture. ICD-9-CM Code: _733.82_

   Cause: fracture, tibia. ICD-9-CM Code: _905.4_

15. Osteoporosis due to previous poliomyelitis.

   Residual: osteoporosis. ICD-9-CM Code: _733.00_

   Cause: poliomyelitis. ICD-9-CM Code: _138_

16. Flaccid hemiplegia affecting dominant side due to cerebrovascular accident 4 months ago.

   Residual and cause flaccid hemiplegia, dominant side, CVA.

   ICD-9-CM Code: _438.21_

Assign ICD-9-CM code(s) to the following diagnoses:

17. Acute and chronic bronchitis.

   ⊛ ICD-9-CM Code(s): _466.0, 491.9_

18. Acute and chronic oophoritis.

   ⊛ ICD-9-CM Code(s): _614.0, 614.1_

19. Acute pyelonephritis due to *E. coli*.

   ⊛ ICD-9-CM Code(s): _590.10, 041.49_

⊛ User to decide number of codes necessary to correctly answer the question.
Odd-numbered answers are located in Appendix B, while the full answer key is only available in the TEACH Instructor Resources on Evolve.

20. Gastroenteritis due to Norwalk virus.

    🌐 ICD-9-CM Code(s): _008.63_

21 and 22 NO code

21. Impending respiratory failure.

    🌐 ICD-9-CM Code(s): _NO code_

22. Threatened shock, patient hypotensive.

    🌐 ICD-9-CM Code(s): _458.9_

23. Pneumonia due to *Hemophilus influenzae*.

    🌐 ICD-9-CM Code(s): _482.2_

24. Streptococcal pharyngitis.

    🌐 ICD-9-CM Code(s): _034.0_

25. Systemic lupus erythematosus with associated nephritic syndrome.

    🌐 ICD-9-CM Code(s): _710.0, 583.81_

Fever, cough - pneumonia

🌐 **User to decide number of codes necessary to correctly answer the question.**
**Odd-numbered answers are located in Appendix B, while the full answer key is only available in the TEACH
Instructor Resources on Evolve.**

CHAPTER 11

Chapter-Specific Guidelines (ICD-9-CM Chapters 1-8)

PRACTICAL

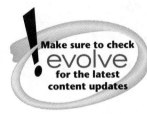

Using the ICD-9-CM, code the following:

1. Tinea pedis.

   ICD-9-CM Code: __110.4__

2. Chronic hepatitis C.

   ICD-9-CM Code: __571.40__

3. Mycobacterium pulmonary infection.

   ICD-9-CM Code: __031.0__

4. Acute prostatitis due to streptococcus.

   ICD-9-CM Codes: __601.0__ , _____

5. Hypokalemic syndrome.

   ICD-9-CM Code: __276.8__

6. Malignant neoplasm of the tail of the pancreas, primary.

   ICD-9-CM Code: _____

7. Infection due to group B streptococcus.

   ICD-9-CM Code: __041.02__

8. Mixed hyperlipidemia.

   ICD-9-CM Code: _____

9. Immunoglobulin G deficiency.

   ICD-9-CM Code: __279.03__

Odd-numbered answers are located in Appendix B, while the full answer key is only available in the TEACH Instructor Resources on Evolve.

10. Tumor abdomen, uncertain behavior.

    ICD-9-CM Code: _____

11. Diabetic retinopathy, type 2, controlled.

    ICD-9-CM Codes: __250.50__, __362.01__

12. Hepatocellular adenoma.

    ICD-9-CM Code: _____

13. Vitamin B12 deficiency.

    ICD-9-CM Code: __266.2__

14. Gangrene, left great toe, due to diabetes mellitus, type 1.

    ICD-9-CM Codes: _____, _____

15. Vitamin D-resistant rickets.

    ICD-9-CM Code: __275.3__

16. Thrombocytopenia.

    ICD-9-CM Code: _____

17. Wermer's syndrome.

    ICD-9-CM Code: __258-01__

18. Active state of childhood autism.

    ICD-9-CM Code: _____

19. Atypical bipolar affective disorder.

    ICD-9-CM Code: __296.7__

20. Chronic lymphadenitis.

    ICD-9-CM Code: _____

21. Streptococcal septicemia.

    ICD-9-CM Code: __038.0__

22. Toxic shock syndrome.

    ICD-9-CM Code: _____

Odd-numbered answers are located in Appendix B, while the full answer key is only available in the TEACH Instructor Resources on Evolve.

23. Chronic schizophrenia, paranoid type.

    ICD-9-CM Code: _295.32_

24. Carpal tunnel syndrome.

    ICD-9-CM Code: _____

25. Tobacco abuse.

    ICD-9-CM Code: _305.1_

26. Pneumococcal meningitis.

    ICD-9-CM Code: _____

27. Panic attack, without agoraphobia.

    ICD-9-CM Code: _300.01_

28. Parkinson's disease.

    ICD-9-CM Code: _____

29. Peripheral retinal edema.

    ICD-9-CM Code: _362.83_

30. Ménière's disease in remission.

    ICD-9-CM Code: _____

31. Total traumatic cataract.

    ICD-9-CM Code: _366.22_

32. Chronic follicular conjunctivitis.

    ICD-9-CM Code: _____

33. Sensorineural hearing loss, right side.

    ICD-9-CM Code: _389.15_

34. Malignant hypertensive heart disease, with heart failure.

    ICD-9-CM Codes: _____, _____

35. A 62-year-old male admitted to the hospital with acute subendocardial myocardial infarction.

    ICD-9-CM Code: _410.70_

Odd-numbered answers are located in Appendix B, while the full answer key is only available in the TEACH Instructor Resources on Evolve.

36. Arteriosclerotic cardiovascular disease, unspecified.

    ICD-9-CM Codes: _____, _____

37. Primary pulmonary hypertension.

    ICD-9-CM Code: __416.0__

38. Fibrosis of the pericardium.

    ICD-9-CM Code: _____

39. Paroxysmal supraventricular tachycardia.

    ICD-9-CM Code: __427.0__

40. Chronic diastolic heart failure.

    ICD-9-CM Code: _____

41. Stenosis of the renal arteries.

    ICD-9-CM Code: __440-1__

42. Saddle embolus in abdominal aorta.

    ICD-9-CM Code: __444.0__

43. Chronic lymphangitis.

    ICD-9-CM Code: __457.2__

44. Acute frontal sinusitis.

    ICD-9-CM Code: _____

45. Abscess of the vocal cords.

    ICD-9-CM Code: __478.5__

46. Chronic tonsillitis and adenoiditis.

    ICD-9-CM Code: __474.02__

47. Acute exacerbation of chronic obstructive bronchitis.

    ICD-9-CM Code: __491-21__

48. Abscess of the lung.

    ICD-9-CM Code: __513.0__

49. ASHD of native coronary artery and COPD.

    ICD-9-CM Codes: __414.01__, __496__

Odd-numbered answers are located in Appendix B, while the full answer key is only available in the TEACH Instructor Resources on Evolve.

50. Candidal endocarditis.

ICD-9-CM Code: __112.81__

51. Pneumonia due to staphylococcus aureus.

ICD-9-CM Code: __482.41__

52. Bacteremia due to pseudomonas.

ICD-9-CM Codes: __790.7__ , __041.7__

53. Type 2 cerebral poliomyelitis with dysphonia.

ICD-9-CM Codes: __045.02__ , __784.42__

54. Malignant ascites, primary site unknown.

ICD-9-CM Codes: __199.1__ , __789.51__

55. Progressive malignant anemia.

ICD-9-CM Code: __281.0__

Remember the ☙ symbol means the answer may be one code or more than one code.

56. Alcoholic delirium tremens due to dependence on alcohol.

☙ ICD-9-CM Code(s): __291.0 , 303.90__

57. Organic personality syndrome.

☙ ICD-9-CM Code(s): __310.1__

58. Transient visual loss.

☙ ICD-9-CM Code(s): __368.12, None__

59. Bilateral otitis media.

☙ ICD-9-CM Code(s): __382.9__

60. Migraine due to menstruation.

☙ ICD-9-CM Code(s): __346.40, None__

61. Retained foreign body of the lens.

☙ ICD-9-CM Code(s): __360.63, ~~V~~ V90.89__

☙ **User to decide number of codes necessary to correctly answer the question.**
Odd-numbered answers are located in Appendix B, while the full answer key is only available in the TEACH Instructor Resources on Evolve.

62. Type 2 diabetic mononeuropathy of the legs.

 ICD-9-CM Code(s): 250.60, 355.8

63. Diarrhea due to paracolon bacillus.

 ICD-9-CM Code(s): 008.47

64. Mobitz II atrioventricular block.

 ICD-9-CM Code(s): 426.12, None

65. Dissecting abdominal aortic aneurysm.

 ICD-9-CM Code(s): 441.02

429.4, 428.9, V45.81, None, None

66. Cardiac insufficiency 6 months after coronary artery bypass surgery.

 ICD-9-CM Code(s): E878.2   V45.81

67. Raynaud's syndrome with gangrene of right index finger.

 ICD-9-CM Code(s): 443.0, 785.4

68. Ulcerated internal hemorrhoids.

 ICD-9-CM Code(s): 455.2, None

69. Deep vein thrombophlebitis of the femoral vein.

 ICD-9-CM Code(s): 451.11

70. Viral pneumonia.

 ICD-9-CM Code(s): 480.9, None

71. Intrinsic obstruction of the eustachian tube.

 ICD-9-CM Code(s): 381.62

72. Elevated blood pressure in a patient with hypertension.

 ICD-9-CM Code(s): 401.9, None

73. Lung nodule, solitary.

 ICD-9-CM Code(s): 793.11

74. Hemochromatosis, hereditary.

 ICD-9-CM Code(s): 275.01, None

 User to decide number of codes necessary to correctly answer the question.
Odd-numbered answers are located in Appendix B, while the full answer key is only available in the TEACH Instructor Resources on Evolve.

REPORTS

Toward the end of this textbook, you will find a section titled Reports, which contains original reports. Read the reports indicated below and supply the appropriate ICD-9-CM codes on the following lines:

75. Report 7

    🌑 ICD-9-CM Code(s): __214.8__

76. Report 9

    🌑 ICD-9-CM Code(s): __174.9__

77. Report 19

    🌑 ICD-9-CM Code(s): __513.0__

78. Report 20

    🌑 ICD-9-CM Code(s): __198.82, 199.1__

79. Report 34

    🌑 ICD-9-CM Code(s): __455.0, 455.3__

80. Report 39   V05 43

    🌑 ICD-9-CM Code(s): __278.01, 571.8__

81. Report 42

    🌑 ICD-9-CM Code(s): __374.30, 368.46__

82. Report 44

    🌑 ICD-9-CM Code(s): __202.81 375.15, V43.1__

🌑 **User to decide number of codes necessary to correctly answer the question.**
Odd-numbered answers are located in Appendix B, while the full answer key is only available in the TEACH Instructor Resources on Evolve.

CHAPTER 12

Chapter-Specific Guidelines (ICD-9-CM Chapters 9-17)

PRACTICAL

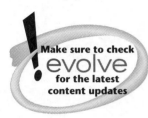
Make sure to check **evolve** for the latest content updates

Using the ICD-9-CM, code the following:

1. Acute prostatitis due to streptococcus.

   ICD-9-CM Codes: __601.0__ , __041.00__

2. Aphthous stomatitis.

   ICD-9-CM Code: _____

3. Chronic gastric ulcer with perforation.

   ICD-9-CM Code: _____

4. Hiatal hernia with obstruction.

   ICD-9-CM Code: _____

5. Constipation.

   ICD-9-CM Code: _____

6. Biliary cirrhosis.

   ICD-9-CM Code: _____

7. Phimosis.

   ICD-9-CM Code: _____

8. Pyelitis due to tuberculosis.

   ICD-9-CM Codes: _____, _____

9. Amenorrhea.

   ICD-9-CM Code: _____

Odd-numbered answers are located in Appendix B, while the full answer key is only available in the TEACH Instructor Resources on Evolve.

10. A 24-year-old woman at 28 weeks' gestation has hypothyroidism.

    ICD-9-CM Codes: _____ , _____

11. A 26-year-old woman at 30 weeks' gestation with quadruplets.

    ICD-9-CM Code: __651.23__

12. Cellulitis left foot and ankle due to staphylococcus.

    ICD-9-CM Codes: _____ , _____ ,

    _____

13. Systemic lupus erythematosus.

    ICD-9-CM Code: __710.0__

14. Decubitus ulcer of the sacrum.

    ICD-9-CM Codes: _____ , _____

15. Winter itch.

    ICD-9-CM Code: __698.8__

16. Hidradenitis suppurative.

    ICD-9-CM Code: _____

17. Arthritis due to ulcerative colitis.

    ICD-9-CM Codes: __556.9__ , __713.1__

18. Osteoarthritis of the cervical spine.

    ICD-9-CM Code: _____

19. Calcaneal spur.

    ICD-9-CM Code: __726.73__

20. Bunion right big toe.

    ICD-9-CM Code: _____

Remember the ⊛ symbol means the answer may be one code or more than one code.

21. Acute osteomyelitis left patella due to staphylococcus.

    ⊛ ICD-9-CM Code(s): __730.06__

⊛ User to decide number of codes necessary to correctly answer the question.
Odd-numbered answers are located in Appendix B, while the full answer key is only available in the TEACH Instructor Resources on Evolve.

22. Newborn female delivered in the hospital by cesarean delivery with evidence of cleft palate and cleft lip.

    🔗 ICD-9-CM Code(s): V30.01, 749.20

23. Chronic osteomyelitis of the hip.

    🔗 ICD-9-CM Code(s): 730.15

24. Hepatomegaly.

    🔗 ICD-9-CM Code(s): _____

25. Epistaxis.

    🔗 ICD-9-CM Code(s): 784.7

26. Proteinuria.

    🔗 ICD-9-CM Code(s): _____

27. Nausea and vomiting.

    🔗 ICD-9-CM Code(s): 787.01

28. Polydipsia.

    🔗 ICD-9-CM Code(s): _____

    2 785.1   3 E854.0 , 969-01

29. Palpitations due to overdose of monoamine oxidase. (accident)

    🔗 ICD-9-CM Code(s): 969.01, 785.1, E854.0

30. Fracture, right clavicle.

    🔗 ICD-9-CM Code(s): _____

31. Sprain, left ankle.

    🔗 ICD-9-CM Code(s): 845.00

32. Abrasion, right elbow.

    🔗 ICD-9-CM Code(s): _____

33. First- and second-degree burn, forehead.

    🔗 ICD-9-CM Code(s): 941.27

34. Concussion.

    🔗 ICD-9-CM Code(s): _____

🔗 **User to decide number of codes necessary to correctly answer the question.**
Odd-numbered answers are located in Appendix B, while the full answer key is only available in the TEACH Instructor Resources on Evolve.

35. Foreign body (penny) in stomach.

    ICD-9-CM Code(s): _____

36. Contusion, left hip.

    ICD-9-CM Code(s): _____

37. Traumatic amputation, right foot without complications.

    ICD-9-CM Code(s): _____

38. Posterior dislocation of elbow, closed.

    ICD-9-CM Code(s): _832.02_

39. Traumatic amputation of the left arm just above the elbow.

    ICD-9-CM Code(s): _____

40. A patient develops gastrointestinal bleeding while taking Motrin as
    prescribed for abdominal cramping. (Hint: Three conditions need to be
    coded. You will need to consult the *Physicians' Desk Reference* or do an
    internet search to find out what Motrin is called in its generic form.)

    Ibuprofen 3

    ICD-9-CM Code(s): _578.9, 789.00, E935.6_

41. A patient is admitted with nausea, weakness, sweating, and tachycardia
    following a gastrectomy. A diagnosis of dumping syndrome is made.

    a. The condition here is dumping syndrome. What is the code for this
       condition?

       ICD-9-CM Code: _____

    b. Why is code 997.4, gastrointestinal complications, not correct to
       assign?

       _____

42. Acute renal failure develops in a patient following a cardiac
    catheterization and the patient is admitted for dialysis.

    a. There are two conditions in the case. What are they?

       _____

    b. What are the two codes for these conditions?

       ICD-9-CM Codes: _____, _____

 User to decide number of codes necessary to correctly answer the question.
**Odd-numbered answers are located in Appendix B, while the full answer key is only available in the TEACH
Instructor Resources on Evolve.**

43. A patient died from an accidental overdose of heroin. What are the codes?

    ICD-9-CM Codes: _____, _____,

    _____

44. A patient is lethargic with severe abdominal cramping and vomiting following an accidental ingestion of 5 tablets of Tylenol with codeine and a bottle of vodka. There are nine codes for this case:

    a. Codeine, poisoning.

       ICD-9-CM Codes: 956.09 , E850.2

    b. Acetaminophen, poisoning.

       ICD-9-CM Codes: 965.4 , E850.4

    c. Alcohol, beverage, poisoning.

       ICD-9-CM Codes: 980.0 , E860.0

    d. Lethargy.

       ICD-9-CM Code: 780.79

    e. Vomiting.

       ICD-9-CM Code: 787.03

    f. Cramp, abdominal, unspecified site.

       ICD-9-CM Code: 789.00

45. Positive occult blood in stools.

    ICD-9-CM Code: 792.1

46. Bacteremia due to pseudomonas.

    ICD-9-CM Code(s): _____

47. First-degree sunburn.

    ICD-9-CM Code(s): _____

48. Contusion of the buttock after slipping on the ice.

    ICD-9-CM Code(s): _____

User to decide number of codes necessary to correctly answer the question.
Odd-numbered answers are located in Appendix B, while the full answer key is only available in the TEACH Instructor Resources on Evolve.

49. Stiffness of the knee.

   🔗 ICD-9-CM Code(s): _____

50. Dehiscence of the internal wires after sternotomy.

   🔗 ICD-9-CM Code(s): _____

51. Congenital splenomegaly causing fevers.

   🔗 ICD-9-CM Code(s): _____

52. Peptic ulcer, bleeding.

   🔗 ICD-9-CM Code(s): _____

53. Impacted wisdom tooth.

   🔗 ICD-9-CM Code(s): _____

54. Colostomy malfunction.

   🔗 ICD-9-CM Code(s): _____

55. Allergic gastritis secondary to aspirin intake, aspirin prescribed for arthritis.

   🔗 ICD-9-CM Code(s): _____

56. Endometriosis of the ovary and round ligament.

   🔗 ICD-9-CM Code(s): _____

57. Chronic prostatitis due to staphylococcus.

   🔗 ICD-9-CM Code(s): _____

58. Stress urinary incontinence, female.

   🔗 ICD-9-CM Code(s): _____

59. Benign prostatic hypertrophy.

   🔗 ICD-9-CM Code(s): _____

60. Pain of the ribs.

   🔗 ICD-9-CM Code(s): _____

🔗 User to decide number of codes necessary to correctly answer the question.
Odd-numbered answers are located in Appendix B, while the full answer key is only available in the TEACH Instructor Resources on Evolve.

61. Term pregnancy, delivered live born, with pre-eclampsia and fetal distress.

    🌐 ICD-9-CM Code(s): _____

62. Impetigo of eyelid.

    🌐 ICD-9-CM Code(s): _____

63. Systemic lupus erythematosus with lung involvement.

    🌐 ICD-9-CM Code(s): _____

64. Marble bones.

    🌐 ICD-9-CM Code(s): _____

65. Arthritis of the hip, status post hip fracture 5 years ago.

    🌐 ICD-9-CM Code(s): _____

66. Localized osteoarthritis of the wrist.

    🌐 ICD-9-CM Code(s): _____

67. Patient comes into the ER unconscious. *main term*

    🌐 ICD-9-CM Code(s): _____

68. Deep cut on the finger embedded with dirt.

    🌐 ICD-9-CM Code(s): _____

69. Obstructive jaundice.

    🌐 ICD-9-CM Code(s): _____

70. Respiratory distress.

    🌐 ICD-9-CM Code(s): _____

71. Left lower quadrant abdominal tenderness.

    🌐 ICD-9-CM Code(s): _____

72. Pathological fracture of two vertebrae.

    🌐 ICD-9-CM Code(s): _____

73. Splinter of the left palm of the hand.

    🌐 ICD-9-CM Code(s): _____

🌐 **User to decide number of codes necessary to correctly answer the question.**
Odd-numbered answers are located in Appendix B, while the full answer key is only available in the TEACH Instructor Resources on Evolve.

74. Second-degree burn of the hand due to an accident caused by a fire.

    🔮 ICD-9-CM Code(s): _____

75. Accidental overdose of ibuprofen.

    🔮 ICD-9-CM Code(s): _____

76. Second-degree burn of the arm caused by hot water.

    🔮 ICD-9-CM Code(s): _____

77. Late effect secondary to intracranial head injury 1 year ago.

    🔮 ICD-9-CM Code(s): _____

78. Occlusion of renal dialysis graft.

    🔮 ICD-9-CM Code(s): _____

79. Abrasion of leg without infection.

    🔮 ICD-9-CM Code(s): _____

80. Wood splinter in the fingertip.

    🔮 ICD-9-CM Code(s): _____

81. Concussion with 2-hour loss of consciousness.

    🔮 ICD-9-CM Code(s): _____

82. Respiratory arrest of the newborn.

    🔮 ICD-9-CM Code(s): _____

83. Epigastric abdominal pain.

    🔮 ICD-9-CM Code(s): _____

84. Findings of elevated glucose tolerance test.

    🔮 ICD-9-CM Code(s): _____

🔮 **User to decide number of codes necessary to correctly answer the question.**
Odd-numbered answers are located in Appendix B, while the full answer key is only available in the TEACH Instructor Resources on Evolve.

REPORTS

Toward the end of this textbook, you will find a section titled Reports, which contains original reports. Read the reports indicated below and supply the appropriate ICD-9-CM codes on the following lines:

85. Report 6

    🌐 ICD-9-CM Code(s): __709.2__

86. Report 8

    🌐 ICD-9-CM Code(s): _____

87. Report 10

    🌐 ICD-9-CM Code(s): __952.04, E815.0__

88. Report 11

    🌐 ICD-9-CM Code(s): _____

89. Report 12

    🌐 ICD-9-CM Code(s): __707.05, 707.24__

90. Report 13

    🌐 ICD-9-CM Code(s): _____

91. Report 14

    🌐 ICD-9-CM Code(s): __659.71, 660.41__

92. Report 15

    🌐 ICD-9-CM Code(s): _____

93. Report 28

    🌐 ICD-9-CM Code(s): _____

94. Report 31

    🌐 ICD-9-CM Code(s): _____

95. Report 32

    🌐 ICD-9-CM Code(s): _____

🌐 **User to decide number of codes necessary to correctly answer the question.**
Odd-numbered answers are located in Appendix B, while the full answer key is only available in the TEACH Instructor Resources on Evolve.

96. Report 33

    935.2

    🔗 ICD-9-CM Code(s): 608.83, 935.0

97. Report 35

    🔗 ICD-9-CM Code(s): _____

98. Report 36

    🔗 ICD-9-CM Code(s): _____

99. Report 38

    🔗 ICD-9-CM Code(s): _____

100. Report 41

    🔗 ICD-9-CM Code(s): _____

101. Report 43

    🔗 ICD-9-CM Code(s): _____

🔗 **User to decide number of codes necessary to correctly answer the question.**
Odd-numbered answers are located in Appendix B, while the full answer key is only available in the TEACH
Instructor Resources on Evolve.

CHAPTER 13

Introduction to the CPT and Level II National Codes (HCPCS)

THEORY

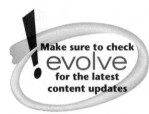

Without the use of reference material, complete the following:

There were six index location methods presented in Chapter 13. List any four of the methods.

1. service or procedure
2. anatomic site
3. condition or disease
4. synonym

Match the appendix with the information it contains:

5. D Appendix E   a. Modifier -63 Information on Infants <4 kg

6. A Appendix F   b. Moderate Sedation

7. B Appendix G   c. Product Pending FDA Approval

8. C Appendix K   d. Modifier -51 exempt

9. You would expect to find the CPT code 71010 in what section of the CPT manual?

   Radiology

10. What is the report called that a physician dictates to show that an unusual or rare procedure is performed?

    special reports

11. What association publishes the CPT?

    AMA

12. When you see the symbol ▲ in front of a code, you know what about the code?

   changed or modified

13. What type of code has the full code description? _section_

14. What type of code has only a portion of the code description?

   subsection

15. What would providers enter on the insurance form to show payers which services or procedures were performed?

   codes and/or _modifiers_

16. The use of a coding system allows you to communicate not only

   quickly, but also _correctly_ .

17. The first edition of the CPT was published in what year? _1966_

18. The updated CPT manual is available for purchase in what month?

   annually

19. A standard for communicating health care data, as represented in CPT, was necessary to address requirements of this 1996 act:

   Health insurance

   portability and _accountability_ Act.

20. What does the symbol of a circle with a line through it () placed before a CPT code indicate about the code?

   modifier 51 exempt

Match the following administration methods for drugs:

21. _G_ OTH   a. Subcutaneous

22. _D_ IT   b. Inhalant solution

23. _F_ IV   c. Various routes

24. _E_ IM   d. Intrathecal

25. _A_ SC   e. Intramuscular

26. _B_ INH   f. Intravenous

27. _C_ VAR   g. Other routes

Odd-numbered answers are located in Appendix B, while the full answer key is only available in the TEACH Instructor Resources on Evolve.

PRACTICAL

With the use of the CPT manual section Guidelines, identify the following unlisted codes:

Radiology

28. Clinical brachytherapy __77799__

29. Therapeutic radiology clinical treatment planning __77299__

30. Therapeutic radiology treatment management __77499__

Pathology and Laboratory

31. Surgical pathology procedure __88399__

32. Urinalysis procedure __81099__

Medicine

33. Allergy/clinical immunological service __95199__

34. Special dermatological service __96999__

35. Dialysis procedures, inpatient or outpatient __90999__

Odd-numbered answers are located in Appendix B, while the full answer key is only available in the TEACH Instructor Resources on Evolve.

CHAPTER 14

Modifiers

THEORY

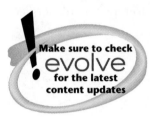

Make sure to check
evolve?
for the latest
content updates

Without the use of reference material, answer the following:

1. What appendix in the CPT manual contains a complete list of all modifiers?

   appendix A

2. What is the word that means assigning multiple codes when one code would do?

   BI-lateral

3. What is the term that describes the services provided to a patient by the physician before surgery?

   pre-op

4. What is another term for the time after the surgery that the physician provides services to the patient?

   post-op

5. Do all third-party payers recognize all modifiers as listed in the CPT manual?

   yes

6. What is the term that describes two physicians working together in the completion of a procedure when each has the same level of responsibility?

   Assistant

Odd-numbered answers are located in Appendix B, while the full answer key is only available in the TEACH Instructor Resources on Evolve.

PRACTICAL

Using the CPT, ICD-10-CM and/or ICD-9-CM manuals, indicate the modifiers and diagnoses that would be reported for the following:

7. A patient is admitted and has bilateral arthroscopy of the knees due to Baker's cysts.

   Modifier: _-50_

   ICD-10-CM Codes: _____, _____

   (ICD-9-CM Code: _____)

8. Ben Carter, surgical resident, assists Dr. Wells, chief cardiologist, in a coronary artery bypass procedure due to coronary arteriosclerosis of a native artery. What modifier would be submitted to report Ben's services in the teaching hospital?

   Modifier: _- 80_

   ICD-10-CM Code: _____

   (ICD-9-CM Code: _____)

9. Dr. Wells began surgery for right knee replacement due to severe osteoarthritis on an 86-year-old female with controlled hypertension. The patient was satisfactorily anesthetized and the site opened to view. Shortly thereafter, the patient's blood pressure dropped significantly, and the physician was unable to stabilize the patient. The procedure was discontinued.

   Modifier: _- 53_

   ICD-10-CM Codes: _____, _____

   (ICD-9-CM Codes: _____, _____)

10. The patient is a 10-month-old boy who fell while trying to walk across the kitchen floor at his home. He suffered an open wound to his bottom lip. Sutures are necessary but due to the patient's age and excessive movement general anesthesia is needed.

    Modifier: _- 23_

    ICD-10-CM Codes: Diagnosis: _____

    External Cause W Code: _____

    External Cause Y Code Place of Occurrence: _____

    (ICD-9-CM Codes: Diagnosis: _____

Odd-numbered answers are located in Appendix B, while the full answer key is only available in the TEACH Instructor Resources on Evolve.

E Code Cause: _____

E Code Place of Occurrence: _____)

11. A radiological examination of the gastrointestinal tract was ordered by a third-party payer for a confirmation of Crohn's disease (regional enteritis) of the large bowel. Crohn's was confirmed.

    Modifier: ‾ 22 _____

    ICD-10-CM Code: _____

    (ICD-9-CM Code: _____)

12. Anesthesia provided by the ENT physician during a tympanoplasty for repair of a tympanic membrane perforation.

    Modifier: ‾ 47 _____

    ICD-10-CM Code: _____

    (ICD-9-CM Code: _____)

13. A patient is seen at the direction of Workers' Compensation for a complete physical examination for insurance certification.

    Modifier: ‾ 92 _____

    ICD-10-CM Code: _____

    (ICD-9-CM Code: _____)

14. The patient returns to the operating room by same physician for removal of deep pins during the postoperative period, due to complication (dislodged) after an open repair of a humerus fracture.

    Modifier: ‾ 78 _____

15. A patient has a surgical procedure on Tuesday, and later that day the physician must take the patient back to the operating room to repeat (redo) a coronary bypass, due to complications of initial procedure.

    Modifier: ‾ 78 _____

16. The patient underwent a bilateral tympanoplasty.

    Modifier: ‾ 50 _____

17. If you must use two or more modifiers to describe a service, you would use which modifier to indicate this circumstance?

    Modifier: ‾ 99 _____

18. A surgeon performs a procedure on a neonate weighing 9 kg; the procedure was extremely complicated. What modifier would you use to indicate this service, which has an increased level of complexity?

    Modifier: ___-63___

19. Dr. Storely performed cataract surgery on 10/31/2011 and Dr. Jones provided postoperative care following discharge. What modifier would you use to indicate the postoperative care following discharge?

    Modifier: ___-55___

20. Dr. Merideth serves as an assistant surgeon to Dr. Taylor. What modifier would you add to the procedure code to indicate Dr. Merideth's status during the procedure?

    Modifier: ___-80___

21. The third-party payer requires the use of HCPCS/National modifiers; the surgeon performed a surgical procedure on the patient's left thumb. What Level II modifier would indicate the left thumb?

    Modifier: ___FA___

22. What Level II modifier indicates the upper left eyelid?

    Modifier: ___E1___

Odd-numbered answers are located in Appendix B, while the full answer key is only available in the TEACH Instructor Resources on Evolve.

80

Evaluation and Management (E/M) Services

THEORY

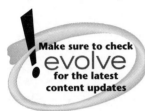

Make sure to check evolve **for the latest content updates**

Without the use of reference material, complete the following:

1. __C__ Consultation

2. __D__ Admission

3. __A__ Office visit

4. __G__ Newborn care

5. __E__ Established patient

6. __F__ Inpatient

7. __B__ New patient

8. __H__ Outpatient

a. A face-to-face encounter in an office between the physician and patient

b. One who has not received professional service from the physician or another physician in the exact same specialty and subspecialty in the same group within the last 3 years

c. Advice or opinion from one physician to another physician

d. One who has been formally admitted to an acute health care facility

e. One who has received professional service from the physician or another physician in the exact same specialty and subspecialty in the same group within the last 3 years

f. Attention to an acute illness or injury that results in hospitalization

g. Evaluation and determination of care for a newborn infant

h. One who has not been formally admitted to a health care facility

Odd-numbered answers are located in Appendix B, while the full answer key is only available in the TEACH Instructor Resources on Evolve.

The four types of medical decision making, in order of complexity from most to least complex, are as follows:

9. High

10. moderate

11. low

12. Straightforward

13. Complexity of medical decision making is based on three

    elements.

List the five types of presenting problems from the most risk and least recovery to least risk and most recovery:

14. High

15. moderate severity

16. minor severity

17. self limited

18. low severity

19. Counseling and coordination of care are what kind of factors in most

    cases? counseling

20. Time that is used as a guide for outpatient services is what kind of time?

    contributory

    Inpatient time spent at the bedside or nursing station during or after

    the visit is what kind of time? global period

21. The patient's medical record will reflect the number of systems examined by a brief statement of the findings.

22. A discussion with a patient and/or family concerning one or more of the following areas: diagnostic results, impressions and/or recommended diagnostic studies; prognosis; risks and benefits of treatment; instructions for treatment; importance of compliance with treatment; risk factor reduction; and patient and family education is

    counceling.

23. The history is the past information the patient tells the physician.

24. There is no distinction made between the new and established patients

    in this service department of a hospital: _False_

25. Those services rendered by a physician whose opinion or advice is requested by another physician or agency in the evaluation and/or

    treatment of a patient is a(n) _Consultation_, whereas the physician who has primary responsibility for the patient in the hospital

    is called _attending_.

26. When critically ill patients in medical emergencies require the constant attendance of the physician (e.g., cardiac arrest, shock, bleeding, and respiratory failure) to stabilize them, what kind of care is needed?

    emergency care

27. When care is provided for similar services (e.g., hospital visits) to the same patient by more than one physician on the same day for different

    conditions, the care is _concurrent_.

28. What is the name for the assumption of the total or specific care of a patient from one physician to another that does not constitute a

    consultation? _Physcian care_

29. An inventory of body systems obtained through questioning to identify signs and/or symptoms that the patient may be experiencing is a(n)

    review of _systems_.

30. If the physician who is standing by does so for 25 minutes, can he or she round the time up to 30 minutes for reporting purposes?

    _NO_

PRACTICAL

Office or Other Outpatient Services and Hospital Inpatient Service

With the use of the CPT manual, complete the following:

31. Analyze this case in which the patient record states: 40-year-old male patient (new) is evaluated for contusion of a finger. The history and examination were problem focused.

    a. Diagnosis and management options for contusion of finger. (Options can be minimal, limited, multiple, or extensive.) Diagnosis and

       management options: __minimal__

       Data to review to provide service. (Data can be minimal/none, limited, moderate, or extensive.) Only data available are current

       information obtained during the visit. Data: __moderate__

    b. Risks if left untreated. (Risk can be minimal, low, moderate, or high.)

       Risks: __low__

    c. All three of the elements have been met to qualify this patient for

       what level of decision making complexity? _____

       __Straightforward__

    d. The patient record indicates that a problem focused history and examination were done. When this is combined with the level of decision-making complexity you arrived at for this patient, what is

       the correct CPT code for the case? Code: __99219__

32. A patient who was on observation status for 48 hours is discharged from the hospital. The patient was being observed after a motor vehicle accident for subdural hematoma, subsequently ruled out. Code only the discharge services and diagnosis.

    CPT Code: __99210__

    ICD-10-CM Codes: _____, _____

    (ICD-9-CM Codes: _____, _____)

33. Initial observation of a patient was for upper abdominal pain, dizziness, and anemia. A comprehensive history and examination was performed. Moderate complexity decision making was conducted to admit the patient to observation to treat and rule out causes of the patient's anemia.

    CPT Code: __99219__

Odd-numbered answers are located in Appendix B, while the full answer key is only available in the TEACH Instructor Resources on Evolve.

34. A 16-year-old female is being admitted by her family practice physician with a 2-week history of fatigue and fever. It has been progressively getting worse. She is suffering from dehydration. The physician performs a comprehensive history to look for explanations for her fatigue, including recent activity level and recent sleep habits. A detailed examination is performed and she is diagnosed with mononucleosis and admitted for treatment.

    CPT Code: _99219_____

    ICD-10-CM Codes: _____, _____

    (ICD-9-CM Codes: _____, _____)

35. A 56-year-old male with an established history of ASHD of native arteries and past stent placement is admitted through the emergency room with acute onset of chest pain. An EKG was performed and troponin levels taken. Both showed evidence of the patient having an acute inferior wall myocardial infarction. The cardiologist performs a comprehensive history, with the chief complaint, 4 from the history of present illness (HPI), a complete review of systems (ROS), and past, family, and social history (PFSH). The history includes the information that the pain started a week ago but last night worsened. Also on a scale of 1 to 10, he rated the pain an 8. It was also discovered that the patient has not been attending regular appointments in the clinic setting. A comprehensive examination was performed along with high-complexity medical decision making (MDM), including management of the patient's acute MI and reviewing data of the medical history of the patient. He was taken immediately to the cardiac catheterization lab to look for the source for the patient's MI.

    CPT Code: _99223_____

    ICD-10-CM Codes: _____, _____, _____

    (ICD-9-CM Codes: _____, _____,

    _____)

36. The patient is a 34-year-old established patient seen in the clinic by her dermatologist. She is followed for extensive psoriasis involving her scalp, trunk, and arms. It has now worsened and spread to her palms, and she is now also complaining of joint pain. The spread to her hands has made it difficult to do many of her day-to-day tasks. A detailed history and examination are performed. The examination includes inspection of the affected areas in addition to bending and rotation of joints. A long discussion took place regarding a change in her medications to try to gain better control of her psoriasis and slow down the systemic progression. Topical and systemic treatment was decided on.

    CPT Code: _99218_____

    ICD-10-CM Codes: _____, _____

    (ICD-9-CM Codes: _____, _____)

Odd-numbered answers are located in Appendix B, while the full answer key is only available in the TEACH Instructor Resources on Evolve.

37. A 2-year-old boy with bacterial pneumonia is hospitalized and has had 5 days of antibiotic therapy. Today the child developed a fever of 101° F with a mild rash on his torso. In a subsequent hospital visit, the attending physician performed a problem focused history and examination. The MDM complexity was low.

CPT Code: __99231__

ICD-10-CM Code: _____

(ICD-9-CM Code: _____)

38. The patient is a 52-year-old male from out of state visiting his daughter. He left his medications for his benign hypertension at home and is now here in the clinic in need of a prescription. A problem focused history and examination is performed and a prescription is given to the patient.

CPT Code: __99 230__

ICD-10-CM Code: _____

(ICD-9-CM Code: _____)

Consultation Services

39. A 47-year-old female was sent by her family practice physician for an office consultation with a gynecologist. The patient has been suffering with moderate pelvic pain, a heavy sensation in her lower pelvis, and marked discomfort during sexual intercourse. In a detailed history, the gynecologist noted the location, severity, and duration of her pelvic pain and related symptoms. In the review of systems, the patient had positive findings related to her gastrointestinal, genitourinary, and endocrine body systems. The physician noted that her medical history was noncontributory to the present problem. The detailed physical examination centered on her gastrointestinal and genitourinary systems, with a complete pelvic examination. The physician ordered laboratory tests and a pelvic ultrasound to determine uterine fibroids, endometritis, or other internal gynecological pathology. The MDM complexity was moderate.

CPT Code: __99243__

ICD-10-CM Codes: _____, _____

(ICD-9-CM Codes: _____, _____)

40. A 38-year-old female has severe low back pain due to a trauma injury she experienced as a factory worker 4 years ago. The chronic pain has become almost unbearable, and her internal medicine physician cannot go any further with her treatment. An initial outpatient consultation is requested and the patient is sent to see the pain management specialist for suggestions to control the chronic pain. A comprehensive history is taken, including all of the pertinent information regarding her injury. During the comprehensive examination the patient's gait and

Odd-numbered answers are located in Appendix B, while the full answer key is only available in the TEACH Instructor Resources on Evolve.

movement were observed. Moderate-complexity decision making is performed, including different treatment options. A separate note is dictated to show the requesting physician what results were found during the visit and the decision on treatment of her pain.

CPT Code: _99240_

ICD-10-CM Codes: _____ , _____

(ICD-9-CM Codes: _____ , _____)

41. An inpatient urological consultation is performed for a 32-year-old female who recently had an elective abortion performed on an outpatient basis. The woman has been admitted with a high fever, pelvic pain, and dysuria. During a detailed history, the urologist notes in the history of present illness that the patient's symptoms began about 2 days after the abortion and progressed to the acute phase, which she is in at the present time. The location of the pain is in the lower abdomen and rated 9 on a scale of 1 to 10. She reports the quality of the pain to be sharp and stabbing. In the review of systems, the physician notes positive responses in 5 of the 12 body systems investigated. The urologist notes a negative medical history related to urinary symptoms other than a mild cystitis about 10 years ago. The detailed physical examination performed by the urologist centers on the genitourinary system and gastrointestinal system in significant detail. The medical decision making is low. Given the patient's past surgical procedure and physical findings at the present, the consultant considers the diagnoses of pyelonephritis, cystitis, pyelitis, and endometritis.

CPT Code: _99253_

42. A 46-year-old male is admitted to the hospital with a progressive staphylococcal pneumonia that is not responding to treatment. A request is made for the infectious disease physician on staff to render his opinion for treatment. The patient is seen in initial inpatient consultation. An expanded problem focused history and examination are performed. After looking at the sputum cultures, the physician decides on the most effective antibiotic for treatment. The decision making is straightforward.

CPT Code: _99251_

ICD-10-CM Code: _____

(ICD-9-CM Code: _____)

43. The initial consulting physician subsequently sees a 55-year-old patient injured at work when he fell from a house roof and struck his head. The patient had a right frontal parietal craniotomy 6 days previously and is recovering rapidly. The initial consultation was requested regarding a possible drug reaction that produced a rash on the upper torso. The consultant recommended a medication change, but after 48 hours the patient had no improvement. The physician re-evaluates for other possible causes of the rash. An expanded problem focused interval

history and a physical examination were performed. The MDM complexity was moderate.

CPT Code: _99232_

ICD-10-CM Code: _____

(ICD-9-CM Code: _____)

44. A 44-year-old patient, with chronic mastoiditis, was seen in consultation by the ENT specialist in the office. Her physician was inquiring as to the advantages of surgery versus continued antibiotic treatment when an acute flare comes on. The ENT specialist recommends surgery because of the increasing severity with each acute flare. She is fearful of the surgery because of the need to go under general anesthetic and a fear of permanent hearing loss. The physician performs an expanded problem focused history to include the duration of this problem and how many acute flares a year the patient experiences. An expanded problem focused examination and straightforward decision making is completed. It is determined that with the number of acute flares a year and the increasing severity of each case that surgery is recommended. The patient's fears are laid to rest and the patient decides to go ahead with the surgery.

CPT Code: _99320_

ICD-10-CM Code: _____

(ICD-9-CM Code: _____)

45. This is a follow-up visit on a 28-year-old male who is admitted with the diagnosis of headaches. The patient is subsequently seen because the physician needs to follow up on test results that weren't back yet at the initial consultation. This will help to find a possible cause of the headaches and course of treatment. A problem focused history and examination and low-complexity decision making is made after viewing the CT results. The diagnosis of tension headaches was made and treatment options discussed.

CPT Code: _99231_

ICD-10-CM Code: _____

(ICD-9-CM Code: _____)

46. An 83-year-old patient is seen at the local nursing home. The patient suffers from severe COPD. Routine labs were drawn on the patient by her primary doctor and her blood sugar came back abnormal. Fasting glucose was then taken and was high. The endocrinologist was asked to render an opinion on a possible diagnosis of diabetes. A problem focused history and examination and straightforward decision making were made. Diabetes was diagnosed and treatment started. The endocrinologist contacted the primary physician and discussed treatment of the patient. Report services for the endocrinologist only.

Odd-numbered answers are located in Appendix B, while the full answer key is only available in the TEACH Instructor Resources on Evolve.

CPT Code: _99240_

ICD-10-CM Code: _____

(ICD-9-CM Code: _____)

47. A patient is sent to a general surgeon by her family physician for an opinion and recommendation for surgical repair of a recurrent femoral hernia, right. A brief problem focused history of present illness and a problem focused examination of the affected body area and organ system are performed in the office. The MDM complexity was straightforward.

CPT Code: _99241_

ICD-10-CM Code: _____

(ICD-9-CM Code: _____)

48. A pulmonologist is asked, by the patient's primary physician, to see a 14-month-old boy who was admitted to the hospital with respiratory distress, cough, and fever. A comprehensive history is taken from the parents because this is an infant. It was determined that the patient does attend a day care facility. The cough and fever have been present for approximately 5 days. The infant started having trouble breathing this morning. The patient is intubated. Pneumonia due to respiratory syncytial virus is the definitive diagnosis. A comprehensive examination is performed along with moderate decision making. More tests will follow. A copy of his dictation will be sent to the primary physician.

CPT Code: _99360_

ICD-10-CM Code: _____

(ICD-9-CM Code: _____)

49. Office neurosurgery consultation is requested by the primary physician for a 32-year-old man on workers' compensation who is unable to work because of displacement of intervertebral lumbar disc with myelopathy. Two previous surgical repairs have been unsuccessful in relieving the patient's pain. The patient has been unable to return to his employment as a bricklayer. He complains of radiating pain throughout the buttocks and leg, with numbness throughout the leg and foot. Reflexes are minimal to nonexistent. A comprehensive history and physical examination are performed. MDM complexity was high due to the prior surgeries and continued complaints.

CPT Code: _99245 – 32_

ICD-10-CM Code: _____

(ICD-9-CM Code: _____)

Odd-numbered answers are located in Appendix B, while the full answer key is only available in the TEACH Instructor Resources on Evolve.

Emergency Department Services, Nursing Facility, Domiciliary, and Home Services

50. A patient presents to the emergency department after being involved in a motor vehicle accident. The patient was wearing a seat belt. The vehicle rolled numerous times. The patient's head struck the side window. The patient is unresponsive and is intubated. A history was unable to be obtained because of the patient's unresponsiveness. What history is available comes from the paramedics and patient's record. A comprehensive examination reveals the abdomen to be quite swollen with extensive bruising around the lower abdomen caused by the seat belt. High-complexity decision making was involved and the patient was rushed to the operating room.

    CPT Code: __99342__

51. A male patient presents to the emergency department with a wrist sprain sustained in a softball game when the patient slid into home, striking his hand on home plate. The patient is in apparent pain with a swollen wrist, which he is unable to flex. An expanded problem focused history and physical examination are done. Radiographs show a Colles' fracture of the distal radius. The MDM complexity was low.

    CPT Code: __99282__

    ICD-10-CM Codes: _____, _____, _____

    (ICD-9-CM Codes: _____, _____,

    _____)

52. An 88-year-old female's family physician comes to the nursing facility to perform the resident's annual assessment. A detailed interval history is taken with some information from the patient, but because of her limited cognitive abilities, most of the information is gathered from the nurses and past records. A comprehensive multisystem physical examination is performed, which includes extensive body areas and related organ systems. The MDM complexity was moderate because multiple diagnoses must be considered for this patient, who has senile dementia, diabetes, hypertension, hypothyroidism, and recurrent transient ischemic attacks. The creation of a new treatment plan is required because some of the patient's conditions have worsened.

    CPT Code: __99308__

    ICD-10-CM Codes: _____, _____,

    _____, _____, _____

    (ICD-9-CM Codes: _____, _____,

    _____, _____, _____)

Odd-numbered answers are located in Appendix B, while the full answer key is only available in the TEACH Instructor Resources on Evolve.

53. This is a home visit on an elderly gentleman, previously unknown to me, who is complaining of edema in his lower extremities. Pain is associated with this. An expanded problem focused history and examination are performed and low complexity decision making. Jobst stockings are prescribed.

    CPT Code: __99342__

    ICD-10-CM Code: _____

    (ICD-9-CM Code: _____)

54. Subsequent follow-up care is provided for the 82-year-old male nursing facility patient with Alzheimer's disease. The resident has responded well to some new medications and appears to have recovered some of his cognitive abilities without behavioral disturbances. The physician performs a problem focused history and physical examination on his neurological problem and orders the current treatments continued. The MDM complexity is low.

    CPT Code: __99321__

    ICD-10-CM Codes: _____, _____

    (ICD-9-CM Codes: _____, _____)

55. Subsequent follow-up care is provided for the patient who was transferred to a skilled nursing facility from an acute care hospital after partial recovery from a stroke. The patient has developed periods of extreme dizziness and mental confusion. A detailed interval history is gathered, and a detailed physical examination of the affected body systems is performed. Given the possibility that a new stroke could have occurred or that other neurological problems have developed, new orders are written, and the physician plans to return the next day to evaluate the patient's condition again. The MDM complexity is moderate.

    CPT Code: __99309__

    ICD-10-CM Codes: _____, _____, _____

    (ICD-9-CM Codes: _____, _____,

    _____)

56. The physician provides services to a resident of a rest home for an ulcerative sore on the heel and midfoot. Given the fact that the patient is in reasonably good health and is not diabetic, the physician focuses his attention on the right lower extremity during the problem focused physical examination. The physician knows the resident well and performs a brief HPI and ROS during a problem focused history. The resident thinks the sore is from new shoes, and the physician agrees

with that conclusion. Topical antibiotic cream is ordered, and the new shoes are sent to the cobbler to be stretched. The MDM complexity is straightforward.

CPT Code: __99234__

ICD-10-CM Code: _____

(ICD-9-CM Code: _____)

57. The physician provides services to a new patient who is in a custodial care center. The patient is 43 years old and is paraplegic, with severe infected stasis ulcers. The physician performs a detailed history and examination and prescribes an antibiotic. The MDM was straightforward.

CPT Code: __99324__

Prolonged Services and Preventive Medicine Services

58. An established patient is seen in the office for a new problem that requires a comprehensive history and examination. The MDM complexity is high, and the physician spends 40 minutes with the patient. However, the patient has numerous concerns, and the physician spends an additional hour and 50 minutes in prolonged direct patient contact.

CPT Codes: __99350__ , __99321__ ,

__99351,__

59. A 44-year-old asthmatic patient (new) is scheduled for a routine office visit for a complaint of severe headaches. The physician provides a comprehensive history and examination. The MDM complexity was high. Toward the end of the visit, the patient develops severe breathing complications, and the physician spends the next hour and 30 minutes administering treatment.

CPT Codes: __99205__ , __99354__ ,

__99355__

60. A 64-year-old man arrives at his appointment with his family physician for his annual physical examination. The patient has no new complaints and all of his medications remain the same. He is told to follow up in 1 year or sooner if necessary.

CPT Code: __99231__

Services from Throughout the E/M Section

61. A new patient is seen in the office for a variety of medical problems. The patient has insulin-dependent diabetes mellitus with complicating eye and renal problems. She also has hypertensive heart disease with episodes of congestive heart failure. Her peripheral vascular disease has

Odd-numbered answers are located in Appendix B, while the full answer key is only available in the TEACH Instructor Resources on Evolve.

worsened, and she can walk only a block before she is crippled with extreme leg pain. The patient reports that a new problem has surfaced: throbbing headaches with radiating neck pain. To manage and investigate the multiplicity of problems, the physician performs a comprehensive history and physical examination. A complete review of systems is performed, as is an update to her complete past, family, and social history. The physician has to take a multitude of factors into consideration because this patient's problems are highly complex.

CPT Code: _99205_

62. A new patient is seen in the office complaining of a sore throat and reports a low-grade fever for the past 4 days. The physician performs an expanded problem focused history and an expanded problem focused examination of the respiratory and lymphatic system. The physician's impression was acute pharyngitis and straightforward decision making was performed. Amoxicillin was prescribed.

CPT Code: _99324_

ICD-10-CM Code: _____

(ICD-9-CM Code: _____)

63. This is a 32-year-old female patient admitted for observation after an allergic reaction to her pain medication. She is alert and oriented, but has severe pruritus and shortness of breath. A detailed history and examination is performed after she takes medication for the pruritus; the breathing improved and the patient was discharged from observation on the same day. _pg. 17 starts - pg. 18_

CPT Code: _99234_

ICD-10-CM Codes: _____, _____,

_____

(ICD-9-CM Codes: _____, _____,

_____)

64. The patient was admitted to the hospital 3 days ago with severe dehydration and hyponatremia. The patient is now being discharged. Discharge takes 30 minutes.

CPT Code: _99205_

ICD-10-CM Codes: _____, _____

(ICD-9-CM Codes: _____, _____)

Odd-numbered answers are located in Appendix B, while the full answer key is only available in the TEACH Instructor Resources on Evolve.

65. A family practice physician who is treating a 20-year-old man (inpatient) for bronchitis calls in a urologist to examine the patient, who has requested a circumcision. The consultant performs a problem focused history and problem focused physical examination and determines that there is no urgency for the surgical procedure. The physician's decision making is fairly straightforward, and he recommends that the patient have the procedure done as an outpatient at a later date.

CPT Code: _99251_

66. A physician visits a 75-year-old female in the extended nursing facility as part of her annual assessment. The physician completes a detailed interval history with a comprehensive, head-to-toe physical examination. The physician reviews and affirms the medical plan of care developed by the multidisciplinary care team at the nursing facility. The patient's condition is stable; her hypertension and diabetes (type 2) are in good control and she has no new problems. The physician has limited data to review and few diagnoses to consider. The MDM complexity was low.

CPT Code: _99284_

ICD-10-CM Codes: _____, _____

(ICD-9-CM Codes: _____, _____)

67. A 67-year-old female is admitted with severe exacerbation of her COPD. The patient is now in respiratory failure and CHF. The patient is intubated and unconscious; 155 minutes of critical care time was spent at bedside and coordinating care for this patient.

☺ CPT Code(s): _99291_

☺ ICD-10-CM Code(s): _____

(☺ ICD-9-CM Code(s): _____)

68. Henry Green, an established patient, came into the office for his yearly physical examination. Henry is 72 and in good health.

CPT Code: _99283_

ICD-10-CM Code: _____

(ICD-9-CM Code: _____)

☺ **User to decide number of codes necessary to correctly answer the question.**
Odd-numbered answers are located in Appendix B, while the full answer key is only available in the TEACH Instructor Resources on Evolve.

REPORTS

Toward the end of this textbook, you will find a section titled Reports, which contains original reports. Read the reports indicated below and supply the appropriate CPT and/or ICD-9-CM code(s) on the following lines:

69. Report 1

    CPT Code: ___99283___

    ICD-10-CM Codes: _____, _____,

    _____

    (ICD-9-CM Codes: _____, _____,

    _____)

70. Report 2

    CPT Code: ___99284___

    ICD-10-CM Codes: _____(secondary neoplasm),

    _____ (primary neoplasm), _____ (vena

    cava syndrome), _____ (catheter complication),

    _____ (hypertension), _____ (nerve pain)

    (ICD-9-CM Codes: _____, _____,

    _____, _____, _____,

    _____)

71. Report 3

    CPT Code: ___99212___

    ICD-10-CM Code: _____

    (ICD-9-CM Code: _____)

72. Report 4

    CPT Code: ___99211___

73. Report 5

    CPT Code: ___99232___

Odd-numbered answers are located in Appendix B, while the full answer key is only available in the TEACH Instructor Resources on Evolve.

Anesthesia

THEORY

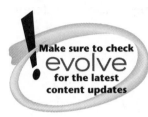

Make sure to check
evolve
for the latest
content updates

Without the use of reference material, answer the following:

1. What two words describe a decreased level of consciousness that does not put patients completely to sleep and that allows the patients to breathe on their own during a surgical procedure? __moderate__
   __(conscious) sedation__

2. What do the initials CRNA stand for?
   __certified registered nurse anesthetist__

3. CMS publishes an annual list of __base unit__ values for anesthesia codes.

4. The "M" in the anesthesia formula stands for __modifying__ unit.

5. What is the term that describes the services provided to a patient by the physician before surgery?
   __pre-op__

6. What is another term for the time after the surgery when the physician provides services to the patient?
   __post-op__

7. The __base__ factor for the locale is multiplied by the number of base units in the procedure plus the time units to determine the price of the anesthesia service.

8. This modifier indicates that a CRNA service with medical direction by a physician was provided. __-QX__

Odd-numbered answers are located in Appendix B, while the full answer key is only available in the TEACH Instructor Resources on Evolve.

PRACTICAL

With the use of the CPT manual, identify the following physical status modifiers:

9. Patient with a severe systemic disease that is a constant threat to life.

   Modifier: __P4__

10. Normal healthy patient.

    Modifier: __P1__

11. Patient with a severe systemic disease.

    Modifier: __P3__

12. Declared brain-dead patient whose organs are being removed for donor purposes.

    Modifier: __P6__

13. Patient with mild systemic disease.

    Modifier: __P2__

14. Moribund patient who is not expected to survive without the operation.

    Modifier: __P5__

Locate anesthesia procedures in the CPT manual index under the entry "Anesthesia" and then subtermed by the anatomic site. Write the CPT index location on the line provided (e.g., Anesthesia, Thyroid). Then locate the code identified in the anesthesia section of the CPT manual. Choose the correct code and write the code on the line provided.

15. Diagnostic arthroscopic procedure of knee joint.

    Index location: __knee and popliteal area__

    CPT Code: __01380__

16. Radical hysterectomy.

    Index location: __obstetric__

    CPT Code: __01962__

17. Corneal transplant.

    Index location: __Head__

    CPT Code: __00144__

Odd-numbered answers are located in Appendix B, while the full answer key is only available in the TEACH Instructor Resources on Evolve.

18. Cesarean delivery only.

    Index location: _Obstetric_

    CPT Code: _01961_

19. Otoscopy used in procedure for middle ear.

    Index location: _Head_

    CPT Code: _00120_

20. Transurethral resection of the prostate.

    Index location: _perineum_

    CPT Code: _00914_

21. Anesthesia for a cardiac catheterization patient having mild systemic disease.

    CPT Code: _01920-P2_

22. Anesthesia for a myringotomy on a healthy 5-year-old patient.

    CPT Code: _00961_

Assign the diagnosis code(s) for Questions 23–26.

23. Diverticulitis of colon with hemorrhage.

    ICD-10-CM Code: _____

    (ICD-9-CM Code: _____)

24. Atherosclerosis of coronary artery bypass graft utilizing internal mammary artery.

    ICD-10-CM Code: _____

    (ICD-9-CM Code: _____)

25. Toxic diffuse goiter with thyrotoxic crisis.

    ICD-10-CM Code: _____

    (ICD-9-CM Code: _____)

26. Mitral valve regurgitation as a late effect of Fen-Phen, taken as prescribed, initial encounter.

    ICD-10-CM Codes: _____, _____

    (ICD-9-CM Codes: _____, _____)

REPORTS

Toward the end of this textbook, you will find a section titled Reports, which contains original reports. Read the reports indicated below and supply the appropriate CPT anesthesia codes on the following lines:

27. Report 7

    CPT Code: ___00400___

28. Report 41

    CPT Code: ___00130___

29. Report 44

    CPT Code: ___00140___

30. Report 83

    CPT Code: ___00140___

CHAPTER 17

Surgery Guidelines and General Surgery

THEORY

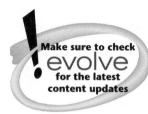

Without the use of reference material, answer the following:

1. The more complex subsections referred to in the text were Integumentary, Musculoskeletal, Respiratory, Cardiovascular, Digestive, ____Femal____ and ____genital____.

2. The information in the ____surgical____ contains information that is necessary to correctly code in the section, and the information is not repeated elsewhere.

3. Notes may appear before subsections, subheadings, ____categories____, and subcategories within the CPT manual.

4. When a note is present, that note must be read and ____understood____ if the coding is to be accurate.

5. Within the Surgery Guidelines, the ____unlisted____ procedure codes are presented in a list by anatomic site.

6. According to the CPT manual, "Pertinent information [in the ____general____ report] should include an adequate definition or description of the nature, extent, need, time, effort, and equipment necessary to provide the service."

7. There are minor and ____major____ procedure designations for the purposes of a surgical package.

8. If a breast biopsy and mastectomy of the left breast were performed during the same operative session, would both procedures be reported?

   ____-59____

9. If a breast biopsy and right knee operation were performed during the same operative session, would both procedures be reported?

   ____yes____

Odd-numbered answers are located in Appendix B, while the full answer key is only available in the TEACH Instructor Resources on Evolve.

10. The CPT manual describes the surgical package as including one related preoperative E/M service, the operative procedure, and immediate

    ___surgical___ care.

11. Local infiltration is considered ___local___ anesthesia.

12. This term means a worsening as described in the text.

    ___problem___

13. This type of anesthesia is not part of the surgical package.

    ___general___

14. The predefined number of days before and after a surgical procedure are

    referred to as the ___global___ period.

15. What is the CPT code that reports a surgical tray? ___99070___

16. What is the HCPCS code that reports a surgical tray?

    ___99070___

17. According to the Medicare guidelines, a surgical package includes the

    treatment of complications by the ___same___ physician.

18. At an office visit, a decision for surgery was made. The surgical procedure was scheduled 21 days later. Would the office visit service be:
    a. reported separately
    b. included in the surgical procedure

19. Splitting open of the surgical wound is ___dehiscene___.

20. Inclusion or exclusion of a procedure in the CPT manual implies health insurance coverage or no health insurance coverage.

    True or False? ___F___

PRACTICAL

With the use of a CPT manual, answer the following:

21. The code range in the Surgical section is ___10021___ to
    ___69990___.

22. The subsection that follows the Digestive System is the
    ___respiratory___ System.

23. What type of microscope has a subsection of the Surgery section?
    ___operating___

24. The difference between 10021 and 10022 is that one is with
    ___local___ ___general___ and one is without it.

25. According to the parenthetical information following code 10022, for a percutaneous needle biopsy other than fine needle aspiration, see
    ___42400___ for salivary gland.

26. According to the Surgery Guidelines, codes designated as
    "___general___ ___local___" should not be reported in addition to the code for the total procedure or service of which it is considered an integral component.

27. According to the Surgery Guidelines, follow-up care for
    ___theraputic___ surgical procedures includes only that care which is usually a part of the surgical procedure.

28. According to the Surgery Guidelines, the code range for Maternity Care and Delivery is ___42400___ - ___40799___.

29. According to the Surgery Guidelines, this is the code for unlisted procedures of the lip. ___40799___

30. According to the Surgery Guidelines, this is the code for unlisted procedures of the urinary system. ___40799___

Integumentary System

THEORY

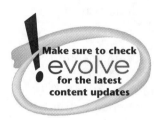

Integumentary System Terminology

Match the following terms to the correct definitions:

1. __B__ Dermis

2. __D__ Epidermis

3. __i__ Subcutaneous

4. __G__ Incision and drainage

5. __A__ Abscess

6. __J__ Cyst

7. __F__ Debridement

8. __H__ Paring

9. __C__ Biopsy

10. __E__ Shaving

a. Localized collection of pus that will result in the disintegration of tissue over time

b. Second layer of skin holding blood vessels, nerve endings, sweat glands, and hair follicles

c. Removal of a small piece of living tissue for diagnostic purposes

d. Outer layer of skin

e. Horizontal or transverse removal of dermal or epidermal lesions, without full-thickness excision

f. Cleansing of or removing dead tissue from a wound

g. To cut and withdraw fluid

h. Removal of thin layers of skin by peeling or scraping

i. Tissue below dermis, primarily fat cells that insulate the body

j. Closed sac containing matter or fluid

Odd-numbered answers are located in Appendix B, while the full answer key is only available in the TEACH Instructor Resources on Evolve.

Match the following terms to the correct definitions:

11. __A__ Excision

12. __D__ Benign

13. __I__ Malignant

14. __G__ Repair

15. __C__ Skin graft

16. __H__ Tissue transfer

17. __E__ Destruction

18. __B__ Mast-

19. __F__ Cryosurgery

a. Full-thickness removal of a lesion that may include simple closure

b. Prefix meaning breast

c. Transplantation of tissue to repair a defect

d. Not progressive or recurrent

e. Killing of tissue, possibly by electrocautery, laser, chemical, or other means

f. Destruction of lesions using extreme cold

g. Pertains to suturing a wound

h. Piece of skin for grafting that is still partially attached to the original blood supply and is used to cover an adjacent wound area

i. Used to describe a cancerous tumor that grows worse over time

20. If multiple lesions are treated, the most complex lesion is listed first and the others are usually listed using modifier:
    a. -50
    b. -51
    c. -47
    d. -99

21. This condition is chronic abscessing and subsequent infection of a sweat gland.
    a. folliculitis
    b. hyperhidrosis
    c. miliaria
    d. hidradenitis

22. An example of a corn or callus is a benign:
    a. hyperkeratotic skin lesion
    b. lipoma or dermatofibroma
    c. nevi or dysplastic nevi
    d. dermoid cyst or nevi or dysplastic nevi

PRACTICAL

Using the CPT and ICD-10-CM/ICD-9-CM manuals, code the following services:

23. Joan, an established patient, comes into the office to have an intermediate repair of a 2.6 cm wound on her right arm. A surgical tray was used.

    CPT Codes: ___12032___ , ___99070___

    ICD-10-CM Code: _____

    (ICD-9-CM Code: _____)

24. Rita, an established patient, has a 16.2 cm simple repair of the cheek. A surgical tray is used.

    CPT Codes: ___19082___ , ___99070___

    ICD-10-CM Code: _____

    (ICD-9-CM Code: _____)

25. Lisa, an established patient, has a percutaneous biopsy with stereotactic image guidance for a left breast mass. A surgical tray was used. The pathology report later indicated a neoplasm of uncertain behavior.

    CPT Codes: ___19081-LT___ , ___99070___

    ICD-10-CM Code: _____

    (ICD-9-CM Code: _____)

26. What code would be used to report Mr. Jones's visit to Dr. Green 2 weeks after major surgery?

    CPT Code: ___99071___

    ICD-10-CM Code: _____

    (ICD-9-CM Code: _____)

27. Excision axillary hidradenitis, complex repair.

    CPT Code: ___11451___

    ICD-10-CM Code: _____

    (ICD-9-CM Code: _____)

28. Debridement; 16 sq. cm. subcutaneous tissue and muscle due to a diabetic foot ulcer.

    CPT Code: ___11042___

    ICD-10-CM Codes: _____ , _____

    (ICD-9-CM Codes: _____ , _____)

Odd-numbered answers are located in Appendix B, while the full answer key is only available in the TEACH Instructor Resources on Evolve.

29. Removal of tissue expander without insertion of prosthesis.

    CPT Code: 11971

30. Excision of abscessed pilonidal cyst; complicated.

    CPT Code: 11042

    ICD-10-CM Code: _____

    (ICD-9-CM Code: _____)

31. Removal of Norplant contraceptive capsule.

    CPT Code: 11976

    ICD-10-CM Code: _____

    (ICD-9-CM Code: _____)

32. Debridement of four fingernails due to onychomycosis.

    CPT Code: 11403

    ICD-10-CM Code: _____

    (ICD-9-CM Code: _____)

33. Excision of 4 cm benign lesion of face (most resource intensive) and excision of 3 cm benign lesion of neck.

    🕸 CPT Code(s): 11444

    🕸 ICD-10-CM Code(s): _____

    (🕸 ICD-9-CM Code(s): _____)

34. Excision of a 2.5 cm malignant lip lesion and two malignant lesions of the skin of the chest, each 1.5 cm in diameter.

    🕸 CPT Code(s): 12073 X2

    🕸 ICD-10-CM Code(s): _____

    (🕸 ICD-9-CM Code(s): _____)

35. Destruction by laser of three premalignant actinic keratoses facial lesions.

    🕸 CPT Code(s): 17000

    🕸 ICD-10-CM Code(s): _____

    (🕸 ICD-9-CM Code(s): _____)

🕸 User to decide number of codes necessary to correctly answer the question.
Odd-numbered answers are located in Appendix B, while the full answer key is only available in the TEACH Instructor Resources on Evolve.

36. Destruction of 4.0 cm malignant lesion of the eyelid.

    ✪ CPT Code(s): __12074__

    ✪ ICD-10-CM Code(s): _____

    (✪ ICD-9-CM Code(s): _____)

37. Suzanne Osterland, a 4-year-old, is brought to the office by her father. Suzanne was playing on the swing set at the playground when she fell approximately 5 feet from the top step of the play set. When she fell, she struck her leg on a birdbath rim and then on the playground gardener's pail with several garden forks protruding over the rim, sustaining 12.9 cm, 3.1 cm, and 2.1 cm lacerations of the lower right leg, requiring deep-layered closure accomplished after subcutaneous tissue debridement of 18 sq. cm.

    CPT Codes: __12073__, __11042-51__

    ICD-10-CM Codes: _____, _____ (W code),

    _____ (W code), _____ (Y code)

    (ICD-9-CM Codes: _____, _____ (E code),

    _____ (E code), _____ (E code),

    _____ (E code))

38. Electrosurgical destruction of a 1.0 cm malignant lesion of the neck.

    ✪ CPT Code(s): __17001__

    ✪ ICD-10-CM Code(s): _____

    (✪ ICD-9-CM Code(s): _____)

39. Cryosurgical destruction of 10 flat warts on the hand.

    ✪ CPT Code(s): __17110__

    ✪ ICD-10-CM Code(s): _____

    (✪ ICD-9-CM Code(s): _____)

40. Laser destruction of multiple malignant lesions, as follows: 3.4 cm on right hand, 2.1 cm on left hand, 5.2 cm on right hand, 4.3 cm on left hand, 0.3 cm on right eyelid, 0.5 cm on left eyelid.

    ✪ CPT Code(s): __12073__

    ✪ ICD-10-CM Code(s): _____

    (✪ ICD-9-CM Code(s): _____)

✪ **User to decide number of codes necessary to correctly answer the question.**
Odd-numbered answers are located in Appendix B, while the full answer key is only available in the TEACH Instructor Resources on Evolve.

41. Debridement of back for extensive eczematous skin, 20% body surface.

    🏵 CPT Code(s): <u>11000, 11001</u>

    🏵 ICD-10-CM Code(s): _____

    (🏵 ICD-9-CM Code(s): _____)

42. Bilateral blepharoplasty of upper eyelid due to ptosis.

    🏵 CPT Code(s): <u>16010</u>

    🏵 ICD-10-CM Code(s): _____

    (🏵 ICD-9-CM Code(s): _____)

43. Initial, local treatment, first-degree burn, of back of hand, 5% body surface. The burn was caused by steam from a pipe at his home that accidentally was connected improperly.

    🏵 CPT Code(s): <u>16000</u>

    🏵 ICD-10-CM Code(s): _____

    (🏵 ICD-9-CM Code(s): _____)

44. Mohs micrographic surgery of arm for a poorly defined malignant neoplasm, first stage, 4 tissue blocks.

    🏵 CPT Code(s): <u>21540</u>

    🏵 ICD-10-CM Code(s): _____

    (🏵 ICD-9-CM Code(s): _____)

45. Mastotomy with drainage of deep abscess.

    🏵 CPT Code(s): <u>19020</u>

    🏵 ICD-10-CM Code(s): _____

    (🏵 ICD-9-CM Code(s): _____)

🏵 User to decide number of codes necessary to correctly answer the question.
Odd-numbered answers are located in Appendix B, while the full answer key is only available in the TEACH Instructor Resources on Evolve.

REPORTS

Toward the end of this textbook, you will find a section titled Reports, which contains original reports. Read the reports indicated below and supply the appropriate CPT and ICD-10-CM/ICD-9-CM codes on the following lines:

46. Report 6

    ☻ CPT Code(s): __19121__

    ☻ ICD-10-CM Code(s): _____

    (☻ ICD-9-CM Code(s): _____)

47. Report 7

    ☻ CPT Code(s): __21554__

    ☻ ICD-10-CM Code(s): _____

    (☻ ICD-9-CM Code(s): _____)

48. Report 8

    ☻ CPT Code(s): __15941__

    ☻ ICD-10-CM Code(s): _____

    (☻ ICD-9-CM Code(s): _____)

49. Report 9

    ☻ CPT Code(s): __19120 - RT__

    ☻ ICD-10-CM Code(s): _____

    (☻ ICD-9-CM Code(s): _____)

50. Report 11

    ☻ CPT Code(s): __19210__

    ☻ ICD-10-CM Code(s): _____

    (☻ ICD-9-CM Code(s): _____)

51. Report 12

    ☻ CPT Code(s): __15940__

    ☻ ICD-10-CM Code(s): _____

    (☻ ICD-9-CM Code(s): _____)

☻ **User to decide number of codes necessary to correctly answer the question.**
Odd-numbered answers are located in Appendix B, while the full answer key is only available in the TEACH Instructor Resources on Evolve.

CHAPTER 19

Musculoskeletal System

THEORY

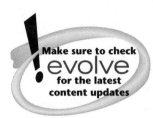

Make sure to check
evolve
for the latest
content updates

Musculoskeletal Terminology

Without the use of reference material, match the following terms to the correct definitions:

1. __D__ Closed treatment
2. __F__ Open treatment
3. __J__ Percutaneous
4. __I__ Fracture
5. __B__ Dislocation
6. __E__ Manipulation
7. __C__ Fixation
8. __A__ Skeletal traction
9. __H__ Soft tissue
10. __K__ Arthroplasty
11. __G__ Arthrodesis

a. Application of force to a limb with the use of a pin, screw, wire, or clamp attached to the bone

b. Displacement of a bone from its normal location in a joint

c. The application of pins, wires, screws, and so on to immobilize; these can be placed externally or internally

d. Fracture treatment when site is not surgically opened and visualized or reduction

e. Word used interchangeably with reduction to mean the attempted restoration of a fracture or joint dislocation to its normal anatomic position

f. Fracture site that is surgically opened and visualized

g. Surgical immobilization of a joint

h. Tissues (fascia, connective tissue, muscle, etc.) surrounding organs and other structures

i. Break in a bone

j. Fixation considered neither open nor closed; fracture is not visualized, but fixation is placed across the fracture site under x-ray imaging

k. Reshaping or reconstructing a joint

Odd-numbered answers are located in Appendix B, while the full answer key is only available in the TEACH Instructor Resources on Evolve.

Without the use of reference material, answer the following:

12. Would a biopsy code usually include the administration of any necessary local anesthesia? Yes or No? ___NO___

13. What is arthrocentesis? ___aspiration of a joint___

14. What is a uniplane fixation device? ___The fracture treatment___

    _____

15. What is the name of the graft that is taken from the upper thigh area where the fascia is the thickest? ___facia lata graft___

16. What type of stimulation often is used to promote healing of a slow-healing fracture? ___osteoarthritis___

17. What is fast becoming the surgical method of choice for many musculoskeletal procedures today? ___arthroscopy___

18. What is the term that describes the use of tape applied to the body to provide support or limit motion? ___strapping___

19. Do you bill for the removal of a cast that your physician applied? Yes or No? ___NO___ Why or why not? ___the removal is part of the cast service___

20. What two words describe when elastic wrap or tape is fastened to the skin or wrapped around a limb and weights are then attached to the wraps or tape? ___skin traction___

21. What is the primary difference between the excision codes found in the Musculoskeletal System subsection and the excision codes found in the Integumentary System subsection? ___The extent___

    _____

    _____

PRACTICAL

With the use of the CPT and ICD-10-CM/ICD-9-CM manual(s), code the following:

(local period)

22. John is returning to the physician's office 2 weeks postsurgery for an application of a <u>new</u> long leg cast. The patient required surgery due to a traumatic fracture of the lower leg.

    CPT Code: _29345 – 58_

    ICD-10-CM Codes: _____, _____

    (ICD-9-CM Codes: _____, _____)

23. Julie Mason, age 5 years, is coming in today to have her long-arm cast removed and replaced with a short-arm cast for 3 weeks. The patient sustained a Torus fracture of the upper end of the radius and is 1 week postop.

    CPT Code: _29075_

    ICD-10-CM Codes: _____, _____

    (ICD-9-CM Codes: _____, _____)

24. Jamie Larson slipped on the ice and twisted her knee when she fell. During diagnostic arthroscopy, a buckle handle tear of the medial and lateral meniscus was seen and repaired.

    CPT Code: _28048_

    ICD-10-CM Codes: _____, _____, _____

    (ICD-9-CM Codes: _____, _____,

    _____)

25. Percutaneous skeletal fixation of closed calcaneal fracture requiring manipulation.

    CPT Code: _28406_

    ICD-10-CM Code: _____

    (ICD-9-CM Code: _____)

Odd-numbered answers are located in Appendix B, while the full answer key is only available in the TEACH Instructor Resources on Evolve.

26. Closed treatment of a pelvic rim fracture; without manipulation.

   CPT Code: ___20614___

   ICD-10-CM Code: _____

   (ICD-9-CM Code: _____)

27. Closed treatment of a single closed metacarpophalangeal dislocation, distal end; with manipulation and without anesthesia.

   CPT Code: __26700___

   ICD-10-CM Code: _____

   (ICD-9-CM Code: _____)

28. Open treatment of a closed traumatic anterior hip dislocation without fixation.

   CPT Code: ___27720___

   ICD-10-CM Code: _____

   (ICD-9-CM Code: _____)

29. Closed treatment of a patellar fracture; no manipulation.

   CPT Code: __27520___

   ICD-10-CM Code: _____

   (ICD-9-CM Code: _____)

30. Closed treatment of a closed patellar dislocation; no anesthesia.

   CPT Code: __20526___

   ICD-10-CM Code: _____

   (ICD-9-CM Code: _____)

31. Manipulation of a knee joint under general anesthesia with application of a traction device. Patient had an anterior dislocation of the tibia, proximal end.

   CPT Code: __27570___

   ICD-10-CM Code: _____

   (ICD-9-CM Code: _____)

Odd-numbered answers are located in Appendix B, while the full answer key is only available in the TEACH Instructor Resources on Evolve.

32. Closed treatment of a closed tarsal bone dislocation without anesthesia.

    CPT Code: ___20661___

    ICD-10-CM Code: _____

    (ICD-9-CM Code: _____)

33. Depressed frontal sinus fracture repaired using open treatment.

    CPT Code: ___21343___

34. Open treatment of a Le Fort I maxillary fracture.

    CPT Code: ___20823___

35. Aspiration and injection of a bone cyst.

    CPT Code: ___20615___

36. Removal of deep screws from a repaired fracture. (The screws are fixation devices.)

    CPT Code: ___20451___

37. Replantation of index finger, including sublimis tendon insertion, following a complete traumatic amputation. Code only the replantation service.

    CPT Code: ___20822___

38. Costochondral cartilage graft.

    CPT Code: ___20660___

39. Therapeutic injection of corticosteroids for medial nerve entrapment (CTS).

    CPT Code: ___20526___

    ICD-10-CM Code: _____

    (ICD-9-CM Code: _____)

40. Aspiration of a shoulder joint.

    CPT Code: ___23929___

41. Removal of a halo that was applied by another physician.

    CPT Code: ___20665___

Odd-numbered answers are located in Appendix B, while the full answer key is only available in the TEACH Instructor Resources on Evolve.

42. Subsequent removal of a short-arm cast by the physician who applied the cast.

    CPT Code: 29705

43. Closed treatment of a mandibular fracture without manipulation.

    CPT Code: 21450

44. Application of a shoulder-to-hip body cast.

    CPT Code: 29035

45. Wedging of a clubfoot cast.

    CPT Code: 29750

46. Application of a short leg splint.

    CPT Code: 29515

47. Strapping of a hip.

    CPT Code: 29520

48. Application of a long-arm splint.

    CPT Code: 29583

49. Strapping of a 40-year-old's thorax.

    CPT Code: 29200

50. Surgical arthroscopy of the temporomandibular joint.

    CPT Code: 29861

51. Application, cast; figure-of-eight.

    CPT Code: 29049

52. Surgical arthroscopy, elbow; limited debridement.

    CPT Code: 24999

53. Diagnostic hip arthroscopy.

    CPT Code: 29860

54. Surgical arthroscopy with lateral meniscus repair of knee.

    CPT Code: 27599

55. Arthroscopic chondroplasty of knee with minimal debridement.

CPT Code: _29877_

56. Endoscopic plantar fasciotomy.

CPT Code: _29840_

57. Release of a transverse carpal ligament of the wrist with surgical endoscopy.

CPT Code: _29848_

58. Arthrocentesis of ganglion cyst of toe joint, both injection and aspiration.

CPT Code: _29861_

ICD-10-CM Code: _____

(ICD-9-CM Code: _____)

59. Excision of maxillary torus palatinus.

CPT Code: _21032_

Odd-numbered answers are located in Appendix B, while the full answer key is only available in the TEACH Instructor Resources on Evolve.

REPORTS

Toward the end of this textbook, you will find a section titled Reports, which contains original reports. Read the reports indicated below and supply the appropriate CPT and ICD-10-CM/ICD-9-CM codes on the following lines:

60. Report 10

    CPT Code: _25601 - LT_

    ICD-10-CM Codes: _____, _____ (E code)

    (ICD-9-CM Codes: _____, _____, _____ (External Cause code))

61. Report 13

    CPT Code: _20610 - RT_

    ICD-10-CM Code: _____

    (ICD-9-CM Code: _____)

62. Report 14

    CPT Code: _27240 - RT_

    ICD-10-CM Codes: _____, _____

    (ICD-9-CM Codes: _____, _____)

63. Report 15

    CPT Code: _25606 - LT_

    ICD-10-CM Codes: _____, _____

    (ICD-9-CM Codes: _____, _____)

64. Report 16

    CPT Code: _27240 - LT_

    ICD-10-CM Codes: _____, _____

    (ICD-9-CM Codes: _____, _____)

Odd-numbered answers are located in Appendix B, while the full answer key is only available in the TEACH Instructor Resources on Evolve.

65. Report 17

CPT Code: _27244-RT_

ICD-10-CM Code: _____

(ICD-9-CM Codes: _____, _____)

66. Report 18

CPT Code: _20610-LT_

ICD-10-CM Code: _____

(ICD-9-CM Code: _____)

CHAPTER 20

Respiratory System

THEORY

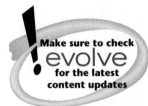

Without the use of reference material, complete the following:

Respiratory Terminology

Match the following terms and prefixes to the correct definitions:

1. __D__ Polyp
2. __H__ Rhino-
3. __K__ Endoscopy
4. __O__ Sinuses
5. __B__ Antrum
6. __L__ Antrotomy
7. __C__ Laryngo-
8. __J__ Bronchoscopy
9. __F__ Thoracentesis
10. __P__ Thoracotomy
11. __M__ Thoracostomy
12. __G__ Thoracoscopy
13. __A__ Lobectomy
14. __I__ Pleura
15. __E__ Pneumo-
16. __N__ Embolectomy

a. Excision of a lobe of the lung
b. Maxillary sinus
c. Prefix meaning larynx
d. Tumor on a pedicle that bleeds easily and may become malignant
e. Prefix meaning lung or air
f. Surgical puncture of the thoracic cavity, usually using a needle, to remove fluids
g. Inspection of the bronchial tree using a bronchoscope
h. Prefix meaning nose
i. Use of a lighted endoscope to view the pleural spaces and thoracic cavity or perform surgical procedures
j. Removal of blockage (embolism) from vessels
k. Inspection of body organs or cavities using a lighted scope that may be placed through an existing opening or through a small incision
l. Covering of the lungs and thoracic cavity that is moistened with serous fluid to reduce friction during respiratory movements of the lungs
m. Cutting into the thoracic cavity to allow for enlargement of the heart or for drainage
n. Cutting through the antrum wall to make an opening in the sinus
o. Cavities within the nasal bones
p. Surgical incision into the thoracic cavity

Odd-numbered answers are located in Appendix B, while the full answer key is only available in the TEACH Instructor Resources on Evolve.

17. What is the name of the item that is placed into the hole in a deviated septum as a repair without surgical grafting?

_____Nasal Button_____

18. What is the name of the surgical procedure for the reshaping of the nose?

_____Lobectomy_____

19. What is the name of the surgical procedure for the rearrangement of the nasal septum often used in patients with a deviated septum?

_____Septoplasty_____

20. This term means destruction by removing, usually by vaporization, chipping, or other erosive process such as laser or cutting:

_____Embolectomy_____

21. Which approach of treating nasal hemorrhage is most difficult to control, posterior or anterior?

_____Posterior_____

22. What term describes washing out of an organ?

_____Debridment_____

23. What are the two different approaches that can be used to perform a

tracheostomy? _____Transtracheal_____ and _____Cricothyroid_____

24. If a surgeon performs a thoracotomy procedure and at the end of the procedure inserts a chest tube for drainage, do you report the insertion of the tube separately? Why?

_____No, done at the same time_____

25. If bilateral destruction of maxillary sinuses is performed, what modifier

would you use? _____50_____

26. Removal of two lobes of a lung is termed a(n)

_____Bronchoscopy_____.

PRACTICAL

With the use of the CPT and ICD-10-CM/ICD-9-CM manuals, complete the following:

27. Endoscopic maxillary antrostomy with removal of granulation tissue.

    CPT Code: 31267

28. Ben is a 5-year-old who swallowed a nickel. Patient needed an indirect laryngoscopy to remove this foreign body.

    CPT Code: 30800

29. Bronchoscopy with transbronchial biopsies of two lobes of the right lung.

    CPT Codes: 31628-RT , 31628

30. Flexible bronchoscopy with brushings.

    CPT Code: 31564

31. Diagnostic flexible fiberoptic laryngoscopy.

    CPT Code: 31575

32. Intranasal biopsy.

    CPT Code: 30150

33. Cauterization of superficial mucosa of bilateral inferior turbinates.

    CPT Code: 30801

34. Primary rhinoplasty with elevation of nasal tip.

    CPT Code: 30152

35. Extensive bilateral removal of nasal polyps, performed in the hospital outpatient department.

    CPT Codes: 30115-50 , 30115

36. Insertion of a septal button.

    CPT Code: 31268

37. Direct, operative, laryngoscopy with biopsy, with use of the operating microscope.

    CPT Code: 31543

Odd-numbered answers are located in Appendix B, while the full answer key is only available in the TEACH Instructor Resources on Evolve.

38. Establishment and subsequent insertion of voice button following construction of a transesophageal fistula.

   CPT Code: _____

39. Arytenoidectomy; external approach.

   🌐 CPT Code(s): _31400_____

40. Laryngoscopy, with stroboscopy.

   🌐 CPT Code(s): _____

41. Nasotracheal catheter aspiration.

   🌐 CPT Code(s): _31720_____

42. Cervical tracheoplasty.

   🌐 CPT Code(s): _____

43. Revision of a tracheostomy scar.

   🌐 CPT Code(s): _31830_____

44. Thoracentesis for aspiration of the pleural space, without image guidance.

   🌐 CPT Code(s): _____

45. Surgical thoracoscopy, with removal of a clot from pericardial.

   🌐 CPT Code(s): _32658_____

46. Double lung transplant with cardiopulmonary bypass.

   🌐 CPT Code(s): _____

47. Repair hernia of the lung through the chest wall.

   🌐 CPT Code(s): _32800_____

48. Open closure of a major bronchial fistula.

   🌐 CPT Code(s): _____

49. Therapeutic fracture of inferior nasal turbinate bone, closed.

   🌐 CPT Code(s): _30930_____

🌐 **User to decide number of codes necessary to correctly answer the question.**
Odd-numbered answers are located in Appendix B, while the full answer key is only available in the TEACH Instructor Resources on Evolve.

50. Sinusotomy, sphenoid, without biopsy for acute sinusitis.

   ✸ CPT Code(s): _____

   ✸ ICD-10-CM Code(s): _____

   (✸ ICD-9-CM Code(s): _____)

51. Tracheostoma revision, simple, without flap rotation due to infection of tracheostomy by cellulitis.

   ✸ CPT Code(s): _37609_____

   ✸ ICD-10-CM Code(s): _____

   (✸ ICD-9-CM Code(s): _____)

52. Bronchial biopsy, bronchoscopic, due to chronic cough.

   ✸ CPT Code(s): _____

   ✸ ICD-10-CM Code(s): _____

   (✸ ICD-9-CM Code(s): _____)

53. Total pneumonectomy due to occupational asbestosis.

   ✸ CPT Code(s): _35452_____

   ✸ ICD-10-CM Code(s): _____

   (✸ ICD-9-CM Code(s): _____)

54. Diagnostic thoracoscopy of the pericardial sac, with biopsy for chronic rheumatic pericarditis.

   ✸ CPT Code(s): _____

   ✸ ICD-10-CM Code(s): _____

   (✸ ICD-9-CM Code(s): _____)

55. Extrapleural resection of the ribs, all stages for deformed ribs, congenital.

   ✸ CPT Code(s): _33513_____

   ✸ ICD-10-CM Code(s): _____

   (✸ ICD-9-CM Code(s): _____)

✸ **User to decide number of codes necessary to correctly answer the question.**
Odd-numbered answers are located in Appendix B, while the full answer key is only available in the TEACH Instructor Resources on Evolve.

56. Carinal reconstruction for lung cancer, primary, malignant.

    ⊛ CPT Code(s): __33640__

    ⊛ ICD-10-CM Code(s): _____

    (⊛ ICD-9-CM Code(s): _____)

57. Instillation, via a catheter, of an agent for pleurodesis for malignant pleural effusion due to ovarian cancer.

    ⊛ CPT Code(s): _33967_____

    ⊛ ICD-10-CM Code(s): _____

    (⊛ ICD-9-CM Code(s): _____)

58. Excision dermoid cyst of the nose, complex.

    ⊛ CPT Code(s): _33641_____

    ⊛ ICD-10-CM Code(s): _____

    (⊛ ICD-9-CM Code(s): _____)

⊛ **User to decide number of codes necessary to correctly answer the question.**
Odd-numbered answers are located in Appendix B, while the full answer key is only available in the TEACH Instructor Resources on Evolve.

REPORTS

Toward the end of this textbook, you will find a section titled Reports, which contains original reports. Read the reports indicated below and supply the appropriate CPT and ICD-10-CM/ICD-9-CM codes on the following lines:

59. Report 19

    ⊛ CPT Code(s): _33641_

    ⊛ ICD-10-CM Code(s): _____

    (⊛ ICD-9-CM Code(s): _____)

60. Report 21

    ⊛ CPT Code(s): _33967_

    ⊛ ICD-10-CM Code(s): _____

    (⊛ ICD-9-CM Code(s): _____)

61. Report 23

    ⊛ CPT Code(s): _33533_

    ⊛ ICD-10-CM Code(s): _____

    (⊛ ICD-9-CM Code(s): _____)

62. Report 24

    ⊛ CPT Code(s): _33961_

    ⊛ ICD-10-CM Code(s): _____

    (⊛ ICD-9-CM Code(s): _____)

⊛ **User to decide number of codes necessary to correctly answer the question.**
Odd-numbered answers are located in Appendix B, while the full answer key is only available in the TEACH Instructor Resources on Evolve.

CHAPTER 21

Cardiovascular System

THEORY

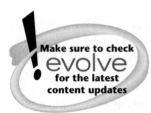

Make sure to check **evolve** for the latest content updates

Cardiovascular Terminology

Without the use of reference material, match the following terms to the correct definitions:

1. _E_ Pericardium

2. _G_ Cardiopulmonary

3. _B_ Bypass

4. _J_ Pacemaker

5. _D_ Single-chamber device

6. _H_ Dual-chamber device

7. _A_ Electrode

8. _K_ Ventricle

9. _I_ Atrium

10. _C_ Cardioverter-defibrillator

11. _F_ Artery

a. Lead attached to a generator that carries the electrical current from the generator to the atria or ventricles

b. To go around

c. Surgically placed device that directs an electrical current shock to the heart to restore rhythm

d. Electrode of the pacemaker is placed only in the atrium or only in the ventricle, but not in both places

e. Membranous sac enclosing the heart and ends of the great vessels

f. Vessel that carries oxygenated blood from the heart to the body tissues

g. Refers to the heart and lungs

h. Electrodes of the pacemaker are placed in both the right atrium and the right ventricle of the heart

i. Chamber in the upper part of the heart

j. Electrical device that controls the beating of the heart by electrical impulses

k. Chamber in the lower part of the heart

Odd-numbered answers are located in Appendix B, while the full answer key is only available in the TEACH Instructor Resources on Evolve.

Match the following terms to the correct definitions:

12. __C__ Vein

13. __J__ Aneurysm

14. __A__ Embolism

15. __D__ Thrombosis

16. __M__ Endarterectomy

17. __I__ Angioplasty

18. __F__ Injection

19. __H__ Catheter

20. __G__ Arteriovenous fistula

21. __N__ Anomaly

22. __K__ Ischemia

23. __B__ Cardiopulmonary bypass

24. __E__ Fistula

25. __L__ Shunt

a. Forcing of fluid into a vessel or cavity

b. Blood bypasses the heart through a heart-lung machine during open heart surgery

c. Vessel that carries deoxygenated blood to the heart from the body tissues

d. Blood clot

e. Abnormal opening from one area to another area within the body or to outside of the body

f. Blockage of a blood vessel by a blood clot or other matter that has moved from another area of the body through the circulatory system

g. Direct communication (passage) between an artery and vein

h. Tube placed into the body to put fluid in or take fluid out

i. Surgical or percutaneous procedure on a vessel to dilate the vessel open, used in treatment of atherosclerotic disease

j. A sac of clotted blood or fluid formed in the circulatory system (e.g., vein or artery)

k. Incision into an artery to remove the inner lining to remove disease or blockage

l. Divert or make an artificial passage

m. Deficient blood supply caused by obstruction of the circulatory system

n. Abnormality

26. The term that describes the procedure in which the surgeon withdraws fluid from the pericardial space by means of a needle inserted into the space is __injection__.

27. Codes for excision of cardiac tumors are divided based on whether the tumor is located __internally__ or __externally__ .

28. What are the names of two devices that are inserted into the body to electrically shock the heart into regular rhythm? __epicardial__ and __transvenous__

29. The two approaches used to insert devices that electrically shock the heart into regular rhythm are __ischemia__ and __fistula__ .

30. If the patient is returned to the operating room for repositioning or replacement of the pacemaker or cardioverter-defibrillator during the global period, modifier __NO__ would be appended to the code.

31. If a physician implanted a pacemaker and 10 days later the patient returns to the same surgeon for removal of sutures, would you charge for the service? Why?

     __NO__ , _____

32. If a patient is seen for a rash on the heel of the foot by the same physician who implanted a pacemaker 20 days earlier, would you bill for the office service for the rash? __NO__

33. When you bill for E/M services unrelated to a pacemaker implantation during the allowable follow-up days, what modifier would you use on the code to alert the third-party payer? __24__

34. What are the four cardiac valves? __vein__ , __ventricle__ , __artery__ , and __atrium__

35. What is the name of the device that can be surgically implanted into the subcutaneous tissue in the upper left quadrant to record heart rhythms when the patient depresses a button?

     __patient-activated event recorder__

36. What arteries feed the heart? __vessels__

37. When a heart artery is clogged and the heart muscle performs at a low level as a result of a lack of blood, the condition is called __reversible__ ischemia.

38. When a heart artery is clogged and the heart muscle dies, the condition

   is called _____local_____ ischemia.

39. A mass of undissolved matter in the blood that is transported by the

   blood current is a(n) _____embolus_____.

40. Local anesthesia, catheter introduction, and injection of

   _____cardioverter_____ _____defibrillator_____ are procedures that are
   included in a vascular injection.

PRACTICAL

Using the CPT and ICD-10-CM/ICD-9-CM manuals, code the following:

41. Valvuloplasty of the aortic valve using transventricular dilation with cardiopulmonary bypass.

    CPT Code: 33403

42. Replacement aortic valve, with cardiopulmonary bypass, with prosthetic valve.

    CPT Code: 33920

43. Valvuloplasty, tricuspid valve, with ring insertion.

    CPT Code: 33463

44. Repair of a coronary arteriovenous fistula, without cardiopulmonary bypass.

    CPT Code: 33960

45. Routine ECG with 12 leads with both the professional and technical components.

    CPT Code: 93000

46. External electrical cardioversion.

    CPT Code: 93010

47. Percutaneous balloon angioplasty; one coronary vessel.

    CPT Code: 92920

48. CPR (Cardiopulmonary resuscitation).

    CPT Code: 37629

49. Electrocardiogram with interpretation and report only.

    CPT Code: 93010

50. Bypass graft of the common carotid-ipsilateral internal carotid artery using synthetic vein.

    CPT Code: 93101

51. Ligation of temporal artery.

    CPT Code: 37609

Odd-numbered answers are located in Appendix B, while the full answer key is only available in the TEACH Instructor Resources on Evolve.

52. Ligation of a common iliac vein.

    CPT Code: _____35530_____

53. Open transluminal balloon angioplasty aorta.

    CPT Code: _____33513_____

54. Coronary artery bypass, single artery, for coronary atherosclerosis of native coronary artery in a transplanted heart.

    CPT Code: _____33260_____

    ICD-10-CM Code: _____

    (ICD-9-CM Code: _____)

55. Coronary artery bypass, four veins, no arteries. Diagnosis of acute coronary insufficiency.

    🌐 CPT Code(s): _____33513_____

    🌐 ICD-10-CM Code(s): _____

    (🌐 ICD-9-CM Code(s): _____)

56. Repair of injury to intra-abdominal blood vessel, inferior vena cava, hepatic vein, with a vein graft.

    🌐 CPT Code(s): _____33961_____

    🌐 ICD-10-CM Code(s): _____

    (🌐 ICD-9-CM Code(s): _____)

57. Percutaneous insertion of an intra-aortic balloon assist device due to initial episode of acute myocardial infarction and cardiogenic shock.

    🌐 CPT Code(s): _____33967_____

    🌐 ICD-10-CM Code(s): _____

    (🌐 ICD-9-CM Code(s): _____)

58. Repair of a traumatic arteriovenous fistula of a lower extremity.

    🌐 CPT Code(s): _____33962_____

    🌐 ICD-10-CM Code(s): _____

    (🌐 ICD-9-CM Code(s): _____)

🌐 **User to decide number of codes necessary to correctly answer the question.**
Odd-numbered answers are located in Appendix B, while the full answer key is only available in the TEACH Instructor Resources on Evolve.

59. Repair congenital atrial septal defect, secundum, with bypass and patch.

    ✿ CPT Code(s): _33641_

    ✿ ICD-10-CM Code(s): _____

    (✿ ICD-9-CM Code(s): _____)

60. Repair of a patent ductus arteriosus by division on a 16-year-old patient.

    ✿ CPT Code(s): _33907_

    ✿ ICD-10-CM Code(s): _____

    (✿ ICD-9-CM Code(s): _____)

61. Reoperation of a one arterial coronary bypass graft and one vein bypass graft for arteriosclerosis of native arteries, 3 months following the initial procedure.

    ✿ CPT Code(s): _33533_

    ✿ ICD-10-CM Code(s): _____

    (✿ ICD-9-CM Code(s): _____)

✿ **User to decide number of codes necessary to correctly answer the question.**

Odd-numbered answers are located in Appendix B, while the full answer key is only available in the TEACH Instructor Resources on Evolve.

REPORTS

Toward the end of this textbook, you will find a section titled Reports, which contains original reports. Read the reports indicated below and supply the appropriate CPT and ICD-10-CM/ICD-9-CM code(s) on the following lines:

62. Report 25

    🔮 CPT Code(s): __33967__

    🔮 ICD-10-CM Code(s): _____

    (🔮 ICD-9-CM Code(s): _____)

63. Report 26

    🔮 CPT Code(s): __33533__

    🔮 ICD-10-CM Code(s): _____

    (🔮 ICD-9-CM Code(s): _____)

64. Report 27

    🔮 CPT Code(s): __33951__

    🔮 ICD-10-CM Code(s): _____

    (🔮 ICD-9-CM Code(s): _____)

🔮 **User to decide number of codes necessary to correctly answer the question.**
Odd-numbered answers are located in Appendix B, while the full answer key is only available in the TEACH Instructor Resources on Evolve.

CHAPTER 22

Hemic, Lymphatic, Mediastinum, and Diaphragm

THEORY

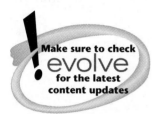

Make sure to check
evolve
for the latest
content updates

Hemic and Lymphatic Terminology

Without the use of reference material, match the following terms to the correct definitions:

1. __k__ Axillary nodes

2. __F__ Splenectomy

3. __E__ Splenoportography

4. __B__ Allogenic

5. __G__ Thoracic duct

6. __H__ Retroperitoneal

7. __D__ Jugular nodes

8. __J__ Cystic hygroma

9. __I__ Cloquet's node

10. __L__ Inguinofemoral

11. __C__ Cannulation

12. __A__ Abscess

a. Behind the sac holding the abdominal organs and viscera (peritoneum)

b. Excision of the spleen

c. Insertion of a tube into a duct or cavity

d. Lymph nodes located next to the large vein in the neck

e. Radiographic procedure to allow visualization of the splenic and portal veins of the spleen

f. Of the same species, but genetically different

g. Collection and distribution point for lymph and the largest lymph vessel located in the chest

h. Congenital deformity or benign tumor of the lymphatic system

i. Also called a gland; it is the highest of the deep groin lymph nodes

j. Term that refers to the groin and thigh

k. Lymph nodes located in the armpit

l. Localization of pus

Odd-numbered answers are located in Appendix B, while the full answer key is only available in the TEACH Instructor Resources on Evolve.

Match the following terms to the correct definitions:

13. __F__ Autologous, autogenous

14. __G__ Aspiration

15. __B__ Stem cell

16. __A__ Transplantation

17. __H__ Lymph node

18. __D__ Lymphadenitis

19. __C__ Lymphangiotomy

20. __E__ Lymphadenectomy

a. Grafting of tissue from one source to another

b. Immature blood cells

c. Incision into a lymphatic vessel

d. Inflammation of a lymph node

e. Excision of a lymph node (or nodes)

f. From oneself

g. Use of a needle and syringe to withdraw fluid

h. Station along the lymphatic system

Mediastinum and Diaphragm Terminology

Match the following terms to the correct definitions:

21. __M__ Mediastinum

22. __I__ Diaphragm

23. __J__ Mediastinotomy

24. __H__ Fundoplasty

25. __D__ Pyloroplasty

26. __E__ Diaphragmatic hernia

27. __L__ Mediastinoscopy

28. __A__ Imbrication

29. __K__ Transthoracic

30. __F__ Transabdominal

31. __G__ Paraesophageal hiatus hernia

32. __C__ Gastroplasty

33. __B__ Vagotomy

a. Overlapping

b. Surgical separation of the vagus nerve

c. Muscular wall that separates the thoracic and abdominal cavities

d. Incision and repair of the pyloric channel

e. Operation on the stomach for repair or reconfiguration

f. Repair of the bottom of an organ or muscle

g. Hernia that is near the esophagus

h. Hernia of the diaphragm

i. Across the abdomen

j. Cutting into the mediastinum

k. Across the thorax

l. Use of an endoscope inserted through a small incision to view the mediastinum

m. The area between the lungs that contains the heart, aorta, trachea, lymph nodes, thymus gland, esophagus, and bronchial tubes

Odd-numbered answers are located in Appendix B, while the full answer key is only available in the TEACH Instructor Resources on Evolve.

PRACTICAL

Using the CPT and ICD-10-CM/ICD-9-CM manuals, code the following:

34. Injection procedure for identification of the sentinel node with intradermal radioisotope injection for the staging of clinically negative axillae in a patient with primary, malignant neoplasm of the central portion of the right breast.

    🔵 CPT Code(s): ___38291_____

    🔵 ICD-10-CM Code(s): _____

    (🔵 ICD-9-CM Code(s): _____)

35. Radical cervical lymphadenectomy for patient with malignant primary cancer of the nipple of the left breast. Pathology findings of the lymphadenectomy were positive.

    🔵 CPT Code(s): ___38720_____

    🔵 ICD-10-CM Code(s): _____

    (🔵 ICD-9-CM Code(s): _____)

36. Drainage of an extensive lymph node abscess. Pathology report indicated *Staphylococcus*.

    🔵 CPT Code(s): ___38240_____

    🔵 ICD-10-CM Code(s): _____

    (🔵 ICD-9-CM Code(s): _____)

37. Autologous bone marrow transplantation for a patient who has acute myelogenous leukemia that has not shown any signs of remission.

    🔵 CPT Code(s): ___38241_____

    🔵 ICD-10-CM Code(s): _____

    (🔵 ICD-9-CM Code(s): _____)

38. Partial splenectomy for a 3-year-old child with sickle cell disease, Hb-C with crisis.

    CPT Code: ___38720_____

    ICD-10-CM Code: _____

    (ICD-9-CM Code: _____)

🔵 **User to decide number of codes necessary to correctly answer the question.**
Odd-numbered answers are located in Appendix B, while the full answer key is only available in the TEACH Instructor Resources on Evolve.

39. Harvesting of bone marrow for transplantation from a father for subsequent transplantation into the daughter. Report only the harvesting service.

CPT Code: _38 230_

ICD-10-CM Code: _____

(ICD-9-CM Code: _____)

40. Repair of laceration of diaphragm by means of abdominal approach.

CPT Code: _38290_

41. Excision of mediastinal cyst.

CPT Code: _39200_

42. Resection of diaphragm with simple repair.

CPT Code: _38230_

43. Preparation of stem (hematopoietic progenitor) cells for transplantation that included thawing of previously frozen cells and washing of the cells.

CPT Code: _38290_

44. Laparoscopic removal of the spleen.

CPT Code: _38231_

45. A radiologist performs lymphoscintigraphy in the radiology department. A few hours later, the patient is taken to the operating room where the general surgeon injects blue dye into the internal mammary lymph node and then excises a sentinel lymph node.

CPT Codes: _78195 - 2_ -26 (for performing both the injection and imaging of the radioisotope in the radiology department [nuclear medicine, lymph nodes]), _38792_ -59 (for injecting the blue dye), and _38530_ (for excision of the sentinel lymph node in the operating room)

Odd-numbered answers are located in Appendix B, while the full answer key is only available in the TEACH Instructor Resources on Evolve.

REPORT

Toward the end of this textbook, you will find a section titled Reports, which contains original reports. Read the report indicated below and supply the appropriate CPT and ICD-10-CM/ICD-9-CM code(s) on the following lines:

46. Report 89

   CPT Code: _38290_

   ICD-10-CM Codes: _____,

   _____ (External Cause code for how accident occurred),

   _____ (Y Code)

   (ICD-9-CM Codes: _____, _____
   (E code for how accident occurred))

CHAPTER **23**

Digestive System

THEORY

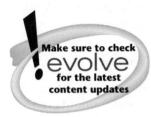

Make sure to check **evolve** for the latest content updates

Digestive Terminology

Without the use of reference material, match the following terms to the correct definitions:

1. __B__ Gloss-

2. __D__ Gastro-

3. __F__ Anastomosis

4. __C__ Hernia

5. __G__ Gastrointestinal

6. __H__ Ostomy

7. __A__ Colostomy

8. __E__ Ileostomy

9. __i__ Jejunostomy

a. Artificial opening between the colon and the abdominal wall

b. Prefix meaning tongue

c. Organ or tissue protruding through the wall or cavity that usually contains it

d. Prefix meaning stomach

e. Artificial opening between the ileum and the abdominal wall

f. Surgical connection of two tubular structures, such as two pieces of the intestine

g. Pertaining to the stomach and intestine

h. Artificial opening

i. Artificial opening between the jejunum and the abdominal wall

Odd-numbered answers are located in Appendix B, while the full answer key is only available in the TEACH Instructor Resources on Evolve.

Without reference material, match the following terms to the correct definitions:

10. __G__ Gastrostomy

11. __i__ Proctosigmoidoscopy

12. __C__ Sigmoidoscopy

13. __E__ Colonoscopy

14. __B__ Cholangiography

15. __H__ Chole-

16. __F__ Hepa-

17. __A__ Incarcerated

18. __D__ Reducible

a. Regarding hernias, a constricted, irreducible hernia that may cause obstruction of an intestine

b. Artificial opening between the stomach and the abdominal wall

c. Radiographic recording of the bile ducts

d. Able to be corrected or put back into a normal position

e. Endoscopic examination of the entire colon that may include part of the terminal ileum

f. Prefix meaning liver

g. Endoscopic examination of the entire rectum and sigmoid colon that may include a portion of the descending colon

h. Prefix meaning bile

i. Endoscopic examination of the sigmoid colon and rectum

PRACTICAL

Using the CPT and ICD-10-CM/ICD-9-CM manuals, code the following:

19. Rigid esophagoscopy with removal of a foreign body.

    CPT Code: _43194_

20. Ligation of an intraoral salivary duct.

    CPT Code: _42831_

21. Transection of esophagus with repair of esophageal varices.

    CPT Code: _43401_

22. Enterotomy of the small intestine for removal of a foreign body.

    CPT Code: _49521_

23. Complicated revision of a colostomy.

    CPT Code: _44345_

24. Frenotomy, labial.

    CPT Code: _42813_

25. Excision of a palate lesion without closure.

    CPT Code: _42104_

26. Removal of a foreign body from the pharynx.

    CPT Code: _43195_

27. Amy is an 18-year-old with severe snoring. She is having an adenoidectomy in order to treat her snoring.

    CPT Code: _42831_

28. Partial colectomy with colostomy.

    CPT Code: _42041_

29. Repair of an incarcerated recurrent inguinal hernia.

    CPT Code: _49521_

30. Surgical laparoscopic placement of a gastric band.

    CPT Code: _43194_

Odd-numbered answers are located in Appendix B, while the full answer key is only available in the TEACH Instructor Resources on Evolve.

31. Full-thickness repair of the vermilion of the lip.

    CPT Code: _40650_

32. Simple repair of 1.6-cm laceration of floor of mouth.

    CPT Code: _49320_

33. Bilateral parotid duct diversion.

    CPT Code: _42507_

34. Surgical laparoscopic repair of a paraesophageal hernia with fundoplasty with implantation of mesh.

    CPT Code: _45060_

35. Biopsy of the stomach by laparotomy.

    CPT Code: _43605_

36. Nontube open ileostomy.

    CPT Code: _41365_

37. Colorrhaphy for multiple perforations of large intestine sustained in auto accident. No colostomy was required.

    CPT Code: _44604_

38. Incision and drainage of perirectal abscess.

    CPT Code: _40650_

39. Diagnostic abdominal laparoscopy.

    CPT Code: _49320_

40. PREPROCEDURE DIAGNOSIS: Screening colonoscopy.

    POSTPROCEDURE DIAGNOSIS: Colon polyps.

    PREMEDICATIONS: Fentanyl 100 mcg and Versed 4 mg.

    PROCEDURE: A colonoscopy was performed to the cecum. The scope was advanced to the cecum under direct vision without any difficulty.

    FINDINGS: The cecum, ascending, transverse, descending, and sigmoid colon was normal. In the descending colon, there was a 2-mm polyp that was biopsied and submitted for histology.

    ASSESSMENT: Diminutive colon polyps.

Odd-numbered answers are located in Appendix B, while the full answer key is only available in the TEACH Instructor Resources on Evolve.

Pathology Report later indicated benign polyps.

CPT Code: _____43605_____

ICD-10-CM Codes: _____, _____

(ICD-9-CM Codes: _____, _____)

41. The patient presented to the emergency department complaining of vomiting coffee-ground material several times within the past 2 hours. He has abdominal pain and has been unable to eat for the past 24 hours. He is dizzy and light-headed. Two stools today have been black and tarry. While in the emergency department, he vomited bright-red blood and some coffee-ground material. A nasogastric tube was inserted and attached to suction with fluoro. An abdominal exam showed a fluid wave consistent with ascites. An IV of lactated ringers was started, and CBC and clotting studies were drawn. A detailed history and physical exam with high-complexity medical decision making were documented. A GI consultant was called and the patient was taken to Endoscopy for further evaluation of upper GI bleeding. Diagnosis: hematemesis, rule out esophageal varices; blood loss anemia (CBC review) acute; ascites. Code the services of the ED physician.

CPT Codes: _____99284-25_____, _____43752_____

ICD-10-CM Codes: _____, _____, _____

(ICD-9-CM Codes: _____, _____,

_____)

REPORTS

Toward the end of this textbook, you will find a section titled Reports, which contains original reports. Read the reports indicated below and supply the appropriate CPT and ICD-10-CM/ICD-9-CM codes on the following lines:

42. Report 22

 ⊛ CPT Code(s): _43920_

 ⊛ ICD-10-CM Code(s): _____

 (⊛ ICD-9-CM Code(s): _____)

43. Report 31

 ⊛ CPT Code(s): _43584_

 ⊛ ICD-10-CM Code(s): _____

 (⊛ ICD-9-CM Code(s): _____)

44. Report 32

 ⊛ CPT Code(s): _43752_

 ⊛ ICD-10-CM Code(s): _____

 (⊛ ICD-9-CM Code(s): _____)

45. Report 33

 ⊛ CPT Code(s): _44143_

 ⊛ ICD-10-CM Code(s): _____

 (⊛ ICD-9-CM Code(s): _____)

46. Report 34

 ⊛ CPT Code(s): _44604_

 ⊛ ICD-10-CM Code(s): _____

 (⊛ ICD-9-CM Code(s): _____)

⊛ **User to decide number of codes necessary to correctly answer the question.**
Odd-numbered answers are located in Appendix B, while the full answer key is only available in the TEACH Instructor Resources on Evolve.

47. Report 35

    ⊛ CPT Code(s): __43752__

    ⊛ ICD-10-CM Code(s): _____

    (⊛ ICD-9-CM Code(s): _____)

48. Report 39

    ⊛ CPT Code(s): __43584__

    ⊛ ICD-10-CM Code(s): _____

    (⊛ ICD-9-CM Code(s): _____)

⊛ **User to decide number of codes necessary to correctly answer the question.**
Odd-numbered answers are located in Appendix B, while the full answer key is only available in the TEACH
Instructor Resources on Evolve.

CHAPTER 24

Urinary and Male Genital Systems

THEORY

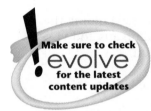

Urinary System Terminology

Without the use of reference material, match the following terms to the correct definitions:

1. __D__ Calculus/calculi

2. __J__ Cystolithectomy

3. __G__ Cystometrogram (CMG)

4. __I__ Endopyelotomy

5. __F__ Exstrophy

6. ____ Nephrectomy

7. __K__ Fulguration

8. __H__ Kock pouch

9. __C__ Lithotripsy

10. __A__ Marsupialization

11. __L__ Nephro-

12. __B__ Nephrostomy

a. With the use of an endoscope, an incision is made to correct stenosis of the ureteropelvic junction

b. Kidney removal

c. Crushing of a gallbladder or urinary bladder stone followed by irrigation to wash the fragment out

d. A concretion of mineral salts, also called a stone

e. Surgical creation of a urinary bladder from a segment of the ileum

f. Condition in which an organ is turned inside out

g. Measurement of the pressures and capacity of the urinary bladder

h. Creation of a channel into the renal pelvis of the kidney

i. Surgical procedure that creates an open pouch from an internal abscess

j. Removal of a calculus from the urinary bladder

k. Use of electrical current to destroy tissue

l. Prefix meaning kidney

Odd-numbered answers are located in Appendix B, while the full answer key is only available in the TEACH Instructor Resources on Evolve.

Without the use of reference material, match the following terms to the correct definitions:

13. __I__ Perivesical

14. __G__ Perirenal

15. __A__ Pyelo-

16. __L__ Pyeloplasty

17. __D__ Pyelostomy

18. __J__ Renal pelvis

19. __F__ Retroperitoneal

20. __K__ Transureteroureterostomy

21. __B__ Ureterolithotomy

22. __E__ Ureterotomy

23. __H__ Urethrocystography

24. __C__ Urethrorrhaphy

a. Prefix meaning renal pelvis

b. Removal of a stone from the ureter

c. Surgical connection of one ureter to the other ureter

d. Surgical creation of an opening into the renal pelvis

e. Suturing of the urethra

f. Behind the sac holding the abdominal organs and viscera (peritoneum)

g. Around the kidney

h. Radiography of the bladder and urethra

i. Around the bladder

j. Funnel-shaped sac in the kidney where urine is received

k. Surgical reconstruction of the renal pelvis

l. Incision into the ureter

Male Genital Terminology

Without the use of reference material, match the following terms to the correct definitions:

25. __C__ Cavernosa-saphenous

26. __A__ Orchiectomy

27. __E__ Hydrocele

28. __F__ Vasogram

29. __B__ Varicocele

30. __D__ Vas deferens

a. Tube that carries sperm from the epididymis to the urethra

b. Swelling of a scrotal vein

c. Creation of a connection between the cavity of the penis and a vein

d. Castration

e. Sac of fluid

f. Recording of the flow in the vas deferens

Odd-numbered answers are located in Appendix B, while the full answer key is only available in the TEACH Instructor Resources on Evolve.

Without reference material, match the following terms to the correct definitions:

31. __D__ Electrodesiccation

32. __A__ Corpora cavernosa

33. __E__ Epididymis

34. __B__ Cavernosography

35. __F__ Cavernosometry

36. __H__ Plethysmography

37. __i__ Hypospadias

38. __G__ Vesiculectomy

39. __C__ Prostatotomy

a. Excision of a seminal vesicle

b. Determining the changes in volume of an organ part or body

c. Incision into the prostate

d. Destruction of a lesion by the use of electrical current radiated through a needle

e. A tube located on the top of the testes that stores sperm

f. Measurements of the pressure in a cavity (e.g., penis)

g. Two cavities of the penis

h. Radiographic measurement of a cavity (e.g., the main part of the penis)

i. Congenital deformity of the urethra in which the urethral opening is on the underside of the penis rather than on the end

Without reference material, match the following terms to the correct definitions:

40. __C__ Lymphadenectomy

41. __B__ Priapism

42. __A__ Chordee

43. __D__ Urethroplasty

44. __F__ Penoscrotal

45. __E__ Spermatocele

a. Surgical repair of the urethra

b. Referring to the penis and scrotum

c. Painful condition in which the penis is constantly erect

d. Excision of lymph node(s)

e. Condition resulting in the penis being bent downward

f. Cyst filled with spermatozoa

Odd-numbered answers are located in Appendix B, while the full answer key is only available in the TEACH Instructor Resources on Evolve.

Without reference material, match the following terms to the correct definitions:

46. __F__ Tumescence

47. __A__ Cavernosa-corpus spongiosum shunt

48. __B__ Cavernosa-glans penis fistulization

49. __D__ Orchiopexy

50. __C__ Vasovasostomy

51. __E__ Vasovasorrhaphy

a. Creation of a connection between a cavity of the penis and the urethra

b. Creation of a connection between a cavity of the penis and the glans penis, which overlaps the penis cavity

c. Reversal of a vasectomy

d. Surgical procedure to release undescended testis

e. Suturing of the vas deferens

f. State of being swollen

Without reference material, match the following terms to the correct definitions:

52. __F__ Epididymectomy

53. __A__ Epididymovasostomy

54. __B__ Vasotomy

55. __D__ Vesiculotomy

56. __E__ Seminal vesicle

57. __C__ Tunica vaginalis

a. Creation of a new connection between the vas deferens and epididymis

b. Creation of an opening in the vas deferens

c. Covering of the testes

d. Incision into the seminal vesicle

e. Glands that secretes fluid that ultimately becomes semen

f. Surgical removal of the epididymis

PRACTICAL

Using the CPT and ICD-10-CM/ICD-9-CM manuals, code the following:

58. Endoscopy for resection of primary malignant renal pelvis tumor through an established stoma.

    CPT Code: 50391

    ICD-10-CM Code: _____

    (ICD-9-CM Code: _____)

59. Aspiration of a solitary, non-congenital renal cyst through percutaneous needle.

    CPT Code: 50390

    ICD-10-CM Code: _____

    (ICD-9-CM Code: _____)

60. Ureteroureterostomy performed for urinary tract obstruction.

    CPT Code: 52441

    ICD-10-CM Code: _____

    (ICD-9-CM Code: _____)

61. Transurethral incision of the prostate to treat benign hypertrophic prostatitis.

    CPT Code: 52450

    ICD-10-CM Code: _____

    (ICD-9-CM Code: _____)

62. Cystourethroscopy due to intermittent hematuria.

    CPT Code: 53271

    ICD-10-CM Code: _____

    (ICD-9-CM Code: _____)

63. Abdominal orchiopexy to release undescended intra-abdominal testes.

    CPT Code: 54650-50

    ICD-10-CM Code: _____

    (ICD-9-CM Code: _____)

Odd-numbered answers are located in Appendix B, while the full answer key is only available in the TEACH Instructor Resources on Evolve.

64. Complicated prostatotomy of prostate cyst.

    CPT Code: __SS 132__

    ICD-10-CM Code: _____

    (ICD-9-CM Code: _____)

65. Closure of nephrocutaneous fistula.

    CPT Code: __SOS20__

66. A steroid injection for urethral stricture using a cystourethroscope.

    ⊛ CPT Code(s): __S4061__

67. Total urethrectomy of a 44-year-old male.

    ⊛ CPT Code(s): __S3215__

68. Circumcision using clamp, routine.

    ⊛ CPT Code(s): __S4150 -52__

    ⊛ ICD-10-CM Code(s): _____

    (⊛ ICD-9-CM Code(s): _____)

69. Excision of Skene's glands.

    ⊛ CPT Code(s): __S3270__

70. Bilateral shunt of corpora cavernosa–saphenous vein for priapism.

    ⊛ CPT Code(s): __S4420__

71. Vasovasorrhaphy.

    ⊛ CPT Code(s): __SS460__

72. Exposure of the prostate for insertion of radioactive substance.

    ⊛ CPT Code(s): __S6410__

73. Surgical reduction of torsion of testis with fixation of contralateral testis.

    ⊛ CPT Code(s): __S4600__

⊛ **User to decide number of codes necessary to correctly answer the question.**
Odd-numbered answers are located in Appendix B, while the full answer key is only available in the TEACH Instructor Resources on Evolve.

74. Distal hypospadias repair with chordee using a V-flap advancement, completed in one stage.

    ⊛ CPT Code(s): __54061__

75. Simple destruction of four lesions of the penis using cryosurgery.

    ⊛ CPT Code(s): __54056__

76. Repair of an incomplete circumcision.

    ⊛ CPT Code(s): __54163__

77. Drainage of a scrotal wall abscess.

    ⊛ CPT Code(s): __55100__

78. Ureterectomy, with repair of the bladder cuff.

    ⊛ CPT Code(s): __50391__

⊛ **User to decide number of codes necessary to correctly answer the question.**
Odd-numbered answers are located in Appendix B, while the full answer key is only available in the TEACH Instructor Resources on Evolve.

REPORTS

Toward the end of this textbook, you will find a section titled Reports, which contains original reports. Read the reports indicated below and supply the appropriate CPT and ICD-10-CM/ICD-9-CM codes on the following lines:

79. Report 36

    ✪ CPT Code(s): _52332 - 50_

80. Report 37

    ✪ CPT Code(s): _52204_

    ✪ ICD-10-CM Code(s): _____

    (✪ ICD-9-CM Code(s): _____)

81. Report 38

    ✪ CPT Code(s): _53445_

    ✪ ICD-10-CM Code(s): _____

    (✪ ICD-9-CM Code(s): _____)

82. Report 81

    ✪ CPT Code(s): _55875 , 77778_

83. Report 82

    ✪ CPT Code(s): _52630_

84. Report 83

    ✪ CPT Code(s): _54640 - LT_

    ✪ ICD-10-CM Code(s): _____

    (✪ ICD-9-CM Code(s): _____)

85. Report 84

    ✪ CPT Code(s): _53852_

✪ **User to decide number of codes necessary to correctly answer the question.**
Odd-numbered answers are located in Appendix B, while the full answer key is only available in the TEACH Instructor Resources on Evolve.

Reproductive, Intersex Surgery, Female Genital System, and Maternity Care and Delivery

THEORY

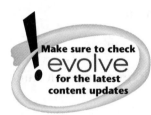

Make sure to check **evolve** for the latest content updates

Female Genital Terminology

Without the use of reference material, match the following terms to the correct definitions:

1. _D_ Vulva
2. _F_ Perineum
3. _H_ Introitus
4. _L_ Vagina
5. _B_ Cervix uteri
6. _E_ Corpus uteri
7. _M_ Oviduct
8. _G_ Salpingo-
9. _C_ Oophor-
10. _I_ Curettage
11. _J_ Dilation
12. _A_ Cystocele
13. _F_ Rectocele

a. Herniation of the bladder into the vagina
b. Rounded, cone-shaped neck of the uterus, part of it protruding into the vagina
c. Prefix meaning ovary
d. External female genitalia, including labia majora, labia minora, clitoris, and vaginal opening
e. Uterus
f. Herniation of the rectal wall through the posterior wall of the vagina
g. Prefix meaning tube
h. Opening or entrance to the vagina
i. Scraping of a cavity using a spoon-shaped instrument
j. Expansion
k. Area between the vulva and anus
l. Canal from the external female genitalia to the uterus
m. Fallopian tube

Odd-numbered answers are located in Appendix B, while the full answer key is only available in the TEACH Instructor Resources on Evolve.

Maternity Care and Delivery Terminology

Without the use of reference material, match the following terms to the correct definitions:

14. _P_ Antepartum

15. _E_ Postpartum

16. _B_ Abortion

17. _G_ Delivery

18. _H_ Cesarean

19. _F_ Ectopic

20. _D_ Version

21. _J_ Amniocentesis

22. _C_ Cordocentesis

23. _L_ Chorionic villus sampling (CVS)

24. _M_ Hysterotomy

25. _O_ Salpingectomy

26. _K_ Oophorectomy

27. _I_ Hysterectomy

28. _A_ Hysterorrhaphy

29. _N_ Tocolysis

30. _Q_ VBAC

a. Turning of the fetus from a presentation other than cephalic (head down) to cephalic for ease of birth

b. Termination of pregnancy

c. Surgical opening through abdominal wall for delivery

d. Before childbirth

e. After childbirth

f. Pregnancy outside the uterus (e.g., in the fallopian tube)

g. Childbirth

h. Incision into the uterus

i. Surgical removal of the uterus

j. Percutaneous aspiration of amniotic fluid

k. Surgical removal of ovary

l. Biopsy of the outermost part of the placenta

m. Suturing of the uterus

n. Repression of uterine contractions

o. Surgical removal of a fallopian tube

p. Vaginal delivery after previous cesarean delivery

q. Procedure to obtain a fetal blood sample, also called a percutaneous umbilical blood sampling

Without the use of reference material, answer the following:

31. Plastic repair of the ___introitus___ is surgical repair of the opening to the vagina.

32. An incision into the vagina to gain access to the pelvic cavity is ___cesarean___.

33. The insertion of a long needle into the back wall of the vagina to gain access to a peritoneal cul de sac abscess is ___colposcope___.

34. A vaginal support device is a(n) ___clamp___.

35. When reporting the service of the introduction of a diaphragm, the cost of the diaphragm is included in the introduction.

    True or (False?) ___False___

36. The term that describes the procedure in which the surgeon strengthens the wall of the weakened vagina by pulling together the weakened vaginal area with sutures is:

    ___chorionic villus sampling___

37. The microscope that is used to view the vagina is a(n) ___colposcope___.

38. The services described in the Manipulation category of the Vagina subheading require this type of anesthesia: ___general___

39. LEEP means ___loop electrode excision procedure___.

40. Endometrial ___amniotic___ is a biopsy of the mucous lining of the uterus.

41. What one procedure represents the majority of the codes in the Corpus Uteri subheading? ___hysterectomy___

42. Hydatidiform mole, also known as a "molar pregnancy," results from genetic abnormalities.

    (True) or False? ___True___

43. A hysterosalpingography would have a component code from what section of the CPT manual? ___Radiology___

44. The first rule of a laparoscopy is that a surgical laparoscopy always includes this type of laparoscopy: _cyrocele_

45. In what subheading would you find the codes to report fallopian tube services?

    oviduct/ovary

46. The three methods of tubal ligation are ligation, _dilation_, and _perineum_.

47. Gestation is divided into three time periods that are termed _trimesters_.

48. The first gestation time period is LMP to week _12_, the second is week _13_ to week 27, and the third is week _28_ to the EDD.

49. What does EDD stand for?

    estimated _date_ of _delivery_

50. Preparation of the cervix for birth or dilation is termed cervical _contractions_.

51. If a physician other than the attending provided only one office visit to a patient before delivery, a code from what section of the CPT manual would be used to report this service? _E/M_

52. The time after delivery is referred to as _postpartum_.

Odd-numbered answers are located in Appendix B, while the full answer key is only available in the TEACH Instructor Resources on Evolve.

PRACTICAL

Using the CPT manual, code the following:

53. Dilation of the vagina under anesthesia.

    CPT Code: 57400

54. Plastic repair of a urethrocele.

    CPT Code: 53275

55. Labial adhesions lysis.

    CPT Code: 56441

56. Simple complete vulvectomy.

    CPT Code: 56625

57. Surgical hysteroscopy with polypectomy and dilatation and curettage.

    CPT Code: 58558

58. Transposition of the left ovary.

    CPT Code: 58825 - LT

59. Bilateral wedge resection of ovaries.

    CPT Code: 58920

60. Therapeutic amniocentesis with amniotic fluid reduction.

    CPT Code: 59001

61. Drainage of a cyst of the left ovary using the vaginal approach.

    CPT Code(s): 58800

62. Surgical treatment of a second-trimester missed abortion.

    CPT Code(s): 59821

63. Cesarean delivery only.

    CPT Code(s): 59514

64. Hysterorrhaphy of a ruptured, pregnant uterus.

    CPT Code(s): 58520

User to decide number of codes necessary to correctly answer the question.
Odd-numbered answers are located in Appendix B, while the full answer key is only available in the TEACH Instructor Resources on Evolve.

65. Fetal contraction stress tests, antepartum.

    🔗 CPT Code(s): __S9020__

66. Radical vaginal hysterectomy.

    🔗 CPT Code(s): __58260__

67. Marsupialization of Bartholin's gland cyst.

    🔗 CPT Code(s): __56440__

68. Excision of Bartholin's gland.

    🔗 CPT Code(s): __56740__

69. Destruction of extensive vaginal lesions.

    🔗 CPT Code(s): __57065__

🔗 **User to decide number of codes necessary to correctly answer the question.**
Odd-numbered answers are located in Appendix B, while the full answer key is only available in the TEACH
Instructor Resources on Evolve.

REPORTS

Toward the end of this textbook, you will find a section titled Reports, which contains original reports. Code only the primary surgery. Read the report indicated below and supply the appropriate CPT and ICD-10-CM/ICD-9-CM code(s) on the following lines:

70. Report 20

    ✺ CPT Code(s): ___59400___

71. Report 28

    ✺ CPT Code(s): ___59401___

    ✺ ICD-10-CM Code(s): _____

    (✺ ICD-9-CM Code(s): _____)

72. Report 29

    ✺ CPT Code(s): ___59 601___

    ✺ ICD-10-CM Code(s): _____

    (✺ ICD-9-CM Code(s): _____)

73. Report 30

    ✺ CPT Code(s): ___59000___

    ✺ ICD-10-CM Code(s): _____

    (✺ ICD-9-CM Code(s): _____)

✺ User to decide number of codes necessary to correctly answer the question.
Odd-numbered answers are located in Appendix B, while the full answer key is only available in the TEACH Instructor Resources on Evolve.

CHAPTER 26

Endocrine and Nervous Systems

THEORY

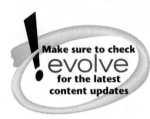
Make sure to check
evolve
for the latest
content updates

Endocrine System Terminology

Match the following terms to the correct definitions:

1. __C__ Isthmus

2. __J__ Isthmus, thyroid

3. __F__ Isthmusectomy

4. __K__ Contralateral

5. __D__ Thyroidectomy

6. __i__ Thyroglossal duct

7. __G__ Thymectomy

8. __A__ Adrenal

9. __H__ Thyroid

10. __E__ Thymus

11. __B__ Parathyroid

a. Glands located on the top of the kidneys that produce steroid hormones

b. Produces a hormone to mobilize calcium from the bones to the blood

c. Connection of two regions or structures

d. Surgical removal of the thyroid

e. Produces hormones important to the immune response

f. Surgical removal of the isthmus

g. Surgical removal of the thymus

h. Part of the endocrine system, a gland that produces hormones that regulate metabolism

i. Tissue connection between right and left thyroid lobes

j. Develops in the embryo stage after the formation of the thyroid gland

k. Affecting the opposite side

Odd-numbered answers are located in Appendix B, while the full answer key is only available in the TEACH Instructor Resources on Evolve.

Nervous System Terminology

Match the following terms to the correct definitions:

12. __C__ Cranium

13. __G__ Skull

14. __A__ Stereotaxis

15. __H__ Laminectomy

16. __E__ Somatic nerve

17. __B__ Sympathetic nerve

18. __F__ Peripheral nerves

19. __D__ Shunt

20. __i__ Central Nervous System

a. A method of identifying a specific area or point in the brain

b. Part of the peripheral nervous system that controls automatic body function; activated under stress

c. That part of the skeleton that encloses the brain

d. Divert or make an artificial passage

e. Twelve pairs of cranial nerves, 31 pairs of spinal nerves, and autonomic nervous system; connects peripheral receptors to the brain and spinal cord

f. Sensory or motor nerve

g. Entire skeletal framework of the head

h. Surgical excision of the lamina

i. Brain and spinal cord

PRACTICAL

Using the CPT manual, code the following:

21. Incision and drainage of an infected thyroglossal duct cyst.

    ⊛ CPT Code(s): _60000_

22. Removal of a complete cerebrospinal fluid shunt system; without replacement.

    ⊛ CPT Code(s): _63746_

23. Suture of the posterior tibial nerve.

    ⊛ CPT Code(s): _64840_

24. Lumbar sympathetic block (left).

    CPT Code: _64818_

25. Microdissection, microrepair ulnar digital nerve left middle finger.

    CPT Codes: _64831_ , _69990_

26. Placement of a dorsal column stimulator with implanted generator, with stereotactic stimulation of spinal cord.

    CPT Code: _63741_

27. Epidural injection of a steroid, caudal.

    CPT Code: _62311_

28. Craniotomy for drainage of an intracranial abscess; infratentorial.

    CPT Code: _61312_

29. Re-operation, skull base surgery, repair of dura mater due to leak of CSF of middle cranial fossa; myocutaneous flap graft.

    CPT Code: _61619_

30. Insertion of a cerebrospinal fluid ventriculoperitoneal shunt for hydrocephalus.

    CPT Code: _62190_

31. Hemilaminectomy, posterior approach, with decompression of two nerve roots and with excision of herniated disc at L1-L2 and foraminotomy at L2-L3.

    CPT Codes: _63030_ , _63035_

⊛ **User to decide number of codes necessary to correctly answer the question.**
Odd-numbered answers are located in Appendix B, while the full answer key is only available in the TEACH Instructor Resources on Evolve.

REPORTS

Toward the end of this textbook, you will find a section titled Reports, which contains original reports. Read the reports indicated below and supply the appropriate CPT and ICD-10-CM/ICD-9-CM codes on the following lines:

32. Report 41

CPT Codes: _____22548_____ (arthrodesis with discectomy),

_____22590_____ (arthrodesis with discectomy), __22600__

(instrumentation), _____20931_____ (allograft),

_____22585_____ (evoked potential)

ICD-10-CM Code: _____

(ICD-9-CM Code: _____)

33. Report 43

🔮 Code(s): __63030 – RT__

🔮 ICD-10-CM Code(s): _____

(🔮 ICD-9-CM Code(s): _____)

🔮 **User to decide number of codes necessary to correctly answer the question.**
Odd-numbered answers are located in Appendix B, while the full answer key is only available in the TEACH Instructor Resources on Evolve.

Eye, Ocular Adnexa, Auditory, and Operating Microscope

THEORY

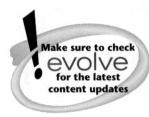

Make sure to check
evolve
for the latest
content updates

Eye and Ocular Adnexa Terminology

Match the following terms to the correct definitions:

1. __A__ Keratoplasty
2. __E__ Evisceration
3. __B__ Enucleation
4. __F__ Exenteration
5. __C__ Cataract
6. __G__ Sclera
7. __D__ Conjunctiva
8. __H__ Uveal
9. __I__ Tarsorrhaphy
10. __J__ Ocular adnexa

a. Surgical repair of the cornea

b. Removal of an eye

c. Opaque covering on or in the lens

d. Lining of the eyelids and covering of the sclera

e. Removal of an organ all in one piece

f. Pulling the viscera outside the body through an incision

g. White outer portion of the eyeball

h. Vascular tissue of the choroids, ciliary body, and iris

i. Suturing together of the eyelids

j. Orbit, extraocular muscles, and eyelid

Match the following terms to the correct definitions:

11. __G__ Anterior segment

12. __C__ Posterior segment

13. __K__ Blephar/o-

14. __L__ Cor/o-

15. __F__ Cyclo/o-

16. __B__ Dacry/o-

17. __D__ Kerat/o-

18. __A__ Ocul/o-

19. __H__ Dacryocyst/o-

20. __E__ Vitre/o-

21. __J__ Astigmatism

22. __I__ Strabismus

a. Prefix meaning eye

b. Prefix meaning tear/tear duct

c. Parts of the eye located behind the lens

d. Prefix meaning cornea

e. Prefix meaning pertaining to the vitreous body of the eye

f. Prefix meaning ciliary body or eye muscle

g. Parts of the eye in the front of and including the lens, orbit, extraocular muscles, and eyelid

h. Prefix meaning pertaining to the lacrimal sac

i. Extraocular muscle deviation resulting in unequal visual axes

j. Condition in which the refractive surfaces of the eyes are unequal

k. Prefix meaning eyelid

l. Prefix meaning pupil

Auditory System Terminology

Match the following terms to the correct definitions:

23. __G__ Aural atresia

24. __J__ Transmastoid antrostomy

25. __N__ Labyrinth

26. __F__ Tympanic neurectomy

27. __H__ Fenestration

28. __B__ Parts of the external ear

29. __i__ Parts of the middle ear

30. __E__ Parts of the inner ear

31. __K__ Mastoid-

32. __D__ Myring-

33. __A__ Audi-

34. __M__ Exostosis

35. __C__ Oto-

36. __D__ Salping(o)-

37. __L__ Apicectomy

a. Prefix meaning hearing

b. Auricle, pinna, external acoustic, and meatus

c. Prefix meaning ear

d. Prefix meaning (eustachian) tube

e. Vestibule, semicircular canals, and cochlea

f. Excision of the tympanic nerve

g. Congenital absence of the external auditory canal

h. Creation of a new opening (e.g., on the inner wall of the middle ear)

i. Malleus, incus, and stapes

j. A bony growth

k. Prefix meaning posterior temporal bone

l. Excision of a portion of the temporal bone

m. Called a simple mastoidectomy, it creates an opening in the mastoid for drainage

n. Inner connecting cavities, such as the internal ear

o. Prefix meaning eardrum

Odd-numbered answers are located in Appendix B, while the full answer key is only available in the TEACH Instructor Resources on Evolve.

PRACTICAL

Using the CPT and ICD-10-CM/ICD-9-CM manuals, code the following:

38. Incision and drainage of conjunctival cysts of left and right eyes.

    🔬 CPT Code(s): __68020-50__

    🔬 ICD-10-CM Code(s): _____

    (🔬 ICD-9-CM Code(s): _____)

39. Optic nerve decompression of the right eye.

    🔬 CPT Code(s): __67570 - RT__

40. Removal of an embedded foreign body of the upper left eyelid.

    CPT Code: __65220 - E1__

    ICD-10-CM Code: _____

    (ICD-9-CM Code: _____)

41. Myringoplasty of the left ear.

    🔬 CPT Code(s): __69620 - LT__

42. Single stage reconstruction of the right external auditory canal for congenital atresia.

    CPT Code: __69310__

    ICD-10-CM Code: _____

    (ICD-9-CM Code: _____)

43. Left stapedectomy with footplate drill out.

    🔬 CPT Code(s): __69661__

44. Excision of a lacrimal sac, left eye.

    🔬 CPT Code(s): __68520 - LT__

🔬 **User to decide number of codes necessary to correctly answer the question.**
Odd-numbered answers are located in Appendix B, while the full answer key is only available in the TEACH Instructor Resources on Evolve.

REPORTS

Toward the end of this textbook, you will find a section titled Reports, which contains original reports. Read the reports indicated below and supply the appropriate CPT and ICD-10-CM/ICD-9-CM codes on the following lines:

45. Report 85

    CPT Code: _66720 – RT_

    ICD-10-CM Code: _____

    (ICD-9-CM Code: _____, _____)

46. Report 86

    ⊛ CPT Code(s): _66724-LT_

47. Report 87

    ⊛ CPT Code(s): _66984 – RT_

48. Report 88

    ⊛ CPT Code(s): _69814– LT_

⊛ **User to decide number of codes necessary to correctly answer the question.**
Odd-numbered answers are located in Appendix B, while the full answer key is only available in the TEACH Instructor Resources on Evolve.

CHAPTER 28

Radiology

THEORY

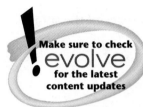

Make sure to check evolve **for the latest content updates**

Match the following terms to the correct definitions:

1. __C__ Anterior (ventral)

2. __E__ Posterior (dorsal)

3. __B__ Superior

4. __F__ Inferior

5. __A__ Medial

6. __D__ Lateral

a. Toward the midline of the body

b. Toward the head or the upper part of the body; also known as cephalad or cephalic

c. In front of

d. Away from the midline of the body (to the side)

e. In back of

f. Away from the head or the lower part of the body; also known as caudad or caudal

Match the following radiographic procedures to the correct structures imaged:

7. __B__ Fluoroscopy

8. __C__ Magnetic resonance imaging (MRI)

9. __F__ Tomography

10. __E__ Xeroradiography

11. __A__ Barium

12. __D__ Biometry

a. Radiographic contrast medium

b. Procedure for viewing the interior of the body using x-rays and projecting the image onto a television screen

c. Photoelectric process of radiographs

d. Application of a statistical method to a biological fact

e. Procedure that uses nonionizing radiation to view the body in a cross-sectional view

f. Procedure that allows viewing of a single plane of the body by blurring out all but that particular level

Odd-numbered answers are located in Appendix B, while the full answer key is only available in the TEACH Instructor Resources on Evolve.

Match the following radiographic procedures to the correct structures imaged:

13. _E_ Arthrography

14. _G_ Cholangiography

15. _i_ Cystography

16. _B_ Discography

17. _H_ Epididymography

18. _A_ Hysterosalpingography

19. _J_ Lymphangiography

20. _F_ Myelography

21. _C_ Urography

22. _D_ Venography

a. Uterine cavity and fallopian tubes

b. Intervertebral joint

c. Kidneys, renal pelvis, ureters, and bladder

d. Bile ducts

e. Joint

f. Veins and tributaries

g. Subarachnoid space of the spine

h. Epididymis

i. Urinary bladder

j. Lymphatic vessels and nodes

PRACTICAL

Using the CPT and ICD-10-CM/ICD-9-CM manuals, answer the following:

23. What is the unlisted diagnostic nuclear medicine code reported for cardiovascular procedures?

    CPT Code: __78499__

24. What is the add-on code for the coronary artery transcatheter placement during coronary intravascular brachytherapy for delivery of the radiation device?

    Code: __73511__

25. The modifier to indicate only the professional component was provided.

    Modifier: __−26__

26. The modifier to indicate only the technical component was provided.

    Modifier: __−26__

27. Supervision and interpretation of angiography, spinal artery, selective. Report radiology service only.

    CPT Code: __75705__

28. Radiological examination of the eye for foreign body.

    CPT Code: __76072__

29. Radiological examination of mastoids, four views per side.

    CPT Code: __70130__

30. Radiological examination of the ribs, unilateral, two views.

    CPT Code: __76604__

31. MRI of the neck, with contrast material.

    CPT Code: __70542__

32. Computed tomography of the thoracic spine, without contrast.

    CPT Code: __70450__

33. Complete hip x-ray study, unilateral, two views.

    CPT Code: __73510__

34. Complete four-view radiological examination of the wrist.

    CPT Code: __70141__

35. Radiological examination of a surgical specimen.

    CPT Code: __76098__

36. An established patient is seen in the clinic office complaining of severe headaches. To diagnose and treat the patient, the physician needs to identify a cause for these headaches. He performs an expanded problem focused history and examination and orders a CT scan of the head. The clinic radiologist performed the x-ray in which contrast was used.

    CPT Codes: __99210__ (physician), __77002__ (radiologist)

37. A new patient is admitted to the hospital on an observation status after a fall at home. A comprehensive history is collected and a general, multisystem comprehensive physical examination is performed. After talking to the patient and relatives and performing the examination, the physician finds that the patient has a number of symptoms that are usually due to an increase in intracranial pressure. The physician considers this patient's problems to be of moderately severe complexity. The MDM complexity is moderate. A CT scan of the brain without contrast is done. Brain lesions are discovered, and the physician advises radiation therapy. The patient is sent to the clinic's radiology department, where an A-scan bilateral ophthalmic biometry by ultrasound is done. The patient later has therapeutic radiology treatment planning that is simple. Later the patient has radiation treatment delivery to a single area up to 5 MeV. The patient continues with weekly radiology therapy management, five treatments.

    CPT Codes: __99219__ , __70450__ , __76516__ , __77261__ , __77402__ , __77427__

38. A new patient is seen in the clinic for an office consult. The patient has a mass in the neck with related pain and dysphagia. The consulting physician performs an expanded problem focused history and examination, and low-complexity decision making. A CT scan of the patient's neck is ordered. This was done with and without contrast.

    ⊛ CPT Code(s): __99242__

39. A patient was admitted to the hospital for removal of a pericardial clot. The physician orders a real-time chest ultrasound. Chest magnetic resonance (proton) imaging is also ordered (without contrast). A pericardiotomy is performed for removal of clot.

    ⊛ CPT Code(s): _76604_

40. Radiological examination, ankle, two views.

    ⊛ CPT Code(s): _70542_

41. X-ray of a 6-month-old's upper arm; 2 views.

    ⊛ CPT Code(s): _73092_

42. Unilateral selective pulmonary angiography, supervision and interpretation. Report radiology service only.

    ⊛ CPT Code(s): _76872-50_

43. Fluoroscopic guidance for needle placement.

    ⊛ CPT Code(s): _77002_

44. Computed tomography guidance for stereotactic localization.

    ⊛ CPT Code(s): _73510_

45. Transrectal ultrasound.

    ⊛ CPT Code(s): _76872_

46. Four-view x-ray of the lumbosacral spine.

    ⊛ CPT Code(s): _73510_

47. Myelography, cervical, radiological supervision and interpretation.

    ⊛ CPT Code(s): _72240_

48. Bilateral screening mammography.

    ⊛ CPT Code(s): _76602_

49. X-ray of the facial bones, 2 views.

    ⊛ CPT Code(s): _70140_

50. TMJ x-ray with mouth open and closed on one side of the mouth.

    ⊛ CPT Code(s): _71004_

⊛ User to decide number of codes necessary to correctly answer the question.

Odd-numbered answers are located in Appendix B, while the full answer key is only available in the TEACH Instructor Resources on Evolve.

51. X-ray of abdomen, single anteroposterior, and additional oblique and cone views.

    🔬 CPT Code(s): ___74010___

52. Placement of a long gastrointestinal tube, including fluoroscopy, radiological supervision and interpretation. Report radiology service only.

    🔬 CPT Code(s): ___74340___

53. Venography, superior sagittal sinus, radiological supervision and interpretation for thrombosis of intracranial venous sinus. Report radiology service only.

    CPT Code: ___75870___

    ICD-10-CM Code: _____

    (ICD-9-CM Code: _____)

54. Magnetic resonance spectroscopy for temporal meningioma, benign.

    CPT Code: ___74000___

    ICD-10-CM Code: _____

    (ICD-9-CM Code: _____)

55. Intravascular ultrasound of a noncoronary vessel, radiological supervision and interpretation due to renal artery stenosis.

    CPT Code: ___75945___

    ICD-10-CM Code: _____

    (ICD-9-CM Code: _____)

56. Venography of unilateral extremity; radiological supervision and interpretation in a patient with end-stage renal disease on hemodialysis. Report radiology service only.

    CPT Code: ___71012___

    ICD-10-CM Codes: _____, _____

    (ICD-9-CM Codes: _____, _____)

Odd-numbered answers are located in Appendix B, while the full answer key is only available in the TEACH Instructor Resources on Evolve.

REPORTS

Toward the end of this textbook, you will find a section titled Reports, which contains original reports. Read the reports indicated below and supply the appropriate CPT and ICD-10-CM/ICD-9-CM codes on the following lines:

57. Report 45

CPT Code: _71010_

ICD-10-CM Code: _____

(ICD-9-CM Code: _____)

58. Report 46

CPT Code: _78450_

ICD-10-CM Code: _____

(ICD-9-CM Code: _____)

59. Report 47

CPT Code: _70480 - 26_

ICD-10-CM Code: _____

(ICD-9-CM Code: _____)

60. Report 48

CPT Code: _74161_

ICD-10-CM Code: _____

(ICD-9-CM Code: _____)

61. Report 49

 ⊛ CPT Code(s): _74000 - 26_

 ⊛ ICD-10-CM Code(s): _____

(⊛ ICD-9-CM Code(s): _____)

⊛ **User to decide number of codes necessary to correctly answer the question.**
Odd-numbered answers are located in Appendix B, while the full answer key is only available in the TEACH Instructor Resources on Evolve.

62. Report 50

    CPT Code(s): __76872-26__

    ICD-10-CM Code(s): _____

    (ICD-9-CM Code(s): _____)

63. Report 51

    CPT Code(s): __70140-26__

    ICD-10-CM Code(s): _____

    (ICD-9-CM Code(s): _____)

64. Report 52

    CPT Code(s): __78582-26__

    ICD-10-CM Code(s): _____

    (ICD-9-CM Code(s): _____)

65. Report 53

    CPT Code(s): __78451-26__

    ICD-10-CM Code(s): _____

    (ICD-9-CM Code(s): _____)

User to decide number of codes necessary to correctly answer the question.
Odd-numbered answers are located in Appendix B, while the full answer key is only available in the TEACH Instructor Resources on Evolve.

CHAPTER 29

Pathology/Laboratory

THEORY

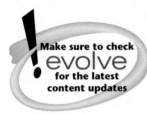

Make sure to check evolve for the latest content updates

Without the use of reference materials, answer the following:

1. In what section of the CPT manual will you find the codes to indicate
   ___surgery___ the service of venipuncture?

2. When a laboratory drug test is qualitative, it measures the
   ___amount___ of the drug.

3. When a laboratory drug test is quantitative, it measures the
   ___presence___ and the ___amount___ of a specific drug.

4. When coding an evocative/suppression test, you may have an E/M code to indicate a prolonged period of time the physician spends with the patient during the testing process or a report of the injection or infusion service. What other service may you need to report?
   ___medicine___

5. A sample of tissue from a suspect area that is examined by a pathologist is a specimen, a block is a frozen piece of the specimen, and a(n)
   ___section___ is a slice of the frozen block.

6. How many levels of surgical pathology are there? ___six___

7. If one breast specimen is received for pathological analysis and the pathologist examines two blocks of the specimen, how many codes would be used to report the service of analysis? ___one___

Odd-numbered answers are located in Appendix B, while the full answer key is only available in the TEACH Instructor Resources on Evolve.

PRACTICAL

Using the CPT and ICD-10-CM/ICD-9-CM manuals, code the following:

8. CARDIAC ENZYMES in a patient newly diagnosed with an acute inferior myocardial infarction.

Ref	Range	Units	12/18/XX
CPK	35-232 IU	69	0.0123
CKMB	0-10	ng/ml	1

CARDIAC MARKERS

12/18/XX	+123 TROPONIN I	<0.3 ng/ml

Troponin I Interpretation

≤0.4 ng/ml for apparently healthy individual

0.5-1.9 ng/ml for clinically Dx non-AMI patients

≥2.0 g/ml reasonably specific for AMI

CPT Codes: CPK, total: __82550__

CKMB (creatine kinase, cardiac fraction):

__82550__

Troponin, quantitative: __84484__

ICD-10-CM Code: _____

(ICD-9-CM Code: _____)

9. GENERAL BLOOD CHEMISTRY in a patient with dehydration, joint pains, and fever.

Ref	Range	Units	10/30/XX 0620	10/27/XX 1855
BUN	7-22	mg/dl		H 37
Sodium	136-145	mmol/L		138
Potassium	3.6-5.5	mmol/L		4.5
Creatinine	0.6-1.3	mg/dl	H 1.9	H 2.4
Uric acid	2.6-6.0	mg/dl	H 9.6	

CPT Codes: BUN: __84520__

Sodium: __84295__

Potassium: __84132__

Creatinine: __82565__

Uric acid: __84550__

ICD-10-CM Codes: _____, _____, _____

(ICD-9-CM Codes: _____, _____,

_____)

10. An 84-year-old monitored for diagnoses of renal failure, anemia, and hypertension.

CPT Codes: Labs include:

Magnesium: _83735_____

Iron: _83540_____

Phosphorus: _84100_____

Total protein serum: _84155_____

ICD-10-CM Codes: _____, _____, _____

(ICD-9-CM Codes: _____, _____,

_____)

11. A 48-year-old female patient with hyperlipidemia, currently on Lipitor.

CPT Codes: Labs include:

Hepatic function: _80076_____

Lipid panel: _80061_____

ICD-10-CM Code: _____

(ICD-9-CM Code: _____)

12. A 20-year-old male in for labs due to chronic asthma.

CPT Codes: Labs include:

Theophylline: _80198_____

ICD-10-CM Code: _____

(ICD-9-CM Code: _____)

13. A 55-year-old male in for labs, digoxin level for chronic atrial fibrillation.

CPT Codes: Labs include:

Digoxin: _80162_____

ICD-10-CM Code: _____

(ICD-9-CM Code: _____)

Odd-numbered answers are located in Appendix B, while the full answer key is only available in the TEACH Instructor Resources on Evolve.

REPORTS

Toward the end of this textbook, you will find a section titled Reports, which contains original reports. Read the reports indicated below and supply the appropriate CPT and ICD-10-CM/ICD-9-CM codes on the following lines:

14. Report 54

    ⚛ CPT Code(s): __88301__

    ⚛ ICD-10-CM Code(s): _____

    (⚛ ICD-9-CM Code(s): _____)

15. Report 55

    ⚛ CPT Code(s): __88305__

    ⚛ ICD-10-CM Code(s): _____

    (⚛ ICD-9-CM Code(s): _____)

16. Report 56

    ⚛ CPT Code(s): __88306__

    ⚛ ICD-10-CM Code(s): _____

    (⚛ ICD-9-CM Code(s): _____)

17. Report 57

    ⚛ CPT Code(s): __88304__

    ⚛ ICD-10-CM Code(s): _____

    (⚛ ICD-9-CM Code(s): _____)

18. Report 58

    ⚛ CPT Code(s): __88300__

    ⚛ ICD-10-CM Code(s): _____

    (⚛ ICD-9-CM Code(s): _____)

⚛ **User to decide number of codes necessary to correctly answer the question.**
Odd-numbered answers are located in Appendix B, while the full answer key is only available in the TEACH Instructor Resources on Evolve.

19. Report 59

   🔘 CPT Code(s): ___88305___

   🔘 ICD-10-CM Code(s): _____

   (🔘 ICD-9-CM Code(s): _____)

20. Report 60

   🔘 CPT Code(s): _88501___

   🔘 ICD-10-CM Code(s): _____

   (🔘 ICD-9-CM Code(s): _____)

21. Report 61

   🔘 CPT Code(s): ___88304___

   🔘 ICD-10-CM Code(s): _____

   (🔘 ICD-9-CM Code(s): _____)

22. Report 62

   🔘 CPT Code(s): __88305___

   🔘 ICD-10-CM Code(s): _____

   (🔘 ICD-9-CM Code(s): _____)

23. Report 63

   🔘 CPT Code(s): ___88307___

   🔘 ICD-10-CM Code(s): _____

   (🔘 ICD-9-CM Code(s): _____)

24. Report 64

   🔘 CPT Code(s): ___88301___

   🔘 ICD-10-CM Code(s): _____

   (🔘 ICD-9-CM Code(s): _____)

🔘 **User to decide number of codes necessary to correctly answer the question.**
Odd-numbered answers are located in Appendix B, while the full answer key is only available in the TEACH Instructor Resources on Evolve.

25. Report 65

    🌐 CPT Code(s): _____88104_____

    🌐 ICD-10-CM Code(s): _____

    (🌐 ICD-9-CM Code(s): _____)

26. Report 66

    🌐 CPT Code(s): _____88100_____

    🌐 ICD-10-CM Code(s): _____

    (🌐 ICD-9-CM Code(s): _____)

27. Report 67

    🌐 CPT Code(s): _____88104_____

    🌐 ICD-10-CM Code(s): _____

    (🌐 ICD-9-CM Code(s): _____)

🌐 **User to decide number of codes necessary to correctly answer the question.**
**Odd-numbered answers are located in Appendix B, while the full answer key is only available in the TEACH
Instructor Resources on Evolve.**

CHAPTER 30

Medicine

THEORY

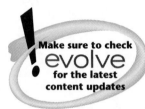

Make sure to check evolve for the latest content updates

Without the use of reference material, match the following terms to the correct definitions:

1. __M__ Aphakia
2. __J__ Echography
3. __H__ Gonioscopy
4. __D__ Hemodialysis
5. __N__ Modality
6. __F__ Nystagmus
7. __i__ Optokinetic
8. __C__ Percutaneous
9. __g__ Phlebotomy
10. __B__ Retrograde
11. __l__ Subcutaneous
12. __K__ Tonometry
13. __a__ Transcutaneous
14. __E__ Tympanometry

a. Entering by way of the skin

b. Moving backward or against the usual direction of flow

c. Through the skin

d. Cleansing of the blood outside the body

e. Procedure for evaluation of middle ear disorders

f. Rapid involuntary eye movements

g. Cutting into a vein

h. Use of a scope to examine the angles of the eye

i. Movement of the eye to objects moving in the visual field

j. Ultrasound procedure in which sound waves are bounced off an internal organ and the resulting image is recorded

k. Measurement of pressure or tension

l. Tissue below dermis, primarily fat cells that insulate the body

m. Absence of the lens of the eye

n. Treatment method

Odd-numbered answers are located in Appendix B, while the full answer key is only available in the TEACH Instructor Resources on Evolve.

Match the following administration methods for drugs:

15. __g__ OTH   a. Subcutaneous

16. __D__ IT   b. Inhalant solution

17. __f__ IV   c. Various routes

18. __E__ IM   d. Intrathecal

19. __a__ SC   e. Intramuscular

20. __B__ INH   f. Intravenous

21. __C__ VAR   g. Other routes

Define the following terms:

22. Oscillating <u>move or swing back and forth at regular speed</u>

23. Audiometry <u>hearing test</u>

24. Tympanometry <u>evaluating middle ear disorders</u>

25. Electrocochleography <u>stimulation of the cochlea to measure electrical activity</u>

26. Orthoptic <u>corrective; in the correct place</u>

27. Angioscopy <u>studying the capillaries of the eyes</u>

28. Electroretinography <u>an eye test, detect abnormal function</u>

29. Anomaloscope <u>a device for detecting color blindness</u>

30. Aphakia <u>absence of the lens of the eye</u>

31. Corneosclera <u>cornea and sclera together forming one organ</u>

32. Cornea <u>transparent layer forming the front of the eye</u>

33. Sclera <u>the thick outer coat of the eye, mostly white and opaque</u>

PRACTICAL

Using the CPT and ICD-10-CM/ICD-9-CM manuals, code the following:

34. Three injections of allergen with the provision of the extract and professional service.

    CPT Code: ___95115___

35. Two photo patch tests.

    CPT Code: ___95052___ × _2_

36. Replacement of contact lenses.

    CPT Code: ___92326___

37. Patient is fitted for bifocal spectacles.

    CPT Code: ___92341___

38. Electro-oculography with interpretation and report.

    CPT Code: ___92270___

39. Optokinetic nystagmus test.

    CPT Code: ___92534___

40. Positional nystagmus test, with recording, five positions.

    CPT Code: ___92532___

41. An esophagus acid reflux test with nasal catheter electrode placement for detection of gastroesophageal reflux.

    CPT Code: ___91034___

42. Peritoneal dialysis with two (repeated) physician evaluations.

    CPT Code: ___90945___

43. Hypnotherapy.

    CPT Code: ___90880___

44. Bernstein test for esophagitis.

    CPT Code: ___91030___

45. Evaluation of auditory rehabilitation status, 1 hour.

    CPT Code: ___92626___

Odd-numbered answers are located in Appendix B, while the full answer key is only available in the TEACH Instructor Resources on Evolve.

46. Family psychotherapy without the patient present.

    CPT Code: _90832_

47. Hemodialysis access flow study to determine blood flow in grafts.

    CPT Code: _90940_

48. Puretone audiometry; air and bone.

    CPT Code: _92553_

49. Insertion of a Swan-Ganz catheter.

    CPT Code: _93503_

50. Electronic analysis for sick sinus syndrome of a single-chamber implantable cardioverter-defibrillator, with reprogramming (in person).

    CPT Code: _92271_

    ICD-10-CM Code: _____

    (ICD-9-CM Code: _____)

51. Ventilation management for assist of breathing; second day for a hospital inpatient. The patient has a diagnosis of acute respiratory failure.

    CPT Code: _94003_

    ICD-10-CM Code: _____

    (ICD-9-CM Code: _____)

52. Training for a prosthetic arm, 45 minutes.

    CPT Code(s): _97761_

53. Conscious sedation provided by the same physician performing the diagnostic test on a 40-year-old patient for 30 minutes.

    CPT Code(s): _99144_

54. GI tract intraluminal imaging.

    CPT Code(s): _91110_

55. Administration of two vaccines.

    CPT Code(s): _90471_

User to decide number of codes necessary to correctly answer the question.

Odd-numbered answers are located in Appendix B, while the full answer key is only available in the TEACH Instructor Resources on Evolve.

56. The patient is being treated for bacterial endocarditis, on IV antibiotic therapy. The patient also has a new onset of ventricular flutter. The cardiologist documents a detailed history, detailed examination, and high medical decision making during this subsequent inpatient encounter.

     ⊛ CPT Code(s): ___94001___

     ⊛ ICD-10-CM Code(s): _____

     (⊛ ICD-9-CM Code(s): _____)

57. The service provided to the patient was an initial episode of care for an acquired atrial septal defect due to acute myocardial infarction of the inferolateral wall. The patient was admitted to the hospital for care.

     ICD-10-CM Codes: _____, _____

     (ICD-9-CM Codes: _____, _____)

58. Arteriosclerosis of legs with intermittent claudication.

     ICD-10-CM Code: _____

     (ICD-9-CM Code: _____)

⊛ User to decide number of codes necessary to correctly answer the question.
Odd-numbered answers are located in Appendix B, while the full answer key is only available in the TEACH Instructor Resources on Evolve.

REPORTS

Toward the end of this textbook, you will find a section titled Reports, which contains original reports. Read the reports indicated below and supply the appropriate CPT and ICD-10-CM/ICD-9-CM codes on the following lines:

59. Report 68

    ☉ CPT Code(s): __99203__

    ☉ ICD-10-CM Code(s): _____

    (☉ ICD-9-CM Code(s): _____)

60. Report 69

    ☉ CPT Code(s): __93503__

    ☉ ICD-10-CM Code(s): _____

    (☉ ICD-9-CM Code(s): _____)

61. Report 70

    ☉ CPT Code(s): __99241__

62. Report 71

    ☉ CPT Code(s): __99251__

63. Report 72

    ☉ CPT Code(s): __None__

64. Report 73

    ☉ CPT Code(s): __92326__

65. Report 74

    ☉ CPT Code(s): __19307 - LT__

    ☉ ICD-10-CM Code(s): _____

    (☉ ICD-9-CM Code(s): _____)

66. Report 75

    ☉ CPT Code(s): __91034__

☉ **User to decide number of codes necessary to correctly answer the question.**

Odd-numbered answers are located in Appendix B, while the full answer key is only available in the TEACH Instructor Resources on Evolve.

67. Report 76

  ⊛ CPT Code(s): __99252-57__

  ⊛ ICD-10-CM Code(s): _____

  (⊛ ICD-9-CM Code(s): _____)

68. Report 77

  ⊛ CPT Code(s): __92770_____

69. Report 78

  ⊛ CPT Code(s): __32554_____

  ⊛ ICD-10-CM Code(s): _____

  (⊛ ICD-9-CM Code(s): _____)

70. Report 79

  ⊛ CPT Code(s): __97760_____

  ⊛ ICD-10-CM Code(s): _____

  (⊛ ICD-9-CM Code(s): _____)

71. Report 80

  ⊛ CPT Code(s): __94060, 94729, 99070__

⊛ User to decide number of codes necessary to correctly answer the question.

Odd-numbered answers are located in Appendix B, while the full answer key is only available in the TEACH Instructor Resources on Evolve.

CHAPTER 31

Inpatient Coding

THEORY

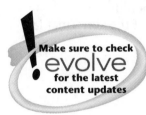

Make sure to check **evolve** for the latest content updates

Without the use of reference material, complete the following:

1. In which setting would an ICD-10-CM/ICD-9-CM procedure code be assigned for a herniorrhaphy?

   ~~Inpatient~~   Outpatient

2. In which setting would documentation in the discharge summary of a suspected condition be coded as if it exists?

   ~~Inpatient~~   Outpatient

3. In which setting would a CPT code be assigned for a cataract extraction?

   Inpatient   ~~Outpatient~~

4. A significant procedure must be performed in an operating room.

   True   ~~False~~

5. The use of a POA indicator is optional.

   True   ~~False~~

6. If a patient is admitted from outpatient surgery for a complication, the reason for the surgery is the principal diagnosis.

   True   ~~False~~

7. When two or more diagnoses equally meet the definition for principal diagnosis, the one that the physician lists first should be assigned as the principal diagnosis.

   True   ~~False~~

Odd-numbered answers are located in Appendix B, while the full answer key is only available in the TEACH Instructor Resources on Evolve.

8. A patient is admitted with syncope. The physician documents that the patient's syncope is due to orthostatic hypotension or bradycardia. Which diagnosis(es) should be reported?
   a. syncope
   b. syncope, orthostatic hypotension, bradycardia
   c. orthostatic hypotension, bradycardia
   d. bradycardia

9. Patient is admitted with right lower quadrant pain and anorexia due to acute appendicitis. Which diagnosis(es) should be reported?
   a. acute appendicitis
   b. right lower quadrant pain, appendicitis
   c. acute appendicitis, anorexia, right lower quadrant pain
   d. anorexia, acute appendicitis

10. If it is documented that the patient has a low magnesium level and magnesium supplements are ordered, the coder should:
   a. query the physician regarding the significance of the abnormal lab value and subsequent treatment
   b. add a code for abnormal lab value
   c. check with supervisor
   d. all of the above

Using Table 31-1 located in the main textbook, answer the following:

11. Altering the route of passage of the contents of a tubular body part is:
   a. alteration
   b. bypass
   c. change device in
   d. control postprocedural bleeding in

12. Cutting into a body part without draining fluids and/or gases from the body part in order to separate or transect a body part is:
   a. alteration
   b. detachment
   c. division
   d. change device in

13. Physical eradication of all or a portion of a body part by the direct use of energy, force, or a destructive agent is:
   a. division
   b. excision
   c. destruction
   d. resection

14. An example of fragmentation is:
   a. lithotripsy
   b. spinal fusion
   c. dermabrasion
   d. cutdown

15. An example of an occlusion type of procedure is:
    a. clamping
    b. clipping
    c. ligation
    d. all of the above

16. ICD-10-PCS will replace CPT codes on Oct 1, 2014.

    True   False

SEQUENCING EXERCISES

Cases of Principal Diagnosis and Other Diagnoses

In the following cases, identify the principal diagnosis and other diagnoses using the ICD-9-CM Official Guidelines for Coding and Reporting. This is a sequencing exercise, not a coding exercise. If there is only one diagnosis, write "none" for Other Diagnoses.

17. Mr. Jones presents to the emergency department with complaints of leg pain, inflammation and swelling of the ankle and calf, and a fever. The day before he had been seen in the physician's office for treatment of cellulitis and was given antibiotics. Mr. Jones was admitted to the hospital for IV antibiotics.

    Principal Diagnosis: _____

    Other Diagnoses: _____

18. Mrs. Beatty was seen in her physician's office with a complaint of shortness of breath and chest pain. Dr. Adams admitted her with a diagnosis of congestive heart failure.

    Principal Diagnosis: _____

    Other Diagnoses: _____

19. Mr. Janes was admitted for colon resection for colon cancer and also had chemotherapy following surgery. Mr. Janes complained of joint pain while in the hospital, and an MRI showed metastases to bone.

    Principal Diagnosis: _____

    Other Diagnoses: _____

20. Mrs. Anderson had a hysterectomy and bilateral oophorectomy for ovarian cancer 1 week ago. It is planned that the patient will undergo chemotherapy. The patient is now admitted with internal hemorrhaging from the surgery site.

    Principal Diagnosis: *postoperative hemorrhage*

    Other Diagnoses: *ovarian cancer*

21. Miss Nelson is admitted for a D&C for menorrhagia. During her preoperative physical examination, the physician notices she has a fever and her lungs are congested. He cancels surgery because the patient shows symptoms of acute bronchitis.

    Principal Diagnosis: _____

    Other Diagnoses: _____

Odd-numbered answers are located in Appendix B, while the full answer key is only available in the TEACH Instructor Resources on Evolve.

22. Jackie Jones was cooking at home and spilled a pot of boiling water on her arms, legs, and stomach. She presented to the emergency department with second-degree burns of the thighs and third-degree burns of the arms and stomach. She was admitted and taken directly to surgery.

Principal Diagnosis: _third-degree burn to arm/stomach_

Other Diagnoses: _second-degree burn thigh_

23. Mr. Anderson regularly sees a physician and is on medication for management of his chronic bronchitis. Last night he was complaining of coughing and difficulty breathing. He was admitted with a diagnosis of chronic bronchitis with acute exacerbation.

Principal Diagnosis: _acute with chronic bronchitis_

Other Diagnoses: _none_

24. Mrs. Smith is at 32 weeks' gestation and complaining of stomach cramps and diarrhea × 36 hours. She is admitted for rehydration with IV fluids and is diagnosed with dehydration and gastroenteritis. Pregnancy is felt to be incidental.

Principal Diagnosis: _dehydration_

Other Diagnoses: _gastroenteritis, pregnancy is reported with a v code for incidental state_

Odd-numbered answers are located in Appendix B, while the full answer key is only available in the TEACH Instructor Resources on Evolve.

PRINCIPAL DIAGNOSIS

Provide the principal diagnosis code, the procedure code, and any additional diagnosis codes for the following:

25. **HISTORY OF PRESENT ILLNESS:** The patient is a 52-year-old male who was involved in an interpersonal altercation at approximately 1:30 in the morning. He presented to the emergency department with complaints of pain and swelling to the right side of the face. The patient had been struck multiple times with the butt end of a handgun. He denied loss of consciousness. The attack was witnessed, and the witnesses also claimed there was no loss of consciousness. He presented with pain and swelling on the right side of his face in the temporal region and in the right eye region. He had a small abrasion on the top of his head and on the right forehead. No lacerations were noted. He had no diplopia. The past medical history and past surgical history were noncontributory. The patient was taking no medications and had no allergies.

HOSPITAL COURSE: Admission x-rays and CT scan revealed a nondisplaced right zygoma fracture and an orbital floor fracture with slight limitation on physical examination of his upward gaze. He was taken to the operating room for exploration and placement of a Silastic implant to the right orbital floor fracture, which was accomplished without difficulty and without complication. The patient tolerated the procedure well. Postoperative course was uncomplicated. He received IV antibiotics throughout his stay in the hospital.

FINAL DIAGNOSIS: Right orbital fracture; right zygoma fracture; abrasion of head.

ICD-10-CM PRINCIPAL DIAGNOSIS and CODE: *Right orbital fracture*

ICD-10-CM OTHER DIAGNOSES and CODES:

_____*802.6*_____, _____*802.4*_____, _____*910.0*_____,

_____*E960.0*_____ *76.79, 76.92*

ICD-10-PCS PROCEDURE CODE: _____

ICD-9-CM PRINCIPAL DIAGNOSIS and CODE:

_____

ICD-9-CM OTHER DIAGNOSES and CODES: _____,

_____, _____

ICD-9-CM PROCEDURE CODE: _____

26. **HISTORY OF PRESENT ILLNESS:** The patient is a 69-year-old, right-handed male who presents with a 4-day history of severe right-sided headache, visual blurring, and diplopia. The patient was seen in the ENT clinic for discharge from his right ear of 2 days' duration, diagnosed to be otitis externa on the day of admission. The patient was subsequently transferred from the clinic to the emergency department. The patient denied a history of seizure, motor or sensory deficit, nausea or vomiting, trauma, or speech difficulties. Past medical history of sinusitis for many years. Current medications are none. Allergies, none.

PHYSICAL EXAMINATION: HEENT: Right pupil 3 mm, nonreactive. Left pupil 2 mm, reactive. Disconjugate gaze present. Right ptosis. Oropharynx clear without lesions. The neck is supple without lymphadenopathy or thyromegaly. Heart: regular rate and rhythm without murmurs or gallops. Lungs clear to percussion and auscultation. The neurological examination: awake, alert, oriented times three, follows three simple commands. Cranial nerves, partial right third nerve palsy with ptosis, 3-mm nonreactive right pupil, right medial gaze with disconjugate extraocular eye movement. Motor is 5/5 throughout without drift. Finger test is within normal limits. The sensory is intact to fine touch and proprioception: cerebral examination within normal limits.

HOSPITAL COURSE: Patient was admitted with suspicion of intracranial aneurysm. On the following day, the patient underwent a three-vessel cerebral angiogram that demonstrated a posterior communicating artery aneurysm and questionable anterior communicating artery aneurysm. The patient underwent a right craniotomy for clipping of right posterior communicating artery aneurysm and anterior communicating artery aneurysm. Postoperatively, the patient was observed in the surgical intensive care unit until his mental status was stabilized. The palsy and ptosis noted preoperatively resolved during the postsurgical course. The patient has been ambulating without assistance and tolerating food well. The patient was also seen by the ENT service during the hospitalization for his otitis externa and their recommendations were followed.

FINAL DIAGNOSES: Right posterior communicating artery aneurysm; anterior communicating artery aneurysm; right otitis externa.

ICD-10-CM PRINCIPAL DIAGNOSIS and CODE: _Right posterior and anterior communicating artery_

ICD-10-CM OTHER DIAGNOSIS and CODE: _____

437.3 aneurysm

ICD-10-PCS PROCEDURE CODE: _____

Right otitis externa

ICD-9-CM PRINCIPAL DIAGNOSIS and CODE: _____

_380.10_

_____

ICD-9-CM OTHER DIAGNOSIS and CODE: _____ _39.51_

ICD-9-CM PROCEDURE CODE: _____

Odd-numbered answers are located in Appendix B, while the full answer key is only available in the TEACH Instructor Resources on Evolve.

Reports

1. EMERGENCY DEPARTMENT REPORT

The patient is a 32-year-old G-5, P-4, female at 36 weeks and 4 days by last menstrual period, who comes in to the emergency room complaining of a 4-day history of urinary frequency and urgency with cloudy urine. She is also complaining of some low back pain × 5 days. She denies burning, itching, pain with urination. She denies fever and chills. She has also had some nausea and vomiting over the same period. She last vomited yesterday. She vomited twice, she states, and, this past Friday, 4 days ago, twice. She has not vomited today. She has had good fluid intake. She has had a slightly decreased appetite, she states. The patient states that she has had some UTIs this pregnancy × 2. Otherwise, she has had an uncomplicated pregnancy.

The patient denies a history of hypertension, diabetes, and pre-eclampsia. She states she has had some irregular contractions, no real contractions today. She denies vaginal bleeding. She denies gush of fluid. She denies abdominal pain. She has had good fetal movement. She has not had headaches, visual changes, or abdominal pain.

PHYSICAL EXAMINATION: Blood pressure 119/66, temperature 36.5, pulse 86, respiratory rate 18. HEENT: Within normal limits. CHEST: Clear to auscultation bilaterally. HEART: Regular rate and rhythm without murmur, rub, or gallop. ABDOMEN: Gravida, nontender. Vertex. EXTREMITIES: The patient has 1+ pitting edema bilaterally to the knee. On cervical examination, the patient was 1-2 cm, long, −1 station. Fetal heart tones are 130's with accels. *(average fetal heart rate is 120-160, so this is not an abnormal rate)* No obvious contractions on the monitor. No flank tenderness to palpation.

LABORATORY DATA: Urinalysis is done and revealed yellow, turbid urine, specific gravity of 1.022, 100 protein, positive nitrite, moderate hemoglobin, large amount of leukocytes, 5-10 red cells, 3+ bacteria, too numerous to count white cells.

ASSESSMENT: This is a 32-year-old, G-5, P-4 at 36 and 4/5 weeks, with a urinary tract infection. The patient was given a prescription for Macrobid 100 mg p.o. b.i.d. × 7 days. She is instructed to follow up with her OB doctor in 2 days for recheck of her urine and her symptomatology. She was given labor precautions. She was advised that, if she develops fevers, back pain, worsening symptomatology, she should come in immediately for evaluation.

2. DISCHARGE SUMMARY

DIAGNOSES include:

1. Chronic pelvic pain secondary to pelvic metastatic clear cell carcinoma of unknown primary location.
2. Vena cava syndrome post placement of Hickman catheter.
3. Anemia due to chronic disease.
4. Hypertension.

HOSPITAL COURSE: The patient is a 78-year-old female whom we have been following in our clinic for hypertension and also chronic pudendal nerve pain. She had been recently diagnosed with pelvic metastatic clear cell carcinoma, which her primary location is unknown at this time. She will be discussing this further after the pathology reports are read. During her hospital stay a Hickman catheter was placed in order to have IV access for pain medication or future cancer therapy. She was also admitted for chronic pain. She did develop swelling of her arms and neck. She was brought to interventional radiology and she did have venography and the Hickman catheter was removed. Her swelling to her arms and neck have decreased greatly. She denies any shortness of breath. No choking sensation as previously noted. Her pain has been managed well with fentanyl patch at 175 mcg. She has also been on IV heparin therapy for anticoagulation following the vena cava syndrome. Today, the patient has been having complaints of nausea. She did get some dexamethasone IV for her nausea, which did improve later this morning. Her blood pressure has been under good control. Her labs today include a WBC of 5.18, hemoglobin 7.8, hematocrit 23.7, protime 14.4, INR 1.5, PTT 39.6, BUN 6, sodium 139, potassium 4.2, CO_2 27.2.

DISCHARGE PLANS:

1. IV heparin is discontinued. She will be switched over to Lovenox 1 mg/kg subcutaneously daily. The patient will have Home Health to help her set up these injections.
2. She will continue with the fentanyl patch 175 mcg for the pain.
3. She will receive 40,000 units subcutaneously of Procrit at the Cancer Center one time per week. We will follow up in 3 days with a CBC and a basic metabolic panel.
4. Follow-up appointment at the Hypertension Center on November 2 at 10:30 in the morning. Will also check CBC and a basic metabolic panel, PTT, PT, and INR before that appointment.
5. Hold potassium supplements for now.
6. She may use Phenergan p.o. 12.5 mg 1-2 tablets p.o. p.r.n. every 6 hours for nausea.
7. She does have a follow-up appointment set up with Dr. Smith on Friday, 10/29/XX, to discuss her pathology results and decide what further treatment is to be done. He will also be discussing plans with Dr. Sticca.

The above plan was discussed with the patient and her husband. They seem to be in agreement. They were encouraged to call our office with any questions or concerns.

DISCHARGE MEDICATIONS:

1. Will continue home medications.
2. Phenergan 12.5 1-2 tabs p.o. p.r.n. every 6 hours for nausea.
3. Lovenox 1 mg/kg subcutaneously every 24 hours. *(treatment for thrombosis—blood clots)*

4. Fentanyl patch 175 mcg to be changed every 3 days. *(analgesic)*
5. Epogen 40,000 units subcutaneously weekly at the Cancer Center. *(treatment for anemia)*

Total time spent with the patient today is 60 minutes.

3. CLINIC CHART NOTE

HISTORY: This 16-year-old female is seen today after falling off a curb and twisting her right ankle. She is normally a patient of Dr. Anderson, who is out of town this week. *(Both physicians are of the same specialty and in the same clinic.)* She states that she has pain surrounding the entire foot and ankle. Seems unable or unwilling to bear weight. *(Problem focused history)*

PHYSICAL EXAMINATION: Ankle and foot examined. Foot is warm to touch. Some swelling and bruising noted around the lateral aspect of the ankle. X-ray is negative for fracture. (Problem focused examination)

IMPRESSION: Sprained right ankle. (MDM complexity straightforward)

PLAN: Elevation; ice to affected area. Weight bearing only as tolerated. Return for follow-up p.r.n.

4. ADMIT INPATIENT

This is a 19-year-old with a living-related donor kidney transplant as of last month and admitted to hospital for possible sepsis.

HISTORY: This patient has type 1 diabetes and had been on dialysis for a number of years before transplantation. She received her mother's kidney on the 14th of last month from the Medical Center Transplant Program in Dallas. She was there this Tuesday for a transplant visit and apparently did not feel well, but they were not certain whether this was a problem or not; but they did go ahead and do blood cultures and called the public health nurse, who was visiting the patient today, and said that one of the cultures was positive for group B strep. The home health nurse called me and stated that the patient has really gone downhill the past few days and was quite fatigued with generalized malaise. Denied cough, fever, or shaking chills but looked poor overall, and the nurse was quite concerned. We recommended she be brought here for evaluation and treatment as an emergency. After arrival here, she was in no acute distress. Initially, she had bibasilar crackles on deep breathing; however, most of these cleared. I cannot hear any significant pulmonary abnormality on auscultation or percussion. Her heart is normal regular rhythm. No significant murmurs, rubs, S3, or S4. Her abdomen is negative. Her left lower-quadrant kidney is nontender. She has no edema and no lateralizing neural sounds. She is a little lethargic. She does not feel warm. Apparently she is afebrile. Her blood pressure is normal, and she is not tachycardic, but she simply does not look well. Past history, social history, and system review are per our recent old chart and noncontributory at present.

MEDICATIONS: See med sheet.

CLINICAL IMPRESSION: One positive group B strep blood culture, significance, and/or etiology to be determined. My impression at this time is probably a significant finding, and I suspect that this will become a progressive syndrome if not treated.

ADDITIONAL DIAGNOSES:

1. Living-related donor kidney transplant
2. Diabetes mellitus type 1
3. Hypertension

PLAN: Repeat culture. Culture urine. Do chest x-ray stat and repeat lab. Will empirically treat pending results at this time.

5. NEPHROLOGY HOSPITAL PROGRESS NOTE

This patient continues to be stable with no new problems. Her cultures remain negative, and she remains afebrile. Her clearance is pending, but she certainly has settled down nicely. The main problem we are having is with her diabetic management. It simply is not working with the former twice a day of 70/30 insulin plus a nighttime Lantus. I think we should go one way or the other, and we will go to Humalog before each meal, starting with an estimated dose of 15 per meal and 40 of Lantus in the evening, and we will titrate from there. We will get Accu-Cheks before each meal to reflect the previous meal's dose of Humalog and adjust it accordingly. Other than that, tomorrow we will review her case with infectious disease with regard to the duration of her antibiotic therapy. Thus far, our cultures have remained negative; however, the positive group B strep is not the type of typical contaminant you get in a blood culture, and we must take it at face value.

Time spent re-evaluating the patient, reviewing the chart, and rearranging diabetic management was 25 minutes; more than half of the time was coordination.

6. OPERATIVE REPORT

PREOPERATIVE DIAGNOSIS: Scar right parietal region.

POSTOPERATIVE DIAGNOSIS: Same.

SURGICAL FINDINGS: 3 × 1 cm elevated scar right parietal region of scalp.

SURGICAL PROCEDURE: Excision scar of scalp.

SURGEON: Dr. Harold Wallingford

ANESTHESIA: General endotracheal anesthesia, plus 2 cc of 1% Xylocaine and 1:100,000 epinephrine.

PROCEDURE: The scalp was prepped with Betadine scrub and solution, draped in the routine sterile fashion. The lesion was anesthetized with 2 cc of 1% Xylocaine with 1:100,000 epinephrine, mostly for the epinephrine effect. After a wait of 4 minutes the lesion was excised, bleeding was electrocoagulated, the wound was closed with vertical mattress sutures of 3-0 Prolene. Surgicel and antibiotic ointment were applied. The patient tolerated the procedure well and left the operating room in good condition.

PATHOLOGY REPORT LATER INDICATED: Benign tissue.

7. OPERATIVE REPORT

PREOPERATIVE DIAGNOSIS: Lipoma left posterior axillary fold.

POSTOPERATIVE DIAGNOSIS: Same.

SURGICAL FINDINGS: 6 cm diameter lipoma attached to latissimus dorsi muscle.

PROCEDURE PERFORMED: Excision of lipoma left posterior axillary fold.

ANESTHESIA: General endotracheal anesthesia with 5 cc 1% Xylocaine with 1 : 100,000 epinephrine injected along the incision line.

COMPLICATIONS: None.

SPONGE AND NEEDLE COUNT: Correct.

DRAINS: One #10 Jackson Pratt.

DESCRIPTION OF PROCEDURE: The patient's posterior arm was prepped with Betadine scrub and solution and draped in the routine sterile fashion. About 5 cc of 1% Xylocaine with 1 : 100,000 epinephrine were injected along the incision line. Dissection was carried down to the site of the lipomatous mass, which was dissected free of the skin and dissected free of the muscle using sharp dissection with very little bleeding. Bleeding was electrocoagulated. Because of the size of the pocket, we inserted a drain and brought it out through a separate stab wound incision using a #10 Jackson Pratt drain. The wound was then closed, effectively closing the dead space with interrupted 2-0 Monocryl, subcuticular 3-0 Monocryl, and a few twists of 4-0 Prolene. Dressing consisted of Kerlix fluffs, Elastoplast, a clavicle strap, and a sling. The patient tolerated the procedure well and left the area in good condition.

PATHOLOGY REPORT LATER INDICATED: See Report 60.

8. OPERATIVE REPORT

PREOPERATIVE DIAGNOSIS: Pyogenic granuloma, sinus tract, buttock.

POSTOPERATIVE DIAGNOSIS: Multiple sinus tracts, one extending inferiorly about 7 × 3 cm in diameter, one extending to the right approximately 4 × 3 cm, and one 4 × 3 cm extending to the left of 4 × 3 cm.

SURGICAL FINDINGS: As above, plus (benign) granulation tissue present in a capsule of multiple sinus tracts. Sinus tracts measured a total of about 15 × 8 cm in their total dimensions.

SURGICAL PROCEDURE: Partial unroofing of sinus tracts. *(This is a full-thickness debridement.)*

ANESTHESIA: General endotracheal.

DESCRIPTION OF PROCEDURE: The patient was intubated and turned in the prone position. A probe was inserted in the sinus cavity, and dissection was carried down to this. I encountered a piece of chronically infected granulation tissue coming out of a hole, in which I stuck the probe, but this continued for a distance longer than the probe and accordingly, I put my finger in this and this extended down the length of my index finger *(i.e., about 7-8 cm by about 3 cm in width)*. I left this intact, because this would necessitate extensive dissection of 15 sq. cm. of subcutaneous tissue and we have no blood on this patient at this time. We then unroofed two other sinus cavities, and packed this opened with 2-inch vaginal packing and applied a dressing and Kerlix plus an Elastoplast. Estimated blood loss: 25 cc. The patient seemed to tolerate the procedure well and left the operating room in good condition.

Coder's Query: It is unclear from the documentation exactly what the procedure was that the physician performed. The coder queried the physician and asked for additional information to ensure correct coding. The physician explained that the patient has a recurrent history of pyogenic granuloma of the buttock with sinus tracts that have, as in this instance, required a subcutaneous tissue debridement.

9. OPERATIVE REPORT

PREOPERATIVE DIAGNOSIS: Mass, right breast.

POSTOPERATIVE DIAGNOSIS: Mass, right breast.

OPERATIVE PROCEDURE: Right breast mass excision.

PROCEDURE: With the female patient under general anesthesia, the breast and chest were prepped and draped in a sterile manner. An elliptical incision was made in the central portion of the breast about the palpated mass, including the area of the nipple. This was excised all the way down to the fascia of the breast and then submitted for frozen section. Frozen section revealed a carcinoma of the breast with what appeared to be a good margin all the way around it. We then maintained hemostasis with electrocautery and proceeded to close the breast tissue using 2-0 and 3-0 chromic. The skin was closed using 4-0 Vicryl in a subcuticular manner. Steri-Strips were applied. The patient tolerated the procedure well and was discharged from the operating room in stable condition.

PATHOLOGY REPORT LATER INDICATED: Primary, malignant neoplasm.

10. OPERATIVE REPORT

PREOPERATIVE DIAGNOSIS: Neck injury, closed posterior cord syndrome caused by a fracture due to a motor vehicle accident.

POSTOPERATIVE DIAGNOSIS: Same as preoperative.

PROCEDURE PERFORMED: Placement of halo crown and vest.

ANESTHESIA: Local.

SURGICAL INDICATIONS: This 56-year-old patient was in a motor vehicle accident, hitting a tree. He was the driver and appears to have sustained a cervical spinal cord fracture at C1–4. He could not be placed in a neck collar because he has a short, thick neck and also because he had a tracheostomy tube. The patient would not be stabilized with traction as he has a distraction injury. It was indicated to place him in a halo vest and crown to immobilize his neck.

PROCEDURE: The hair was shaved behind both ears. There was a sterile prep done along the forehead region and the region behind both ears. The halo crown was then positioned and stabilized with the three positioners anteriorly and two laterally. I then injected Xylocaine behind both ears and along the supraorbital ridge laterally. I then placed the four pins and torqued them to 8 pounds per sq inch. The hexagonal lock nuts were then tightened. The patient tolerated this well without any apparent complications. The halo vest was then connected to the crown. The crown was placed. A large vest was used but this was still too small for the patient, and on the right side the vest had to be tied with string until some permanent straps could be fashioned by orthotics. During the placement of the vest, I maintained the neck in neutral position and at no time was there any rotation or flexion or extension of the neck.

11. OPERATIVE REPORT

PREOPERATIVE DIAGNOSIS: Bulky free flap, right heel.

POSTOPERATIVE DIAGNOSIS: Same.

SURGICAL FINDINGS: 10.5 × 8.5 cm area of redundant fat of flap of right heel.

PROCEDURE PERFORMED: Defatting of flap of right heel with excision of redundant skin (benign).

ANESTHESIA: General endotracheal anesthesia.

POSITION: Prone.

ESTIMATED BLOOD LOSS: Negligible.

DESCRIPTION OF PROCEDURE: The patient was intubated and turned into prone position. The right foot and lower leg were prepped with Betadine scrub and solution and was draped in the routine sterile fashion. The medial aspect of the flap was elevated excising the old scar in the process, and the flap was elevated to about 60% of its extent to include all of the redundant fat that was within the flap. We removed about 1.5 cm thickness of flap from the bottom of the flap and left a layer of padding of about a cm on the bed. Hemostasis was secured, and then we closed the wound with a combination of plain 3-0 Prolene and horizontal mattress sutures and some horizontal half mattress sutures of 3-0 Prolene. We dressed the wound temporarily with Kerlix and Kling. Dr. Miller will then proceed with his portion of the procedure.

12. OPERATIVE REPORT

PREOPERATIVE DIAGNOSIS: Ischial pressure ulcer with massive ischioperineal and buttock sinus.

POSTOPERATIVE DIAGNOSIS: Same.

FINDINGS: There was a 2 cm open surgical ulcer extending down and connecting with an 8 × 30 cm diameter granulation-lined sinus cavity.

SURGICAL PROCEDURE: Excision of left ischial ulcer with total excision of 8 × 30 cm sinus of the buttock, perineal, and ischial areas.

ANESTHESIA: General endotracheal.

ESTIMATED BLOOD LOSS: 400 ml.

FLUIDS: 2 liters Ringer's lactate.

DRAINS: None.

COMPLICATION: None.

SPONGE AND NEEDLE COUNTS: Correct.

DESCRIPTION: The patient was intubated and turned in the right lateral decubitus position. I injected about 10 ml of 1% Xylocaine with 1:100,000 epinephrine around the surface ulcer, and made incisions down to the granulation tissue, keeping this intact. I opened the skin over the extent of the sinus tracts proximally and distally, trying to keep this in line with a potential Y-V advancement flap, and with some difficulty and remarkable bleeding around what appeared to be the sacrum, I was able to remove virtually intact the entire ulcer, covered with chronically infected granulation tissue. This granulation tissue was poor quality and had an unhealthy appearance. A piece of this was dropped in a culture tube as was a piece of what appeared to be the sacrum, which was quite sclerotic and consistent with an osteomyelitis of the sacrum. Following this extensive removal of the ulcer, I cauterized all of the bleeding and did a stick-tie on one of the bleeders with 2-0 Vicryl. I then sprayed the base with topical thrombin, packed the wound open with 2-inch vaginal packing soaked in 5/10th percent metronidazole, and then put several #2 Prolene sutures to keep the packing in place and to help seal off the wound from the fecal contamination. I put a Vi-Drape over this and then dressed it with Kerlix fluffs, ABD pads, and Elastoplast. The patient tolerated the procedure well and left the area in good condition.

PATHOLOGY REPORT LATER INDICATED: See Report 62.

13. OPERATIVE REPORT

PROCEDURE: Steroid injection.

INDICATIONS: Left shoulder bursitis, rotator cuff syndrome.

PROCEDURE: This procedure was done in the procedure area in the outpatient department of the hospital. After obtaining consent, area of the left shoulder was prepped in the usual fashion with Betadine. 6 cc of 1% lidocaine with 1 cc of Kenalog was injected in the left subacromial bursa without difficulty. The patient tolerated the procedure well without immediate complications. There was moderate relief of pain afterward. The patient was advised to call me if she gets any signs of infection, such as fever, chills, erythema, or swelling. She will call me in 3 days and tell me how she is doing.

14. OPERATIVE REPORT

PREOPERATIVE DIAGNOSIS: Deltoid muscle pain and swelling, myositis.

POSTOPERATIVE DIAGNOSIS: Same.

PRELIMINARY NOTE: This patient was brought down to the operating room on the ventilator, and we used the operating room because of this.

OPERATIVE NOTE: With the patient in the supine position we prepped and draped the left deltoid region. After infiltration with 0.5% Marcaine with epinephrine, a vertical incision was made over the palpated muscular belly. Sharp dissection was carried down to the muscle belly and then we freed up a segment of muscle. We did infiltrate the ends of the muscle away from where we were taking our biopsy with the Marcaine. A segment of muscle was then isolated between clamps and then we excised the segment of muscle and submitted it immediately to the histology department for proper processing. The ends of the muscle were ligated using 2-0 chromic and then the muscular fascia was brought together using 2-0 chromic. Subcutaneous tissue was closed using 2-0 chromic and then the skin was closed using 4-0 nylon in running mattress fashion. A sterile dressing was applied. The patient tolerated the procedure well and was discharged from the operating room in stable condition. At the end of the procedure all sponges and instruments were accounted for.

PATHOLOGY REPORT LATER INDICATED: See Report 59.

15. OPERATIVE REPORT

PREOPERATIVE DIAGNOSIS: Left distal radius fracture.

POSTOPERATIVE DIAGNOSIS: Same.

PROCEDURE PERFORMED: Closed reduction and pinning of closed left distal radius fracture.

COMPLICATIONS: None.

INDICATIONS: This is a 31-year-old female who fell yesterday down a flight of stairs, fracturing her left wrist. She has been stabilized in the intensive care unit throughout the day today. Her injuries include a comminuted intra-articular left distal radius fracture, displaced.

The patient's x-rays are consistent with a displaced comminuted intra-articular distal radius fracture. This is an unstable fracture and requires reduction and probable pinning versus open reduction and internal fixation.

Prior to the procedure, I spoke with the patient regarding her left wrist. We discussed management options in detail, and I recommended proceeding with a closed reduction versus pinning versus ORIF of her left distal radius. The procedure, alternatives, risks, benefits, and expected rehab course were discussed in detail. She understood the implications of surgery and wished to proceed.

PROCEDURE: The patient was brought to the operating room and placed supine on the operating room table. She underwent general anesthesia. The left wrist was initially examined under fluoroscopic guidance. There was comminution and intra-articular involvement. There was dorsal tilt of 30 degrees, shortening, and angulation. We performed a closed reduction with longitudinal traction, manipulation at the fracture, and volar flexion. We obtained a near anatomic reduction with maintenance of radial length and inclination. Additionally, there was neutral tilt. However, with release of traction, there was some instability to the fracture with some residual collapse. Subsequently, the left upper extremity was prepped and draped in standard surgical fashion. Under fluoroscopic guidance, a closed reduction was again obtained. Two separate 0.062 K-wires were placed through the radial styloid, across the main fracture, and into the more proximal shaft. Both of these screws had good fixation in the bone.

Final fluoroscopic views were obtained confirming a near anatomic reduction. The pins were then cut off 1 cm above skin level. The pin sites were dressed with Xeroform gauze and adequately padded. The left upper extremity was then placed into a well-padded and molded long arm cast with the wrist in neutral, forearm neutral, and elbow 90 degrees.

The patient was awakened from anesthesia and tolerated the procedure well. She was transferred back to the recovery room in stable condition. There were no intraoperative complications for the wrist portion of the procedure.

16. OPERATIVE REPORT

PREOPERATIVE DIAGNOSIS: Degenerative joint disease, medial compartment plus old meniscal tear.

POSTOPERATIVE DIAGNOSIS: Posterior horn tear, old, medial meniscus; diffuse grade 3-4 chondromalacia, medial femoral condyle 0-90 degrees; and grade 4 chondromalacia, superior half of the patella.

PROCEDURE PERFORMED: Arthroscopy and partial arthroscopic meniscectomy, right knee.

OPERATIVE PROCEDURE: After suitable general anesthesia had been achieved, the patient's right knee was prepped and draped in the usual manner. Before prepping, a thigh tourniquet was applied; after draping, it was inflated to 300 mm Hg. No inflow cannula was used. Arthroscope was inserted through an anteromedial portal. The lateral compartment was examined. Everything looked good. Examination of the notch revealed some inflated synovial tissue, which was cauterized with a radiofrequency probe. Examination of the medial compartment revealed a horizontal cleavage tear and flap tear of the posterior horn of the medial meniscus. Using a combination of punch and shaver, the unstable meniscus was excised and contoured. The tibial surfaces revealed a small area of water by the anterior horn of the meniscus. Femoral surfaces showed diffuse wear of grade 3 with occasional areas of grade 4 chondromalacia from 0 to 90 degrees. Examination of the patellofemoral joint revealed very good looking articular surfaces on the inferior half of the patella in the trochlea. However, there was essentially bare bone on the superior half of the articular surface.

The knee joint was then thoroughly irrigated, and the arthroscope removed. Stab wounds were closed with 3-0 nylon. A dressing was then applied. Tourniquet was released, after which good circulation was noted to return to the foot. The patient tolerated the procedure well and returned to the recovery room in stable condition.

PATHOLOGY REPORT LATER INDICATED: Benign meniscus tissue and bone chips.

17. OPERATIVE REPORT

PREOPERATIVE DIAGNOSIS: Intertrochanteric/subtrochanteric fracture, closed, right hip.

POSTOPERATIVE DIAGNOSIS: Intertrochanteric/subtrochanteric fracture, right hip.

PROCEDURE PERFORMED: Open reduction internal fixation of intertrochanteric/subtrochanteric fracture, right hip.

ANESTHESIA: Spinal.

FINDINGS: The patient had a displaced comminuted intertrochanteric/subtrochanteric fracture of her right hip. We were able to align this fairly well and hold this in place with a dynamic hip screw device.

PROCEDURE: While under spinal anesthetic, the patient was placed in the supine position on the fracture table, where gentle traction was applied to the right leg and the left leg was abducted. We visualized the fracture using the C-arm image intensifier. We were satisfied with the position and then prepped the patient's right hip with Betadine and draped it in a sterile fashion. She was given 1 g of Kefzol intravenously preoperatively.

We then created a longitudinal incision over the lateral aspect of the right hip and carried the dissection down through the subcutaneous tissue. The fascia was incised longitudinally, and we reflected the vastus lateralis anteriorly, exposing the lateral aspect of the femoral shaft. We were able to palpate the fracture and found that it was significantly displaced. We attempted to reduce this. We then drilled a 9/64-inch hole in the lateral aspect of the femoral shaft through which we advanced a guide pin into the femoral head at an angle of 135 degrees to the femoral shaft. We then passed a reamer over this and reamed to a depth of 110 mm and inserted a 100-mg lag screw into the femoral head. We attempted to position this lag screw in the center of the femoral head as best as possible as seen in both the AP and lateral views.

We then attached a 135-degree four-hole side plate and secured this plate to the femoral shaft using four cortical screws. We then released the traction of the leg and inserted a compressing screw into the end of the lag screw. The resultant fixation appeared to be quite satisfactory. We again used the C-arm image intensifier to evaluate the fracture and found it to be very acceptable.

We then thoroughly irrigated the area with saline and placed a Hemovac drain deep to the fascia. We then closed the fascia using 0 Vicryl and the subcutaneous tissue with 2-0 Vicryl. The skin was closed using skin staples. A sterile Xeroform dressing was applied, and the patient was then taken from the operating room in good condition breathing spontaneously. The final sponge and needle counts were correct. She will be continued on IV Kefzol for at least 24 hours.

18. OPERATIVE REPORT

PREOPERATIVE DIAGNOSIS: Comminuted fracture, right olecranon process of the ulna.

POSTOPERATIVE DIAGNOSIS: Comminuted fracture, right olecranon process of the ulna.

PROCEDURE PERFORMED: Open reduction internal fixation, right olecranon fracture.

ANESTHESIA: General.

FINDINGS: The patient had a markedly comminuted displaced fracture of his right olecranon. He had involved a significant portion of the articular surface. We were able to reassemble the major fragments; however, we did have to debride some of the articular cartilage from the joint, which resulted in a defect in the articular cartilage of some significance.

PROCEDURE: While under a general anesthetic, the patient was placed in supine position on the operating room table, where his right arm was prepped with Betadine and draped in a sterile fashion. We used an Esmarch bandage to exsanguinate the arm, and a tourniquet on the limb was inflated to 250 mm Hg. The total tourniquet time ended up being 43 minutes.

We created a longitudinal incision over the posterior aspect of the elbow, skirting to the radial side of the olecranon. We carried the dissection down through the subcutaneous tissue and easily identified the fracture site as the periosteum was torn over this area. We used suction to irrigate the hematoma. Several pieces of articular cartilage lay in the joint, which we debrided, and there was some other cancellous bone, which we debrided as well because it was laying loose in the joint. We then thoroughly irrigated the area with saline to look for any remaining loose fragments. We held this in place with a towel clip as we drilled a transverse hole through the ulna, perhaps 2.5 cm distal to the fracture site. We passed an 18-gauge wire through this transverse tunnel through the ulna, and then we passed two smooth Steinmann pins across the fracture site. We started the Steinmann pins from the proximal fragment and drilled across the fracture site into the distal ulnar shaft. After we had completed the second Steinmann pin across the fracture site, we passed the 18-gauge wire in a figure-of-eight fashion across the fracture site and around the Steinmann pins. We then tightened this with a Harris wire tightener. The combination of the Steinmann pins and the figure-of-eight wire seemed to secure the fracture quite nicely. There was no movement of the fracture site with placing the elbow through a range of motion. We left the Steinmann pins long until we had obtained an intraoperative x-ray confirming an acceptable alignment of the fragment. The x-rays did confirm a significant loss of the articular cartilage; however, it was elected to accept this because the fragments appeared to be relatively stable clinically.

We then bent the Steinmann pins at 90 degrees and cut them off and then taped the Steinmann pins so that they were buried into the triceps muscle. We placed the elbow through a range of motion and found that no crepitus was noted. The fracture appeared to be in good condition, and we therefore irrigated the area with saline and closed the subcutaneous tissue using 2-0 Vicryl and the skin with 3-0 nylon. A Xeroform dressing was applied, and a long-arm splint was applied with the elbow flexed about 60 degrees. He was taken from the operating room in good condition and breathing spontaneously. Tourniquet released after 43 minutes of tourniquet time, and we released this just after the x-rays. He was given IV Kefzol preoperatively and will be continued on IV Kefzol for 24 hours postoperatively as well. The final sponge and needle counts were correct.

19. OPERATIVE REPORT

PREOPERATIVE DIAGNOSIS: Left lung abscess.

POSTOPERATIVE DIAGNOSIS: Same.

PROCEDURE PERFORMED: Left upper lobectomy with decortication and drainage.

INDICATIONS: This 52-year-old female with radiographic evidence of a left upper lobe abscess was admitted the evening before surgery with tension pneumothorax treated with double-lumen intubation and a chest tube. She was subsequently dialyzed to improve hemodynamics and oxygenation and was felt to be as optimal as possible for her left thoracotomy.

FINDINGS AT SURGERY revealed a large abscess in the left upper lobe accounting for approximately 70% of the left upper lobe parenchyma. Fibrinopurulent exudate was noted on the left lower lobe and throughout the parietal pleural surfaces. This was removed piecemeal with gradual improvement in the left lower lobe pulmonary expansion.

PROCEDURE: The patient was brought to the operating room and placed in the supine position, and under general intubation with a double-lumen tube that had been placed the night before, the patient was rolled into the right lateral decubitus position with her left side up. A posterolateral thoracotomy was performed. Adhesions were taken down sharply and bluntly and with cautery. Following this, a standard artery first left upper lobectomy was carried out utilizing 0 silk and hemoclips. The left upper pulmonary vein was secured with a single application of the TA-30 vascular stapling machine. The posterior fissure was created with multiple applications of the TIA automatic stapling machine and the bronchus secured with a single application of the TA-30 bronchus stapling machine. Following this, the wound was drained with three 24-French atrium chest tubes and hemostasis obtained with spray Tisseel, Surgicel gauze. The bronchus was sealed with Bio-glue and the wound closed in layers and a sterile compression dressing applied, and the patient returned to the surgical intensive care unit after changing the double-lumen tube to a single-lumen tube. The patient received 3 units of packed cells intraoperatively to maintain hemostasis. Sponge count and needle count correct × 2.

PATHOLOGY REPORT LATER INDICATED: See Report 65.

20. OPERATIVE REPORT   *Biopsy*

Endocervical and Endometrial Biopsy

The patient is a 60-year-old married white female, whose last menstrual period was at age 55. No postmenopausal bleeding. Pap is current. Mammogram is not given.

CHIEF COMPLAINT: Metastatic clear cell carcinoma.

The patient is status post CT-guided transgluteal biopsy of a presacral mass, which returns as metastatic clear cell carcinoma. Biopsy was performed September 17, 20XX. The patient's CT of the abdomen shows the uterus to be slightly enlarged for patient's age but does not mention ascites or ovarian masses.

MEDICATIONS:

1. Citracal.
2. Lanoxin 0.25 mg.
3. Metoprolol 50 mg b.i.d.
4. Multivitamin.
5. Ocuvite.
6. Xanax.

MEDICAL PROBLEMS:

1. Chronic pelvic pain syndrome.
2. Sacroiliac lipoma.
3. Pudendal neuralgia.
4. Hiatal hernia.

FAMILY HISTORY: Negative.

REVIEW OF SYSTEMS: Positive for glasses, high blood pressure, anxiety, depression.

PROCEDURE: Endocervical and endometrial biopsy.

The patient received antibiotic prophylaxis and then the procedure was performed by visualizing the cervix. The cervix was prepped with Betadine, and cytobrush was then used to obtain cervical curetting. The endocervical os was unable to be demonstrated by the Pipelle curette or the uterine sound. The cytobrush was then used to locate the central endometrial canal, and the Pipelle curette was then used to obtain endometrial curetting. Bimanual examination shows the uterus to measure 4 to 6 weeks, anteverted, smooth, mobile. Adnexa negative. Rectal declined. BUS within normal limits.

IMPRESSION: Clear cell carcinoma of unknown origin.

PLAN: Refer the patient to the University of Minnesota for diagnostic workup and treatment. The patient and University of Minnesota will be advised of the results of the biopsies when they become available.

PATHOLOGY REPORT LATER INDICATED: See Report 54.

21. OPERATIVE REPORT

PREOPERATIVE DIAGNOSIS: Atelectasis of the right lower lobe, suspecting either a mucous plug or obstructing cancer.

POSTOPERATIVE DIAGNOSIS: Mildly inflamed airways with some thick secretions. No definite mucous plug was seen, and certainly no cancer was noted.

PROCEDURE PERFORMED: Bronchoalveolar lavage, bronchial brushings, and bronchial washings.

For a detail of drugs used and amounts of drugs used, please refer to the bronchoscopy report sheet.

The patient was in the ICU on the ventilator, intubated, and so we simply used ICU sedation. We put the bronchoscope down the endotracheal tube. We could see the trachea, which appeared okay. The carina appeared normal. In the right and left lungs, all segments were patent and entered, and in the right lower lobe and middle lower lobe, there were increased, thick, tenacious secretions. No definite mucous plug. It did take a little suctioning to dislodge all of the mucus; however, it was not as bad as I thought it would be looking at the x-ray. The area was brushed, washed, and then, to be more specific, because of evidence on chest x-ray of something going on in the periphery, a bronchoalveolar lavage of the right lower lobe is performed. The patient tolerated the procedure well. Specimens were performed. Specimens were sent for appropriate cytological, pathological, and bacteriological studies, and we hope to be able to follow up on that tomorrow.

PATHOLOGY REPORT LATER INDICATED: See Report 66.

22. OPERATIVE REPORT

PREOPERATIVE DIAGNOSIS: Chronic adenotonsillitis and chronic tonsillitis.

POSTOPERATIVE DIAGNOSIS: Chronic adenotonsillitis and chronic tonsillitis.

PROCEDURE PERFORMED: Tonsillectomy and adenoidectomy.

OPERATIVE NOTE: The patient is a 15-year-old woman who was seen in the office and diagnosed with the above condition. Decision was made in consultation with the patient to undergo the procedure.

She was admitted through the same-day department and taken to the operating room, where she was administered general anesthetic by intravenous injection. She was then intubated endotracheally. The Jennings gag was inserted into the mouth and expanded; this was secured to a Mayo stand. Two red rubber catheters were placed through the nose and brought out through the mouth; these were secured with snaps. This was done to elevate the palate. A laryngeal mirror was placed in the nasopharynx. The adenoid tissue was visualized. Using suction cautery, the adenoid tissue was removed in systemic fashion. Once this was completed, the red rubbers were released and brought out through the nose. The right tonsil was grasped with an Allis forceps and retracted medially using a harmonic scalpel, and the capsule was entered bilaterally. The tonsil was removed from its fossa in an inferior fashion, and one small area was cauterized. The left tonsil was then grasped with an Allis forceps and retracted medially. Again, the capsule was identified laterally, and the harmonic scalpel was used to remove the tonsil from its fossa in an inferior to superior fashion. Once this was completed, the bed was inspected, and two small areas were cauterized here. Three tonsillar sponges were soaked in 1% Marcaine with epinephrine; one was placed in the nasopharynx, and one in each tonsil bed. These were left in position for 5 minutes, and at the end of this interval they were removed. The beds were inspected. No further bleeding was noted. The gag was then removed from the mouth. The TMJ joint was checked. The patient was allowed to recover from a general anesthetic and taken to the post anesthesia care unit in stable condition. There were no complications during this procedure.

PATHOLOGY REPORT LATER INDICATED: Benign tonsil and adenoid tissue.

23. OPERATIVE REPORT

PREOPERATIVE DIAGNOSIS: Pleural fluid, unknown cause.

POSTOPERATIVE DIAGNOSIS: Loculated pleural effusion with removal of 40 cc of bloody pleural fluid.

PROCEDURE PERFORMED: Diagnostic thoracentesis.

On ultrasound, the areas were loculated by that method as well as by attempting to draw out fluid. I had to do four different sticks to get 40 cc of fluid and that was about the extent of each pocket. There were four different pockets I entered just in the one general area that was marked by ultrasound. This, of course, was done after marking it with ultrasound, rubbing the area with swabs to sterilize the area, and then using 20 cc of 1% lidocaine for local anesthesia. With a one-pass maneuver, we were able to get into some fluid. At first actually, we did not get any fluid. We moved over about 1 inch, and then we were able to get 10 cc of fluid before the pocket petered out. The next one we got 5 cc, and I had to go to a different pocket to get that. Then in the fourth pocket we were able to get two syringe fulls with 10 cc to get at least 40 cc of fluid. As this was such a tenuous area, I did not put a chest tube in to drain it because I did not think we would get anything that would amount to anything with the small chest tube I had at my command. I think we might need thoracoscopy to break up adhesions and drain it right. Of course, the differential of bloody pleural fluid includes tuberculosis, trauma, cancer, and pulmonary embolus. A V/Q scan would probably be pointless in this particular effort. I think I would wait to see what the cultures are before I went down the pulmonary embolus tree. I will have to get a hold of Dr. Marrot about CT surgery.

PATHOLOGY REPORT LATER INDICATED: See Report 67.

24. OPERATIVE REPORT

PROCEDURE PERFORMED: Fiberoptic bronchoscopy, bronchial biopsy, bronchial washings, bronchial brushings.

PREPROCEDURE DIAGNOSIS: Abnormal chest x-ray.

POSTPROCEDURE DIAGNOSIS: Inflammation in all lobes, pneumonia. With pleural plaquing consistent with possible candidiasis.

The patient was already on a ventilator, so the bronchoscope tube was introduced through the endotracheal tube. We saw 2.5 cm above the carina of the trachea, which was red and swollen, as was the carina. The right lung—all entrances were patent, but they were all swollen and red, with increased secretions. The left lung was even more involved, with more swelling and more edema and had bloody secretions, especially at the left base. This area from the carina all the way down to the smaller airways on the left side had shown white plaquing consistent with possible candidiasis. These areas were brushed, washed, biopsied. A biopsy specimen was also sent for tissue culture, as well as two biopsy specimens sent for pathology. Sheath brushings were also performed. The patient tolerated the procedure well, was still in the ICU, monitored throughout the procedure.

25. CARDIAC CATHETERIZATION REPORT

PROCEDURES PERFORMED: Left-sided heart catheterization, selective coronary angiography, and left ventriculography.

INDICATION: Chest pain and abnormal Cardiolite stress test.

COMPLICATIONS: None.

RESULTS:

I. HEMODYNAMICS: The left ventricular pressure before the LV-gram was 117/1 with an LVEDP of 4. After the LV-gram, it was 111/4 with an LVEDP of 10. The aortic pressure on pullback was 111/17.

II. LEFT VENTRICULOGRAPHY: The left ventriculography showed that the left ventricle was of normal size. There were no significant segmental wall motion abnormalities. The overall left ventricular systolic function was normal with an ejection fraction of better than 60%.

III. SELECTIVE CORONARY ANGIOGRAPHY:

A. RIGHT CORONARY ARTERY: The right coronary artery is a medium to large size dominant artery that has about 80% to 90% proximal/mid eccentric stenosis. The rest of the artery has only mild surface irregularities. The PDA and the posterolateral branches are small in size and have only mild surface irregularities.

B. LEFT MAIN CORONARY ARTERY: The left main has mild distal narrowing.

C. LEFT CIRCUMFLEX ARTERY: The left circumflex artery was a medium size, nondominant artery. It gave rise to a very high first obtuse marginal/intermedius, which was a bifurcating medium size artery that has only mild surface irregularities. The second obtuse marginal was also a medium size artery that has about 20% to 25% proximal narrowing. After that second obtuse marginal, the circumflex artery was a small size artery that has about 20% to 30% narrowing, a small aneurysmal segment. After that, it continued as a small third obtuse marginal that has mild atherosclerotic disease.

D. LEFT ANTERIOR DESCENDING CORONARY ARTERY: The left anterior descending artery was a medium size artery that is mildly calcified. It gave rise to a very tiny first diagonal that has mild diffuse atherosclerotic disease. Right at the origin of the second diagonal, the LAD has about 30% narrowing. The rest of the artery was free of significant obstructive disease. The second diagonal was also a small caliber artery that has no significant obstructive disease.

CONCLUSION:

1. Normal overall left ventricular systolic function
2. Severe single vessel atherosclerotic heart disease

RECOMMENDATIONS: Angioplasty stent of the right coronary artery.

26. CORONARY ARTERY BYPASS SURGERY

PREOPERATIVE DIAGNOSIS: Atherosclerotic heart disease, coronary artery disease with depressed LV function.

POSTOPERATIVE DIAGNOSIS: Same.

PROCEDURE PERFORMED: Single vessel coronary artery bypass grafting, LIMA to LAD, off-pump.

ANESTHESIA: General endotracheal.

SPONGE COUNT, NEEDLE COUNT, INSTRUMENT COUNT: Correct.

ESTIMATED BLOOD LOSS: Approximately 666 cc and CellSaver given back is approximately 287 cc.

DRAINS: Four 19-French round Blake drains, one in the left chest, one in the right chest, one over the heart, and one over the pericardial wall, placed to Pleur-evac suction.

INDICATIONS: The patient is a 62-year-old man who has undergone approximately 12 heart catheterizations in the last several years. He has had recurrent in-stent stenosis of the proximal LAD lesion and also a branch of an OM with disease proximally. The patient is taken to the operating room because of recurrent angina, Class III anginal symptoms.

PROCEDURE: After informed consent was obtained, the patient was taken to the operating room. The patient was properly identified. A Swan-Ganz catheter was placed and a right arterial line was placed. A Foley catheter was inserted. The patient was prepped from his chin to both feet bilaterally. A midline sternotomy was performed. The sternum was divided with the sternal saw and the left internal mammary was harvested in a standard fashion.

Simultaneously, the right greater saphenous vein was harvested beginning in the thigh and extending down to the level of the knee. The vein was adequate for bypass grafting. It was excised. The wound was then closed in layers.

Once the LIMA was nearly completely dissected free, the patient was heparinized. The LIMA was divided distally and noted to have excellent flow. It was tied distally. LIMA bed was examined for bleeding. There appeared to be no bleeding present from the LIMA bed. Attention was then turned to the pericardium. The pericardium was opened. Pericardial stay sutures were placed. The left side of the pericardium was fashioned so that the LIMA could sit nicely to the LAD under the lung. Deep pericardial stitch was placed allowing the heart to be elevated and brought medially. A stay suture was placed around the proximal LAD and around the distal LAD. The octopus stabilizing device was used to stabilize the LAD at its mid portion. The proximal stay suture was placed down on the LAD. The LAD was opened and the LIMA had been fashioned for the anastomosis, and the LIMA to LAD anastomosis was carried out using a 7-0 Prolene in a continuous running fashion using a single knot technique. LIMA pedicle was then sutured down. There appeared to be no leak present from the LIMA anastomosis. The starfish stabilizing device was placed on the apex of the heart. The heart was elevated. The lateral wall of the heart was examined extensively for the OM branch that had some proximal disease in it. This artery was not able to be identified. The heart was covered heavily in fat making it somewhat more difficult, but a thorough examination was carried out. At this point I actually broke scrub, went to the catheterization laboratory, re-examined the heart catheterization, and then went back to the OR again looking for that vessel. It almost could have been acting like a high diagonal vessel as it was a high OM, but again in this territory in this distribution I could not identify that vessel, so only a single vessel LIMA to LAD anastomosis was created and the patient ended up with a single bypass. I think he should do well with just a single bypass.

The surgical sites were all examined for bleeding, and there appeared to be no bleeding present. The patient was reversed with 50 mg of Protamine and four Blake drains were placed, one in the left chest, one in the right chest, one over the heart, and one in the pericardial wall. The patient tolerated the procedure well. The preoperative and postoperative transesophageal echocardiogram looked fine. Sternal wires were placed and then the wound was closed in layers. Initial cardiac index here revealed a cardiac index of approximately 2.4 on low dose nitro drip.

27. OPERATIVE REPORT

PREOPERATIVE DIAGNOSIS: Symptomatic right internal carotid artery stenosis.

POSTOPERATIVE DIAGNOSIS: Symptomatic right internal carotid artery stenosis.

OPERATIVE PROCEDURE:

1. Right carotid thromboendarterectomy with patch placement.
2. Intraoperative electroencephalogram monitoring.

INDICATION: This 30-year-old woman has a tight right internal carotid artery stenosis. She has had an episode of amaurosis fugax. She has some other medical problems that also complicate her overall situation, but she has a significantly tight stenosis that is symptomatic, and I would recommend an endarterectomy for this. The procedure, along with the risks, has been previously discussed with the patient. Please see the clinic notes. We will be doing this with the patient awake. We also will be doing EEG monitoring though because of the patient's overall condition, and if she does not end up needing to be intubated during the middle of the case, we will still be able to monitor her brain activity.

PROCEDURE: This was done with the patient under cervical block. Local anesthesia was also infiltrated (0.5% Marcaine with epinephrine). Dissection was carried down through a cervical oblique incision along the anterior border of the sternocleidomastoid muscle. Dissection was carried down to the carotid artery. The common carotid as well as the internal and external carotid arteries and superior thyroid arteries were all dissected free sharply and circumferentially controlled with vessel loops. The common carotid was controlled with umbilical tape and Rumel tourniquet. The patient was systemically heparinized. ACTs were obtained and followed. The ICA was occluded, then the common and then the external carotid. Arteriotomy was made. The plaque was hemorrhagic and ulcerated. It was quite friable. We were able to dissect this out with Freer elevator. This came out quite nicely. The distal endpoint feathered off nicely, but we did place one single tacking suture at the 6-o'clock position. This was 7-0 Prolene. We then used the Impra carotid patch to close the arteriotomy site. This was done with a CV-7 Gore-Tex suture in a running fashion. We heparinized, backbled, and forebled. Intermittently, we had her move her left hand during the case. After suturing the suture line, we opened up the external carotid and the common carotid. After about 10 heartbeats, we then opened up the internal carotid artery. There was bleeding from needle holes. This was controlled with FloSeal. There was good flow through all the arteries at the end of the procedure by Doppler. A 10-mm flat Jackson-Pratt drain was placed before closure of the wound. Hemostasis was present. At the end of the procedure in the admit room, she was awake and following commands and moving all of her extremities. She went to the recovery room in stable condition. I met with the patient's family postoperatively to discuss the operation.

ADDENDUM: It should be noted that this procedure was done with intraoperative EEG monitoring. No changes were noted in the EEG during the procedure. Clamp time was 40 minutes. A patch closure was used as noted. She was also reversed with 40 mg of protamine at the end of the procedure.

28. OPERATIVE REPORT

INDICATION: Prolonged fetal heart rate deceleration. *(report delivery complicated by fetal heart rate)*

PROCEDURE: Vacuum-assisted vaginal delivery. *(report delivery vacuum assisted)*

COMPLICATIONS: Shoulder dystocia, relieved with McRobert's maneuver. *(report delivery complication due to shoulder presentation)*

PREAMBLE: The patient is a 33-year-old gravida 3, para 2, 38 week, 3 days gestation, admitted from the emergency department secondary to pelvic pain *(not reported because the pain is part of delivery)*. The patient was quite uncomfortable and had artificial rupture of membranes followed by labor progression to full dilation. She then began pushing, and some prolonged fetal heart rate decelerations down to about 90 beats per minute were noted *(supports delivery complicated by fetal heart rate)*. Because of this, a decision was made to proceed with vacuum extraction *(supports delivery vacuum assisted)* to assist in expediting delivery.

PROCEDURE NOTE: Maternal bladder was emptied using straight catheter. Pelvic examination was carried out and the cervix was confirmed to be fully dilated. Fetal vertex was present at +1 station. The small kiwi cup vacuum *(supports delivery vacuum assisted)* was then applied to the fetal vertex. On the second pull, there was one pop off but this was after good descent of the fetal head had been achieved. Baby then delivered and was a live-born male infant. *(report one liveborn with a V code)* There was moderate shoulder dystocia present *(supports delivery complicated by shoulder presentation)* and this was relieved with McRobert's maneuver. The baby was handed off to the NICU team and is currently in the NICU for further observation. Apgar's *(a newborn maturity scoring method)* are not available at this time. Cord blood gas is also pending. After an episiotomy, a second-degree perineal tear still occurred during delivery. *(for ICD-9-CM, report delivery complicated by second degree laceration of perineum with fifth digit "1" to indicate the complication occurred at the time of delivery)* This was repaired using 3-0 chromic in usual manner. The patient tolerated this procedure well. Estimated blood loss during delivery was 200 cc.

29. OPERATIVE REPORT

PREOPERATIVE DIAGNOSES:

1. Intrauterine pregnancy, 39 weeks.
2. Multiparity.
3. Desires permanent sterilization.
4. History of previous cesarean section × 2.

POSTOPERATIVE DIAGNOSES:

1. Intrauterine pregnancy, 39 weeks.
2. Multiparity.
3. Desires permanent sterilization.
4. History of previous cesarean section × 2.

PROCEDURE: Repeat low transverse cervical segment cesarean section with postpartum tubal ligation.

ANESTHESIA: Spinal.

ESTIMATED BLOOD LOSS: 800 cc

URINE OUTPUT: 40 cc

FLUIDS: 3000 cc

COMPLICATIONS: None.

FINDINGS: Viable male infant *(report the outcome of delivery)* weighing 6 pounds 10 ounces with Apgar's of 9 at 1 minute and 10 at 5 minutes.

PROCEDURE: The patient was prepped and draped in a supine position with left lateral displacement of the uterine fundus. Under spinal anesthesia and Foley catheter indwelling, a transverse incision was made in the lower abdomen using the old scar. The fascia was divided laterally. Rectus muscles were divided in the midline. The peritoneum was entered in a sharp manner. The incision was extended vertically. The bladder flap was created using sharp and blunt dissection and reflected inferiorly. The uterus was entered in a sharp manner in the lower uterine segment, and the incision was extended laterally with blunt traction. The head was delivered, the infant was delivered, and the infant was bulb suctioned while the cord was being doubly clamped and divided. The infant was given to the intensive care nursery staff in good condition. The placenta was manually expressed. Uterus was delivered through the abdominal cavity and placed on a wet lap sponge. A dry lap sponge was used to ensure that the remaining products of conception were removed. The cervical os was ensured patent with a ring forceps. The uterus incision was closed with 0 Vicryl in an interlocking suture in two layers with second layer imbricating the first. Figure-of-eight sutures were also placed as required for hemostasis. Operative site was inspected, irrigated, and hemostatic. The bladder flap was reapproximated using 2-0 Vicryl in a continuous suture in the midline. The left tube was identified in its entirety, including the fimbriated end and was grasped at its midportion and elevated. The mesosalpinx was transected using the Bovie. Approximately 3 cm of tube was isolated and excised. The proximal end of the distal portion and the distal end of the proximal portion were ligated with 0 chromic suture. The right tube was identified and ligated in the same fashion. Operative site was inspected and was hemostatic. Uterus was placed back in the midabdominal cavity. Pelvic gutters were irrigated. The anterior peritoneum was reapproximated with 2-0 Vicryl continuous suture. The incision was irrigated. Subcutaneous drain was placed, and the skin was closed with 2-0 silk. Sponges and needles were accounted for at the completion of the procedure. The patient left the operating room in apparent good condition after tolerating the procedure well. The Foley catheter was patent and draining a small amount of clear urine at the completion of the procedure.

30. OPERATIVE REPORT

PREOPERATIVE DIAGNOSIS: Complicated pregnancy with prior cesarean sections.

POSTOPERATIVE DIAGNOSIS: Complicated pregnancy with prior cesarean sections. *(V code for history of obstetrical disorder affecting management of current pregnancy)*

PROCEDURE PERFORMED: Amniocentesis for fetal lung maturity. *(V code for screening, antenatal based on amniocentesis)*

INDICATIONS: The patient is at $38\frac{1}{2}$-weeks' gestation and has had three prior C-sections and hospitalizations for recurrent episodes of pyelonephritis. *(V code for personal history a specified urinary system disorder)* We desired to check fetal maturity so we could expedite delivery if possible.

PROCEDURE: The patient was scanned with ultrasound, and few pockets of amniotic fluid were noted; therefore, we elected to do a suprapubic tap. The abdomen was prepped and draped. Dr. Marco elevated the breech of the infant up out of the pelvis, and we scanned suprapubically and found a nice pocket of amniotic fluid. A single tap was done and 10 cc of clear yellow fluid obtained. This fluid was checked for pH and was deeply blue on Nitrazine, indicating it to be most likely amniotic fluid, not urine. She tolerated this well.

Cytology report later indicated slightly decreased fetal lung maturity based on levels of phosphatidylglycerol, with recommendation to re-evaluate in 10 days. *(abnormal amnion, affecting fetus)*

31. OPERATIVE REPORT

Colonoscopy and Polypectomy

PREOPERATIVE DIAGNOSIS: Hematochezia.

POSTOPERATIVE DIAGNOSIS: Two small polyps in the cecum ascending colon, hot biopsied off. A small rectal polyp, hot biopsied off.

INDICATION: This is a 46-year-old white male with Tourette's and some MR who has had some hematochezia. There are no risk factors with no other symptoms.

PREOPERATIVE MEDICATIONS: Fentanyl 100 mcg IV; Versed 4 mg IV.

FINDINGS: The Pentax video colonoscope was inserted without difficulty to the cecum. The ileocecal valve was identified. The appendiceal orifice was seen. I could not enter the cecum. Just above the valve, there was a small 2- to 3-cm polyp. This was hot biopsied off. There was a sessile 3-mm polyp in the proximal ascending colon, hot biopsied off. Inspection of the remainder of the ascending colon, hepatic flexure, transverse colon, splenic flexure, descending colon, and sigmoid colon, revealed no erythema, ulceration, exudate, friability, or other mucosal abnormalities. The rectum showed a small 2-mm polyp that was hot biopsied off. The patient tolerated the procedure well.

IMPRESSION: Three small polyps, two in the cecum ascending colon area and one on the rectum, hot biopsied off.

PLAN: If these polyps are adenomatous, the patient should return again in 5 years for surveillance.

PATHOLOGY REPORT LATER INDICATED: See Report 56.

32. OPERATIVE REPORT

PREOPERATIVE DIAGNOSIS: Nonhealing duodenal ulcer.

POSTOPERATIVE DIAGNOSIS: Nonhealing duodenal ulcer.

PROCEDURES PERFORMED:

1. Exploratory laparotomy.
2. Partial gastrectomy (antrectomy).
3. Truncal vagotomy.
4. Gastrojejunostomy.
5. Cholecystectomy with intraoperative cholangiogram.

INDICATION: The patient is a 60-year-old female who presented with a nonhealing gastric ulcer. She has had symptoms for about a year. She complains of epigastric pain. Medical therapy with Prilosec failed, as did therapy for *H. pylori*. Biopsy of the ulcer has been done, and it was benign. The patient had a negative workup for gastrinoma. Calcium level was also normal. The patient now presents for exploratory laparotomy and partial gastrectomy. The risks and benefits were discussed with the patient in detail. She understood and agreed to proceed.

PROCEDURE: The patient was brought to the operating room. Her abdomen was prepped and draped in a sterile fashion. A midline umbilical incision was made. The peritoneal cavity was entered. Initial inspection of the peritoneal cavity showed normal liver, spleen, colon, and small bowel. There was an ulcer along the first portion of the duodenum just beyond the pylorus with some scarring. There was also an ulcer in the posterior part of the duodenal bulb, which was penetrating to the pancreas. We started dissection along the greater curvature of the stomach. Vessels were ligated with 2-0 silk ties. There was an enlarged lymph node along the greater curvature of the stomach, which was sent for frozen section. It proved to be a benign lymph node. This was the only enlarged node found during dissection. We then proceeded with truncal vagotomy. The anterior vagus and posterior vagus were identified. They were clipped proximally and distally, and a segment of each nerve was excised and sent for frozen section, and a segment of both vagus nerves was excised and confirmed by frozen section. An incision was made around the gastrohepatic ligament. The mesentery along the lesser curvature of the stomach was dissected. The vessels were ligated with 2-0 silk ties along the lesser curvature of the stomach. A Kocher maneuver was performed to aid mobilization. The pancreas was completely normal. No masses were found in the pancreas. There was penetration of the ulcer in the superior part of the head of the pancreas. Dissection was continued posterior to the stomach. The adhesions posterior to the stomach were taken down. The ulcer was in the posterior segment of the duodenal bulb just beyond the pylorus and it had penetrated the pancreas. All the posterior layer of the ulcer that was left adherent to the pancreas was shaved off. The stomach was divided with the GIA stapler so that the complete antrum would be in the specimen. The duodenum was divided between clamps. The stomach pylorus and first part of the duodenum were sent to pathology for examination. Then the duodenal stump was closed with running suture. Using 3-0 Lembert sutures, the posterior wall of the ulcer was incorporated for duodenal closure. The base of the duodenum was rolled over the ulcer, and it was all-incorporating to the duodenal closure. Our next step was to proceed with cholecystectomy. The gallbladder was separated from the liver, reflected, and taken down, and the gallbladder was divided from the liver with blunt dissection and cautery. The cystic artery was doubly ligated with silk. The cystic duct was identified. The cystic duct and gallbladder junction and gallbladder ducts were identified. Intraoperative cholangiogram was performed showing free flow of bile into the intrahepatic duct and into the duodenum. No leaks were seen. The cystic duct was doubly ligated, and the gallbladder was sent to pathology. The staple line in the proximal stomach was oversewn with 3-0 silk Lembert sutures. A retrocolic isoperistaltic Hofmeister-type gastrojejunostomy was performed on the remaining stomach and loop of jejunum. This was an isoperistaltic end-to-side two-layer anastomosis with 3-0 chromic and 3-0 silk. The stomach was secured to the transverse mesocolon with several interrupted silk sutures to prevent any herniation along the retrocolic space. The anastomosis had a good lumen and good blood supply. There was no twist along the anastomosis. Before the anastomosis was finished, a nasogastric tube was placed along the afferent limb of the jejunum to decompress the duodenum and prevent blow out of the duodenal stump. Extra holes were made in the NG tube to provide adequate drainage. The anastomosis was marked with two clips on each side, and a Jackson-Pratt drain was placed over the duodenal stump. The peritoneal cavity was irrigated until clear. Hemostasis was adequate. The fascia was then closed with interrupted 0 Ethibond sutures. Skin edges were approximated with staples. Subcutaneous tissues were irrigated before closure. Estimated blood loss throughout the procedure was 200 ml. IV fluids: 3400 ml. Urine output: 840 ml.

FINDINGS:
1. Nonhealing benign ulcer in the posterior duodenal bulb penetrating into the head of the pancreas.
2. Partial gastrectomy *(antrectomy performed)* and excision of the pylorus, first portion of the duodenum along with ulcer.
3. Hofmeister-type retrocolic isoperistaltic gastrojejunostomy.
4. Posterior wall of the ulcer that was penetrating into the pancreas incorporated into closure of the duodenal stump.

5. Truncal vagotomy performed with intraoperative frozen section confirming both vagus nerves.
6. Cholecystectomy performed due to chronic cholecystitis with normal intraoperative cholangiogram.
7. Jackson-Pratt drain placed over the duodenal stump.

The items that are to be coded are listed below:

Partial gastrectomy *(antrectomy)* with gastrojejunostomy
Truncal vagotomy
Cholecystectomy with intraoperative cholangiogram

PATHOLOGY REPORT LATER INDICATED: Tissue showed no evidence of carcinoma. The radiologist reported the x-ray with 74300.

33. OPERATIVE REPORT

PREOPERATIVE DIAGNOSIS: Fournier's gangrene.

POSTOPERATIVE DIAGNOSIS: Fournier's gangrene, gastric foreign bodies.

PROCEDURES PERFORMED:

1. Exploratory laparotomy with gastrotomy and removal of gastric foreign body.
2. Placement of 18-French Moss gastrojejunostomy feeding tube.
3. Diverting end-sigmoid colostomy *(Hartmann's procedure)*.

ANESTHESIA: General.

INDICATIONS: This is a 33-year-old patient with Fournier's gangrene who presents today for a diverting colostomy due to wound care and placement of a gastrostomy tube for help with further follow-up feeding. He presents today for exploration. The family understands the risks of bleeding, infection, and postoperative fluid collections and wishes to proceed.

PROCEDURE: The patient was brought to the operating room, placed under general anesthesia, and prepped and draped with Betadine solution. A midline incision was made with a #10 blade and dissection was carried down through subcutaneous tissues using electrocautery. The midline fascia was identified and divided. The posterior sheath and peritoneum were sharply incised, thus allowing entry into the peritoneal cavity. There was some free fluid within the peritoneal cavity but no evidence of any abnormalities. We first identified the stomach and could feel what we felt were some polyps in the stomach. We first placed concentric purse-string sutures along the greater curvature of the stomach, opened up the stomach, and then passed an 18-French Moss gastrojejunostomy tube but were unable to get it down through the pylorus. We could feel these multiple masses in the stomach. We tied the purse-string sutures and inflated the balloon. We then made a small opening in the stomach with electrocautery and retrieved about 20 large what appeared to be vegetable matter and partially digested peppers and pickles. We irrigated with saline and then were able to pass the Moss gastrojejunostomy tube, the distal end, down through the pylorus. We closed the gastrotomy with a running 3-0 Vicryl and an outer layer of 3-0 silk Lembert sutures. We irrigated this area well. We then identified the sigmoid colon, fired a TLC-75 stapler across the sigmoid/descending colon, and then placed a 3-0 Prolene on the rectal stump. We divided the mesentery between right angle clamps and tied the pedicles with 3-0 silk ties. We had a previously marked stomal opening in the left lower quadrant. We grasped this with a Kocher clamp, made an elliptical incision around this, and then divided the anterior sheath of the rectus in cruciate fashion, divided through the rectus muscles, and then opened the posterior sheath and peritoneum. We brought the colon then through this area. There was good mobility of the colon, and the colon was viable. We then irrigated the abdomen with saline, and, once all sponge and needle counts were correct, we closed the midline fascia with a combination of interrupted 0 Vicryl and running 0 PDS. The skin was closed with skin clips. The staple line was then removed from the colon and the colostomy was matured with 3-0 Vicryl sutures. An appliance was placed. All sponge and needle counts were correct. He tolerated this well.

Prior to leaving the operating room, we took down the dressings of his right leg. There was good granulation tissue, which was pink and viable, and we then re-dressed the wound and sent him back to the surgical critical care unit in critical but stable condition.

PATHOLOGY REPORT LATER INDICATED: Idiopathic gangrene. Numerous undigested vegetable matter.

34. OPERATIVE REPORT

PREOPERATIVE DIAGNOSIS: Severe internal and external hemorrhoids.

POSTOPERATIVE DIAGNOSIS: Same.

PROCEDURE PERFORMED: Three quadrant hemorrhoidectomy.

ANESTHESIA: Spinal.

INDICATION: This is a very pleasant female who presents today with severe internal and external hemorrhoids for elective excision. She understands the risks of bleeding, infection, and postoperative fluid collection. She wishes to proceed.

PROCEDURE: The patient was brought to the operating room and placed under spinal anesthesia, prepped, and draped sterilely with Betadine solution. Digital rectal examination was first performed. There were severe external hemorrhoids. Pratt anoscope was inserted. The severest of the hemorrhoids were at the 6-o'clock, 9-o'clock, and 3-o'clock positions. These were each grasped with an Allis clamp, excised in diamond shape fashion. The mucosal defects were closed with running locked 3-0 Vicryl with the suture lines imbricated with 3-0 chromic sutures. This gave us a good closure that was hemostatic. We anesthetized the area with 30 cc of 0.5% Sensorcaine with epinephrine solution and then placed four gauze in the rectal canal. She tolerated this well and was taken to recovery in stable condition.

PATHOLOGY REPORT LATER INDICATED: Benign tissue.

35. OPERATIVE REPORT

PROCEDURE: Placement of CORFLO, feeding tube.

INDICATION: Feeding, patient with gastroparesis.

PROCEDURE: The patient was placed in the sitting position and then tilted to the right with a wedge. CORFLO was placed at the level of 19 cm without any complications. KUB was then done demonstrating the tip of the CORFLO in the third portion of the duodenum. After confirmation of postpyloric position of the CORFLO, the patient was started on Ultracal at 10 cc/hr.

36. OPERATIVE REPORT

PREOPERATIVE DIAGNOSES:

1. Expressed desire of the operating gynecologist to insert indwelling ureteral stents for ease of dissection of the anticipated enlarged adherent uterus.
2. Gynecologic diagnosis of pelvic endometriosis.

POSTOPERATIVE DIAGNOSES: Same.

PROCEDURE PERFORMED: Cystourethroscopy, insertion of bilateral ureteral catheters.

PROCEDURE: After general anesthesia and after the abdomen and genitalia had been prepped and draped in the usual fashion, the patient was placed in the dorsolithotomy position. The genitalia were examined and proved to be essentially unremarkable. The urethra was instrumented with a 24-French panendoscope sheath, and, using the foroblique and right-angle lenses, inspection of the entire vesical cavity showed no indication of any pathologic lesion. There is slight indention and some of the bladder incident to the uterine impression. The two ureteral orifices appear to be essentially unremarkable. The left ureteral orifice was catheterized with a 6-French Whistle Tip catheter with ease. The catheter was advanced to approximately 25 cm on the left side. Attention was then directed to the right side, and the right ureteral orifice was catheterized with a 6-French Whistle Tip catheter. The catheter was placed at approximately 24 cm. The bladder was then entered, Panendoscope sheath was withdrawn. A 18-French 5-ml balloon Foley catheter was then inserted into the bladder and left indwelling to the Foley catheter. The two ureteral catheters were anchored with no. 1 black silk. The two ureteral catheters and the Foley catheters were then connected to straight drainage and the patient was removed from the dorsolithotomy position. Dr. Weasly, the patient's gynecologist, then proceeded with a total abdominal hysterectomy and bilateral salpingo-oophorectomy.

37. OPERATIVE REPORT

PREOPERATIVE DIAGNOSIS: Recurrent transitional cell carcinoma of the bladder.

POSTOPERATIVE DIAGNOSIS: Same.

PROCEDURE PERFORMED: Cystoscopy; multiple random bladder biopsies.

CLINICAL NOTE: This patient has recurrent transitional cell carcinoma of the bladder. He has had BCG bladder instillation to help prevent recurrence. His last instillation was 6 weeks ago. The patient is doing well. He denied any complaints.

PROCEDURE: The patient was given a general endotracheal anesthetic and prepped and draped in lithotomy position. A 24-French resectoscope was passed into the bladder under direct vision. The urethra was normal. Prostate was nonobstructed. Inspection of the bladder demonstrated areas of hyperemia that would be most consistent with BCG changes but might also represent recurrent TCC. These areas were biopsied using a cold-cup biopsy. A 24-French resectoscope loupe was then used to cauterize these areas. Ureteric orifices were identified. Clear urine could be seen effluxing bilaterally.

The patient tolerated the procedure well. A B&O suppository was placed rectally after the end of the procedure. An 18-French Foley catheter was placed to straight drainage. Bimanual examination showed no significant abnormality and the prostate felt normal.

The patient will be scheduled for recheck cystoscopy in three months time providing pathology shows no evidence of recurrent tumor.

ADDENDUM: Total resected and fulgurated area of the bladder was 7 square centimeters.

PATHOLOGY REPORT LATER INDICATED: See Report 55.

38. OPERATIVE REPORT

PREOPERATIVE DIAGNOSIS: Urinary incontinence.

POSTOPERATIVE DIAGNOSIS: Same.

PROCEDURE PERFORMED: Insertion of double cuff artificial urinary sphincter with 25 cc reservoir (multicomponent).

CLINICAL NOTE: This patient has had radiation for prostate cancer. This recurred. He then had cryotherapy. His PSA is undetectable but he has significant urinary incontinence unresponsive to pharmacotherapy. External clamp devices have been unsatisfactory.

PROCEDURE NOTE: The patient was given a spinal anesthetic, prepped and draped in a supine position. A penoscrotal incision was made. A 16-French Foley was placed in the bladder to straight drainage. The urethra was dissected to the level of the bulb. The bulbocavernous muscle was very atrophic and was not dissected off the urethra. A double cuff placement was selected. The urethra was mobilized in two places with a small bridge of tissue between them. These cuffs were incised. Both were incised at 4.5 cm. A reservoir space was created by manual dissection in the left inguinal canal into the retropubic space. The reservoir was placed, cycled, and filled with 25 cc of sterile saline. Both cuffs were placed in the usual fashion. The pump was then placed in the mid-scrotal pouch. Connections were made using a Y connector and straight connectors in the usual fashion. The system was cycled; it worked well. Foley catheter was withdrawn to insure cycling appropriately. Subcutaneous tissues were closed with 3-0 chromic and skin with a 4-0 subcuticular Vicryl stitch. The pump was cycled again and then deactivated; the Foley catheter replaced. The patient tolerated the procedure well and was transferred to the recovery room in good condition. The wounds were thoroughly irrigated with Bacitracin solution.

39. OPERATIVE REPORT

PREOPERATIVE DIAGNOSIS: Morbid obesity.

POSTOPERATIVE DIAGNOSIS: Same.

PROCEDURES: 278.01

1. Laparoscopic Roux-en-Y gastrointestinal bypass.
2. Liver biopsy. (follow up w/ path report)

ANESTHESIA: General.

INDICATION: The patient is a 36-year-old female who presents with morbid obesity, with a current BMI of 46.0. She has gone to the seminars, and we have discussed laparoscopic Roux-en-Y gastrointestinal bypass along with the risk of surgery including bleeding, infection, leakage from the anastomoses, conversion to open procedure, postoperative stenoses of the anastomoses, or bowel obstruction. She understands and wishes to proceed.

PROCEDURE: The patient was brought to the operating room and placed under general anesthesia. A Foley catheter and orogastric tubes were inserted. She was prepped and draped sterilely with Betadine solution. A supraumbilical incision was made with a #15 blade, and dissection was carried down through the subcutaneous tissues bluntly. The patient had an incisional hernia from an old trocar port site. We placed our operative trocar into the abdomen, insufflated the abdomen. There was no damage to the underlying viscera. Under direct vision, we then placed two, midclavicular line, 12-millimeter ports that were just lateral and above the umbilical port. There was a right upper quadrant 12-millimeter port in the anterior axillary line and a left upper quadrant 5-millimeter port in the anterior axillary line. These were all placed under direct vision with no damage to the bowel. The patient had some adhesions of her gastrohepatic ligament to the liver. We took these down using the harmonic scalpel. Before continuing, a needle specimen was obtained from the liver, appropriately marked for pathologic evaluation. We then entered the retrogastric space and placed our taut catheter behind the stomach. We then flipped the omentum up over the top of itself. We elevated the transverse colon and opened the transverse colon where we could see the drain. We identified the ligament of Treitz and fired an Endo-GIA stapler across the bowel, down from the ligament of Treitz. We fired an additional load across the mesentery. We then counted out 100 centimeters of bowel and then performed a stapled side-to-side functional end-to-end anastomosis by opening the bowel on the proximal and distal sides with the harmonic scalpel, firing two loads of the Endo-GIA stapler and closing the anastomosis with an Endo-GIA fired staple line. This gave us a nice anastomosis. We closed the mesenteric defect here with an Ethibond suture and fixed with Laparoties. We then sutured the proximal end to the catheter and flipped the mesentery back down. We then brought the bowel and the catheter up in retrogastric fashion. Next, we identified the angle of His. We opened the angle of His, and we fired five loads of the Endo-GIA stapler across the stomach. We had blown up the 20-cc balloon and had about a 20-cc pouch. Once we had completely transected the stomach, we went above and placed the Bioenteric catheter within the gastric pouch. We passed the snare through it. We made a separate stab incision in the upper abdomen and passed the wire through. We then fed the anvil end of the CEA-21 stapler down through the back of the pharynx down through the esophagus and brought out through our gastric pouch. We then enlarged the left midclavicular line, abdominal port, and placed the CEA-25 stapler through here. We opened the staple line on the bowel that we had brought up after we had removed the taut catheter and placed the CEA stapler into the bowel, brought the spike through, connected the two ends of the CEA, closed it, and fired it. This gave us a nice 21-millimeter circular anastomosis. We completed the anastomosis with the Endo-GIA stapler. We imbricated the staple line with two Ethibond sutures, placed a wad of fat over the last to adhere the fat near our staple line. We tested the anastomosis with air with the bowel clamped, and there was no evidence of a leak. We then placed Hemaseel over this anastomosis, and then once again mobilized the mesentery. We then closed the mesenteric defect where the small bowel had gone in retrogastric fashion with the Ethicon Endo-suture. We once again placed Hemaseel on our small anastomosis. We placed 10 flat Jackson-Pratt drains near our GJ anastomosis, which came on out the left side. We removed the trocar ports under direct vision. We then extended our umbilical incision and reduced the umbilical hernia. We closed the fascial defect with interrupted 0 Prolene sutures. We anesthetized the wounds at all areas with a total of 60 cc of 0.50% Sensorcaine with epinephrine solution. We secured the drains in place with 0 silk sutures and then closed the skin with 3-0 Prolene sutures. Steri-Strips and sterile Band-Aids were applied. All sponge and needle counts were correct. We left the taut catheter and a Penrose drain in the left midclavicular line incision.

All sponge and needle counts were correct. She tolerated this well and was taken to recovery in stable condition.

PATHOLOGY REPORT LATER INDICATED: See Report 63.

40. OPERATIVE REPORT

HISTORY: This patient, who is unknown to me, reports working in the shop at his home grinding metal approximately 5 hours ago. He was wearing safety glasses, but he has noticed a foreign body in his right eye. He reports slight irritation to the eye. Denies blurred vision.

PHYSICAL EXAMINATION: PERLA, fundi without edema. There was no foreign body on lid eversion. Slit lamp shows a foreign body approximately 2 to 3 o'clock on the edge of the cornea. This foreign body appears metallic. There is very small area of rust around the site. Iris is intact. There are no cells in the anterior chamber. Fluorescein dye reveals uptake only over foreign body.

PROCEDURE: Two drops of Alcaine were used in the right eye. Foreign body was removed with an eye spud without difficulty. Slight orange discoloration at the base of cornea, but no definite rust ring visible.

IMPRESSION: Residual corneal abrasion.

DISPOSITION: Foreign body removed from right eye.

41. OPERATIVE REPORT

PREOPERATIVE DIAGNOSIS: Left cervical spondylosis, C5–6, C6–7, with cervical discs.

POSTOPERATIVE DIAGNOSIS: Same.

PROCEDURE PERFORMED: Anterior discectomy and osteophytectomy for decompression at C5–6 and C6–7, with allograft fusion and Zephyr plating.

This case was monitored with sensory evoked potentials throughout the case. There were no changes.

PROCEDURE: Under general anesthesia, the patient was placed in the cervical outrigger. The neck was prepped and draped in the usual manner.

An incision was made parallel to the sternocleidomastoid, and then we got onto the omohyoid and incised this. Then with sharp dissection we got onto the prevertebral fascia, put the Farley-Thompson retractor in, and then I was able to localize the C5–6 and C6–7 interspaces. The plan here was to decompress the nerve roots and get rid of the ridges, the disc, and to fuse and plate. The discectomies were done at C5–6 and C6–7. The ridges were removed, the discs were removed, and then the cartilaginous surfaces were prepared for reception of the bony fusion. At C6–7, a #8 trial was utilized and at C5–6 a #7 trial was utilized with bone. I took off the ridges, I took off the osteophytes, I removed the discs. I got down to the dura on both sides and was satisfied now that the nerve roots were decompressed and I could put the trial in and place the structural bone graft in. This was done at both levels. This having been done, they were countersunk and I then utilized a Zephyr plate from C5 down to C7 and put a screw into C6 as well. This done, a Hemovac drain was placed into the wound. Of course, the plate was locked, and we then closed the wound in layers utilizing 2-0 chromic on the platysma with 2-0 plain in the subcutaneous tissue and 3-0 nylon interrupted mattress sutures on the skin. A dressing was applied. The patient was to wear a collar in the postop period.

PATHOLOGY REPORT LATER INDICATED: Benign bone and tissue.

42. OPERATIVE REPORT

PREOPERATIVE DIAGNOSES:

1. Ptosis, right upper lid.
2. Loss of superior visual field secondary to #1.
3. Superior hemianopia secondary to #1, right eye.

POSTOPERATIVE DIAGNOSES: Same.

PROCEDURE PERFORMED: Fasanella-Servat procedure, right upper lid.

ANESTHESIA: General endotracheal.

INDICATIONS: This 57-year-old white female has had progressively drooping lid on her right for many years which has now reduced her superior visual field in the right eye and has actually limited her vision. After the prior approval and the photos and documentation were obtained, it was noted that the patient did have a 3- to 4-mm ptosis of the right upper lid and we would approach this with a Fasanella-Servat procedure. The risk of infection, hemorrhage and reoperations were discussed.

PROCEDURE: After the patient was placed under suitable general endotracheal anesthesia; the superior tarsal border was then marked with a marking pen and a 15 Bard-Parker blade cut down through skin to the muscle area. The lid was then everted on a Desmarres retractor and two curved mosquitos were then placed with the point central and pointing superiorly when the lid was everted. A 6-0 gut rapid absorbing suture was then started through the skin incision at the superior tarsal border and then a purse string was then woven along the curve tips and then the 3 to 4 mm resection was then obtained and then the serpentine 6-0 gut suture was then approximated without cutting it and brought out through the skin and tied. It was allowed to retract into the knot. There was no bleeding and there was no cut suture. Maxitrol ointment, a Telfa pad, and patch was applied and the patient was sent to the recovery room. There were no complications.

43. OPERATIVE REPORT

PREOPERATIVE DIAGNOSIS: Lumbar radiculopathy secondary to herniated L5-S1 disc.

POSTOPERATIVE DIAGNOSIS: Same.

PROCEDURE PERFORMED: Right L5-S1 hemilaminectomy with excision of herniated L5-S1 disc.

PROCEDURE: The patient was taken to the operating room and placed under general endotracheal anesthesia. He was rotated into the prone position on chest rolls with arms extended over the head. The lumbar region was shaved, prepped, and draped in the usual sterile manner. The proposed vertical midline incision was infiltrated with lidocaine, with epinephrine. The skin was incised and sharp dissection carried through the subcutaneous tissues. The fascia was incised and subperiosteal dissection undertaken at L5-S1. The hemilamina of L5 was then removed in piecemeal fashion. This allowed evaluation of both the L4–5 disc as well as the L5-S1 disc. At L5-S1, moderate-sized disc herniation was immediately evident. The surrounding capsule was incised, and a large fragment of ligamentous degenerative disc was removed. The interspace was then probed, and all degenerative disc material was removed. On completion, the thecal sac and nerve root were noted to be well decompressed at L4–5. The L4–5 level appeared normal. Epidural space was lined with Surgicel and fat graft, and the wound closed in interrupted layers, with 4-0 Vicryl subcuticular stitch for skin. Steri-Strips and sterile dressing were applied to the wound. The patient tolerated the procedure well and was transferred to the recovery room in good condition.

PATHOLOGY REPORT LATER INDICATED: See Report 57.

44. OPERATIVE REPORT

cancer
neoplasm (malignant)

PREOPERATIVE DIAGNOSES:

1. Left orbitonasal mass.
2. Dry eye syndrome.
3. Pseudophakia, both eyes.
4. Computerized tomography confirmed tumor left orbital, left nasal side.

(1) **POSTOPERATIVE DIAGNOSES:** Same with the addition of low-grade lymphoma, left orbit. *(Malignant)*

PROCEDURE: Anterior orbitotomy, debulking and biopsy.

ANESTHESIA: General endotracheal anesthesia.

INDICATION: This 81-year-old white woman has had a progressively enlarging mass of the left superior nasal orbit, which had become quite hard and is attached to the bone. CT shows there has been no bony invasion, and the brain has not been invaded. More than likely, this is a lymphoma, but we want to take the patient for an anterior orbitotomy for debulking and biopsy.

DESCRIPTION OF PROCEDURE: After the patient was prepped and draped in the usual sterile fashion for ophthalmic surgery, the superior sulcus fold was marked out on her medial left upper lid. This was then cut through skin and muscle with the 25 Bard-Parker blade down through the orbital fat pad. It was noted there was some saponified fat and a hard mass that was kind of an orangish-red color and was attached to this. Two specimens were removed and tagged and sent for frozen section, and into the cryo unit with liquid nitrogen down to –80 degrees and was then brought in to remove the rest of the mass. There were some fragments of mass still attached to the nasal wall of the orbit. The frozen section revealed lymphoma, low grade, probably stage I, and since this is radiosensitive and that all of the tumor could not be removed without exenterating the orbit, it was elected to close at this point and treat the rest conservatively. The wound was closed after the remaining tumor was infiltrated with Solu-Medrol 125 mg per ml for a total of 2 ml, after which the wound was closed with interrupted 6-0 black nylon suture and Maxitrol ointment. Telfa pad, patch and shield were applied. The patient was sent to the recovery room. There were no complications.

PATHOLOGY REPORT LATER INDICATED: Lymphoma.

45. RADIOLOGY REPORT

EXAMINATION OF: Chest.

CLINICAL SYMPTOMS: Chest pain.

PORTABLE CHEST, AP SITTING (ONE VIEW), 4:45 PM: Comparisons are made with the previous study of 08/23/XX. The cardiac silhouette is not grossly enlarged for this projection. The mediastinum is not widened. Lung fields are generally clear and expanded to the periphery. Cardiac monitors do superimpose the chest.

CONCLUSION: Generally stable appearance of the chest, unchanged compared with the previous study.

46. RADIOLOGY REPORT

EXAMINATION OF: Biophysical profile.

CLINICAL SYMPTOMS: High blood pressure, estimated gestational age 28 weeks 5 days.

BIOPHYSICAL PROFILE: The placenta is located along the anterior wall. It is heterogeneous in echotexture, grade II. The AFI is 5.4 cm, which is low. Fetal motion noted by the technologist. Heart rate 147 beats per minute. Intrauterine hypoechoic area seen anteriorly within the uterus measures about 2 cm in size and a second similar sized hypoechoic area is located within the uterus. Both findings are presumed fibroids.

They are nonspecific findings, however. Biophysical profile was scored a perfect 8 out of 8.

47. CT SCAN

EXAMINATION OF: CT of orbits.

CLINICAL SYMPTOMS: Left eye pain.

CT OF ORBITS: CT of orbits in axial and coronal planes without contrast. Patient was vomiting therefore contrast was not given.

1. Complete opacification of right aspect of sphenoid sinus.
2. Near complete opacification of right maxillary antrum.
3. Polypoid membrane thickening left maxillary antrum.
4. Scattered membrane thickening throughout a few ethmoidal air cells.
5. Remainder negative.

48. MRA REPORT

EXAMINATION OF: MRA brain.

CLINICAL SYMPTOMS: Third nerve palsy, complete.

MAGNETIC RESONANCE EXAMINATION OF THE ARTERIAL VASCULATURE OF THE POSTERIOR FOSSA AND CIRCLE OF WILLIS REGION was performed utilizing three-dimensional time-of-flight multislab technique. Raw data and selected maximum-intensity projection images were photographed. Additionally, I have personally manipulated the maximum-intensity projections on a computer console in order to view the vasculature from various angulations.

I don't appreciate evidence of aneurysm. In particular, I don't appreciate evidence of aneurysm in the region of the posterior communicating arteries. I have personally reviewed the raw data images.

Bilaterally, there is some signal loss at the origin of the A1 segment of each anterior cerebral artery. This gives the appearance of stenosis. Most probably, this is technical, rather than due to true stenosis, but stenosis is not ruled out.

Internal carotid arteries appear unremarkable. Vertebral arteries are unremarkable. The basilar artery is unremarkable.

Proximal segments of the middle and posterior cerebral arteries appear unremarkable. Posterior communicating arteries are not visualized and are most probably very small.

49. RADIOLOGY REPORT

EXAMINATION OF: X-Ray Abdomen; single view.

CLINICAL SYMPTOMS: Malnutrition.

FINDINGS: A single supine view of the abdomen is submitted for interpretation. The majority of the pelvis and a portion of the left side of the abdomen are excluded from this examination. Feeding tube is identified. The tip overlies the left upper quadrant. Air is present within both small and large bowel, which does not appear distended as visualized on this examination. There is degenerative change and dextroscoliosis of the lumbar spine. Surgical clips overlie the right upper quadrant. Opacity is noted in the left lung base, which may relate to atelectasis or infiltrate. Follow-up is suggested.

50. RADIOLOGY REPORT

EXAMINATION OF: Left foot.

CLINICAL SYMPTOMS: Severe foot pain.

TWO VIEWS, LEFT FOOT: Comparison is made with the most recent films available 10/15/XX. There is diffuse demineralization of the osseous structures of the foot. Soft-tissue swelling is seen. Erosive changes have been previously described involving multiple metatarsophalangeal joints, and these are identified once again today. The differential is not significantly changed compared with the previous examination.

IMPRESSION:

1. Overall there is no significant interval change compared with 10/15/XX. There are extensive demineralization and extensive erosive changes involving the metatarsophalangeal joints and digits as described previously. Large cystic lesion is identified within the calcaneus as previously seen.
2. Diffuse soft-tissue swelling and inferior calcaneal spur.

51. CT REPORT

CT of Abdomen

CLINICAL HISTORY: Increased liver enzyme.

TECHNIQUE: The patient was scanned from the dome of the diaphragm through the iliac crest after administration of oral and intravenous contrast.

COMPARISON: Comparison is made with a previous ultrasound examination dated 11/18/XX.

FINDINGS: Evaluation of the liver demonstrates mildly decreased attenuation to be present throughout the liver diffusely. No focal abnormalities are present within the liver. The spleen, pancreas, kidneys, and adrenal glands appear unremarkable. No enlarged lymph nodes are seen within the abdomen. No abnormal fluid collections are seen within the abdomen. The lung bases appear clear. No pleural effusions are seen.

IMPRESSION:

1. There is diffusely decreased attenuation present within the liver. This suggests the presence of fatty infiltration of the liver. No focal abnormalities are seen within the liver.
2. The remainder of the CT examination of the abdomen appears unremarkable.

52. LUNG SCAN REPORT

EXAMINATION OF: Ventilation-perfusion lung scan.

CLINICAL SYMPTOMS: Shortness of breath.

VENTILATION-PERFUSION LUNG SCAN:

DOSE: 2.0 millicuries of technetium-99m DTPA via aerosol. 6.0 millicuries of technetium-99m MAA IV. Comparison is made with chest radiograph obtained at the same time.

There is inhomogeneity regarding ventilatory scan. This is seen bilaterally. There appears to be elevation of the right hemidiaphragm.

There is decreased perfusion and ventilation along the right posterior lung base. The patient is noted to have pulmonary opacities and pleural effusions on chest radiograph. Small area of decreased perfusion and ventilation noted along the posterior aspect of the left upper lobe. Overall findings indeterminate for pulmonary embolus.

IMPRESSION: Indeterminate probability for pulmonary embolus.

53. MRI REPORT

EXAMINATION OF: Myocardial perfusion imaging.

CLINICAL SYMPTOMS: Chest pain, shortness of breath.

MYOCARDIAL PERFUSION IMAGING: CARDIOLITE HEART IMAGING: SPECT left ventricular myocardial perfusion imaging study was performed in this patient. 29.5 millicuries of technetium-99m sestamibi was injected intravenously at peak stress. The patient had a maximal heart rate of 88%.

Evaluation of the qualitative image series shows the left ventricular myocardium to have a normal uptake of tracer. There is no evidence to suggest myocardial infarction or stress-induced ischemia.

IMPRESSION: Normal Cardiolite heart imaging as described above.

54. FROM OPERATIVE REPORT 20

Cancer

CLINICAL HISTORY: C/C clear cell CA pelvis.

SPECIMEN RECEIVED: A. Endocervical curettings. B. Endometrial biopsy.

GROSS DESCRIPTION:

metastatic
Secondary
primary
Unknown

A. The specimen is labeled with the patient's name and "ecc" and consists of specimen jar with negligible tissue. The specimen is filtered and placed in one cassette.
B. The specimen is labeled with the patient's name and "endometrial" and consists of approximately 1 cc of wispy fragments.

MICROSCOPIC DESCRIPTION:

A. Sections show no tissue after processing.

Sections show fragments of tissue consisting predominantly of endocervical tissue and lower uterine segment. The endometrial glands are lined by 1 to 2 layers of columnar epithelium. Malignant clear cell carcinoma is microscopically identified.

DIAGNOSIS:

A. Endocervical curettings: Malignant clear cell carcinoma identified.

Endometrial biopsy: Scant fragments of endocervical mucosa and lower uterine segment; Grade 3, secondary, malignant endocervix and endometrium clear cell carcinoma, Primary site unknown.

55. FROM OPERATIVE REPORT 37

CLINICAL HISTORY: Bladder cancer.

SPECIMEN RECEIVED: Random bladder biopsy.

GROSS DESCRIPTION: The specimen is labeled with "biopsy" and consists of 3 specimens processed in toto, and random bladder pink-tan tissue biopsies in 1 cassette.

MICROSCOPIC DESCRIPTION: Sections show fragments of bladder mucosa showing vascularization and congestion with mild lymphocytic, plasma cell infiltrates, and lymphoid aggregates. The urothelium varies from normal to moderate to severe dysplasia to carcinoma in situ with full-thickness cytologic atypia and occasional mitoses. One fragment shows grade 2 papillary transitional cell carcinoma. The underlying lamina propria shows reactive fibroblasts with scattered lymphocytic, plasma cell, and eosinophilic infiltrates with admixed multinucleated giant cells. No definitive stromal invasion is identified.

DIAGNOSIS: Random bladder biopsies: Moderate to severe urothelial dysplasia/transitional cell carcinoma in situ and noninvasive grade 2 *(of 3)* papillary transitional cell carcinoma.

56. FROM OPERATIVE REPORT 31

CLINICAL HISTORY: Adenoma.

SPECIMEN RECEIVED: Cecal ascending polyp.

GROSS DESCRIPTION: Received in a container labeled "cecal ascending polyp" are three fragments of tan tissue measuring 0.3 to 0.4 cm diameter. The specimen is totally submitted.

MICROSCOPIC DESCRIPTION: The cecum and ascending mucosal fragments show glands that vary in size and configuration and are lined by uniform epithelial cells. Hyperplasia of the glandular and surface epithelium are prominent with serrated architectures evident.

DIAGNOSIS: Cecum and ascending colon biopsies, mucosal (three): Hyperplastic polyps (three).

57. FROM OPERATIVE REPORT 43

CLINICAL HISTORY: Lumbar herniated disc.

TISSUE RECEIVED: Lumbar disc.

GROSS DESCRIPTIONS: Submitted in formalin, labeled with the patient's name and "lumbar disc" are several irregular fragments of pink-tan ragged tissue measuring approximately 2 × 1.5 × 0.5 cm in aggregate. Submitted in toto.

MICROSCOPIC DESCRIPTIONS: The slide shows several irregular fragments of fibrocartilaginous intervertebral disc material. There are no significant inflammatory infiltrates or evidence of neoplasm.

DIAGNOSIS: Intervertebral disc, lumbar region, discectomy: fragments of intervertebral disc.

58. PATHOLOGY REPORT

SPECIMEN RECEIVED: A. polyps, cecum/sigmoid—adenoma. B. Barrett's esophagus—rule out dysplasia.

GROSS DESCRIPTION: The specimens are received in two containers:

A. In the container labeled "colon biopsy and polyp" are four fragments of tan-pink tissue measuring 0.3 to 0.6 cm diameter. The specimen is totally submitted as "A."
B. In the container labeled "Barrett's esophagus biopsy" are six fragments of tan-gray tissue measuring 0.1 to 0.3 cm diameter. The specimen is totally submitted.

MICROSCOPIC DESCRIPTION:

A. The mucosal fragments of the cecum and sigmoid colon show polypoid architectures with adenomatous features within surface and glandular epithelial sites. The glands vary in size and configuration and are lined by enlarged, mildly pleomorphic cells with elongated hyperchromatic nuclei.

B. The esophageal biopsies demonstrate gastric cardia mucosa exhibiting intestinal metaplasia. The glands vary in size and configuration and have uniform elongated epithelial cells. Separation by a fibrous lamina propria is evident.

DIAGNOSIS:

A. Cecum and sigmoid colon biopsies, mucosal: Adenomatous polyp fragments.

B. Esophageal biopsy: Gastric cardia mucosa with intestinal metaplasia, consistent with Barrett's esophagus.

59. FROM OPERATIVE REPORT 14

SPECIMEN RECEIVED: Muscle biopsy, left deltoid.

INDICATION: Lipoma left posterior axillary fold.

GROSS DESCRIPTION: Received in a container labeled "muscle biopsy left deltoid" is a fragment of brown tissue measuring $0.7 \times 0.5 \times 0.5$ cm. The specimen is totally submitted.

MICROSCOPIC DESCRIPTION: The skeletal muscle of the left deltoid shows normal morphology.

DIAGNOSIS: Muscle biopsy, left deltoid: No pathologic diagnosis.

60. FROM OPERATIVE REPORT 7

CLINICAL HISTORY: Mass of axillary fold.

SPECIMEN RECEIVED: Lipoma from axillary fold.

GROSS DESCRIPTION: The specimen is labeled with the patient's name and "lipoma from axillary fold, intramuscular," which consists of a loosely encapsulated yellow adipose tissue, $8 \times 7.8 \times 1.8$ cm. Sectioning reveals homogeneous yellow adipose tissue throughout. Representative sections in 4 cassettes.

MICROSCOPIC DIAGNOSIS: Mature adipose tissue consistent with lipoma, axillary fold.

61. PATHOLOGY REPORT

CLINICAL DIAGNOSIS AND HISTORY: Cyst.

TISSUE(S) SUBMITTED: Lesion, back.

GROSS DESCRIPTION: Specimen is received in fixative and consists of a $3.3 \times 2.5 \times 2.2$-cm thin-walled cyst containing charcoal, gray-black, friable material.

MICROSCOPIC DESCRIPTION: One microscopic slide examined.

DIAGNOSIS: Follicular cyst, infundibular type, skin of back.

62. FROM OPERATIVE REPORT 12

CLINICAL HISTORY: Left ischial ulcer.

SPECIMEN RECEIVED: Ischial tissue *(left).*

GROSS DESCRIPTION: Received in a container labeled "left ischial tissue" is an irregularly shaped fragment of soft tissue with a small portion containing an ellipse of skin. The specimen measures 18 × 7.5 × 6 cm in greatest dimension. The skin ellipse measures 4.5 × 2.5 × 0.3 cm. A central opening measuring 2 cm in greatest dimension is present. The remainder of the tissue has a nodular solid tan-gray to brown appearance. On sectioning diffuse fibrosis extends through the area. Representative portions are submitted.

MICROSCOPIC DESCRIPTION: The soft tissue of the left ischial region demonstrates extensive diffuse fibrosis with mild infiltrates of mononuclear inflammatory cells. A significant portion of the soft tissue is covered with granular fibrin containing sheets of neutrophils that rest upon a granulation tissue base. The adjacent epidermis shows pseudoepitheliomatous hyperplasia and normal maturation pattern.

DIAGNOSIS: Skin and soft tissue of left ischial region, excision: Granulation tissue, extensive, with diffuse fibrosis and mild chronic inflammation. Ulcer with mild to moderate acute inflammation.

63. FROM OPERATIVE REPORT 39

CLINICAL HISTORY: Morbid obesity.

SPECIMEN RECEIVED: Liver biopsy.

GROSS DESCRIPTION: The specimen is labeled with the patient's name and "liver biopsy" and consists of a 2 cm needle core of greenish tissue.

MICROSCOPIC DESCRIPTION: Sections show liver showing mild fatty change. The portal triads are unremarkable.

DIAGNOSIS: Liver biopsy showing mild fatty change.

condition and anatomic site   condition

64. FROM OPERATIVE REPORT 6

CLINICAL DIAGNOSIS AND HISTORY: Cyst.

TISSUE(S) SUBMITTED: Scalp cyst.

GROSS DESCRIPTION: Specimen is received in fixative and consists of an ovoid, rubbery, gray-white, 2 × 1.3 cm diameter cyst with gray-white laminated, friable contents.

MICROSCOPIC DESCRIPTION: One microscopic slide examined.

DIAGNOSIS: Follicular cyst, isthmus-catagen type (pilar cyst), clinically scalp.

65. FROM OPERATIVE REPORT 19

CLINICAL HISTORY: Left upper lobe abscess—probably secondary aspiration, culture and pseudomonas.

SPECIMEN RECEIVED: Lung, left upper lobe.

GROSS DESCRIPTION: Received in a container labeled "left upper lobe of lung" is a lung upper lobe measuring 17 × 11 × 3.4 cm as a collapsed specimen. The lobe weighs 283 grams. All surfaces have a dull gray yellow exudate that extends over the pleura. The pleura has a wrinkled collapsed appearance. On sectioning the majority of the lung parenchyma is replaced by a necrotic collapsed cyst with a ragged gray-yellow wall. This completely encompasses the vast majority of lung parenchyma with only small portions persisting in the base of the upper lobe. Bronchus and vascular structures are identified and appear unremarkable. Multiple representative sections of lung parenchyma are submitted.

MICROSCOPIC DESCRIPTION: The left upper lobe tissue sections show an extensive area of coagulation necrosis and marked destruction of the pulmonary parenchyma. Sheets of neutrophils are present within fibrin and coagulation necrosis debris. The adjacent lung tissue shows collections of macrophages and inflammatory cells within alveoli. Abundant fibrin debris accompanies the inflammation. Prominent squamous metaplasia is present within the bronchial tree that persists. Extensive interstitial fibrosis within the adjacent lung parenchyma is also present.

DIAGNOSIS: Lung, left upper lobe, resection: Abscess, large, with severe acute inflammation and extensive necrosis. Interstitial fibrosis with chronic inflammation, adjacent lung tissue.

66. FROM OPERATIVE REPORT 21

CLINICAL HISTORY: Atelectasis lung.

GROSS DESCRIPTION: 20 ml of mucoid fluid received in one container.

SPECIMEN RECEIVED: Bronchial washing.

SPECIMEN ADEQUACY: Specimen satisfactory for cytologic evaluation.

DIAGNOSIS: Atypical cells, cannot rule out malignancy.

COMMENTS: Rare groups of mildly atypical squamous cells present, significance and origin unknown. Cytology correlated with accompanying histology specimen. Please see pathology report.

Report amended due to transcription error on original. Discussed with Dr. Green.

67. FROM OPERATIVE REPORT 23

CLINICAL HISTORY: Pleural effusion, unknown cause.

GROSS DESCRIPTIONS: Ten ml bloody fluid received in one syringe.

SPECIMEN RECEIVED: Pleural fluid.

SPECIMEN ADEQUACY: Specimen satisfactory for cytologic evaluation.

DIAGNOSIS: No cytologic evidence of malignancy.

COMMENTS: Specimen shows predominantly lymphocytes.

68. 2/1/XX FAMILY PRACTICE SERVICE, MARK ADAMS, MD

(REPORTS 68 TO 79 ARE FOR THE SAME PATIENT)

This 68-year-old female presents to the office today requesting a complete physical examination. She recently moved to our area and states that she would like to establish with a family practitioner. She has a history of coronary artery disease, status post coronary artery bypass × 3 in 1978. She has been doing well. Gravid 3, para 3, postmenopausal about 20 years. History is also significant for hypertension, controlled by diet. Otherwise no complaints.

PAST MEDICAL HISTORY: Remarkable for conditions stated above.

OPERATIONS:

1. Hysterectomy with bladder repair, 1973
2. Bilateral blepharoplasty
3. D&C × 4

ALLERGIES: None.

MEDICATIONS: Digoxin 0.25 mg, Lasix 40 mg p.o. q.d., estrogen.

TOBACCO: Does not smoke.

ALCOHOL: Occasional.

SOCIAL HISTORY: Homemaker, mother of three. Husband recently transferred to area from California.

FAMILY HISTORY: Mother deceased from heart disease. Father has had multiple strokes. Two brothers, one with polio. Three children, health good. One sister, died of breast cancer at age 35.

REVIEW OF SYMPTOMS: Denies nausea, vomiting, headaches, dysuria, incontinence, dyspnea. Occasional bouts of atrial fibrillation; always converts spontaneously.

HEENT: Wears glasses. Otherwise negative.

RESPIRATORY: Negative.

CARDIOVASCULAR: Negative except as discussed above.

GI/GU: Postmenopausal, on estrogen.

ENDOCRINE: No diabetes or thyroid problems.

MUSCULOSKELETAL: Some arthritis, both hands.

PSYCHIATRIC: Negative.

PHYSICAL EXAMINATION: Reveals a very pleasant elderly female in no distress.

VITALS: Blood pressure is 140/84 right arm sitting position, 150/90 left arm sitting position; pulse 90 and regular.

WEIGHT: 115 lb.

SKIN: No skin lesions are present.

NODES: No lymphadenopathy.

ENT: Negative.

CHEST: Clear to auscultation.

CARDIAC: Reveals a regular rhythm. I did not hear any murmurs or gallops.

BREAST EXAMINATION: Right side free from lumps or masses. Small lump noted in left breast on examination, which is painless, without discharge, without retraction.

ASSESSMENT AND PLAN:

1. History of coronary artery disease, status post coronary artery bypass. No complaints at present, no abnormal findings. Continue medications as previously prescribed.
2. Breast mass on examination. Suggest mammography. If positive, consultation will be requested from surgery.
3. Postmenopausal, continue on estrogen therapy.

69. 2/2/XX JACOB BOND, MD

Patient has bilateral diagnostic mammography that shows normal finding on the right but dense, suspicious area on the left. Suggestion by radiologist is further clinical study.

70. 2/5/XX JACOB BOND, MD

Patient is seen today in the clinic at the request of Dr. Adams for evaluation of suspicious lump in the left breast. Patient states that she does not practice self-breast examination and therefore was unaware of the existing lump. She does state, however, on reflection, that the left breast at times was painful. No nipple discharge or puckering has been noted. Patient states that she has a sister who died of breast cancer in her mid-thirties. No other family history for cancer was noted.

EXAMINATION: Both breasts seem to be symmetrical. No abnormal findings on first view, right breast examination benign. Left breast identifies small lump where calcifications were noted on mammography.

ASSESSMENT: Left breast mass.

PLAN: Although it is difficult to say that this is not a single cyst, I would recommend a breast biopsy at patient's earliest convenience to rule out any possible malignancy. Options to include conservative measures of waiting for further signs, repeat mammography, 6-month breast checks were discussed with patient as well as risks and benefits of biopsy and possible mastectomy if findings are positive. Patient wishes to discuss with her husband and will let me know what she decides.

Thank you for asking me to consult on the care of Mrs. Smith. My recommendations are as above. I will await her further decision if she wishes further care from a surgical standpoint.

71. 2/8/XX JACOB BOND, MD

Phone call from patient wishing to schedule left breast biopsy. Scheduled for 2/10/XX by Dr. Bond.

72. 2/10/XX JACOB BOND, MD (ADMISSION SERVICE)

This patient is a 68-year-old female with chief complaint of left breast mass, admitted for left breast biopsy. The patient has a history of hypertension, coronary artery disease, and coronary artery bypass × 3. She also has a history of hysterectomy and is on estrogen therapy. She was in her usual state of health until a physical examination in early February, which revealed a small mass in the left breast. Mammography reportedly confirmed presence of mass and calcifications. Right breast exhibited no abnormal findings. The patient had menarche at age 12 and has given birth to three children. The patient has a family history positive for one sister with breast carcinoma. Medical history: as stated above for hypertension and CAD.

PHYSICAL EXAMINATION: Reveals a well-developed, well-nourished female in no apparent distress. The vital signs are stable, afebrile. The HEENT examination is within normal limits. The neck is supple, and the trachea is midline. No masses or adenopathy are present. The lungs are clear to auscultation and percussion. The cardiovascular examination is within normal limits. The left breast exhibits the presence of a small mass. The right breast is within normal limits. The right axilla is normal without adenopathy. The left axilla reveals small, less than 1 cm nonfixed, no matted lymph nodes. The abdominal examination is within normal limits. The rectal examination is normal, with guaiac-negative stool present in the vault.

ASSESSMENT: Left breast mass, admitted for breast biopsy and possible mastectomy.

73. 2/10/XX JACOB BOND, MD

Excisional breast biopsy was performed using local anesthesia. Pathology report documented adenocarcinoma of left breast. Patient was taken to operating room, administered general anesthesia, and underwent surgery the same day for mastectomy.

74. 2/10/XX JACOB BOND, MD

PREOPERATIVE DIAGNOSIS: Carcinoma of the left breast.

POSTOPERATIVE DIAGNOSIS: Same.

PROCEDURE PERFORMED: Left total mastectomy and left axillary node dissection. *(This is a modified radical mastectomy.)*

HISTORY: Patient underwent left breast biopsy for suspicious lesion 2/10/XX. Pathology report returned with diagnosis of adenocarcinoma of breast. Patient and her family discussed the benefits of the proposed total mastectomy and the risks, including death. Patient gives her understanding and agrees to proceed with the proposed procedure.

PROCEDURE: With the patient in the supine position under good general endotracheal anesthesia, a folded towel was placed beneath her left scapula and her left arm abducted on a pillow. She was prepped thoroughly with Betadine; the extent of her mastectomy incision was marked with a marking pen. We went about half an inch superior and half an inch inferior to her most medial circum-mammary incision, and it was a transverse incision. The draping was completed with Minnesota Mining drape and sterile paper in the usual manner. The superior flap was raised first. Bleeders on the breast were clamped and bovied; small bleeders on the flap were clamped and tied with 3-0 silk. The superior flap was raised to the clavicle inferior to the rectus sheath, medially to the sternal border, and laterally to the latissimus dorsi. The breast was outlined with a bovie, and then the breast was removed medially and laterally. We were somewhat concerned about involving the pectoralis muscle here, but it did not, and we could not see any invasion to the pectoralis fascia. Perforators were clamped and oversewn with 2-0 silk figure-of-eights. Small bleeders on the pectoralis major were bovied. The breast was allowed to fall laterally. The clavipectoral fascia was taken down. There was an area of scar tissue on the superior lateral portion of the pectoralis major attached to the breast, and we thought this was in the area of the previous biopsy. We had to dissect this off sharply, and it did not appear to be a cancer. Then she had a lot of inflammatory tissue in the axilla, which was rather difficult to define, but we exposed the axillary vein, hemoclipped the small venous tributaries, and dissected the axilla down to the 7th rib, and then took the breast off the serratus by bovie; the lateral chest bleeders were clamped and tied with 3-0 silk. The axilla was inspected, and the long thoracic and thoracodorsal nerve was intact. We left the superior branch of the intercostal brachial. It was dry. The mastectomy site was lavaged out with a liter of sterile water. Small bleeders were bovied. Several bleeders on the flaps were clamped and tied with 3-0 silk. The chest tubes were placed in the axilla and over the pectoralis major and exited laterally inferiorly, and the flaps were brought together without any tension with pulley sutures of 2-0 silk; then the wound was closed with a running 4-0 Prolene vertical mattress suture, removing the pulley sutures as we went. Vaseline dressings and dry dressings were applied.

Estimated blood loss was 400 ml. She tolerated this well. The flaps seemed to be intact. The drains were sewn into place and dry dressings applied. She tolerated the procedure well and was returned to the recovery room in good condition.

75. 2/12/XX JOYCE HARKNESS, MD, CONSULTING PHYSICIAN

CHIEF COMPLAINT: Atrial fibrillation.

Patient is a 68-year-old female, status post left total mastectomy for carcinoma of left breast. She has been doing fairly well postoperatively until this morning when she awoke with complaints of fluttering in the chest. ECG shows periods of rapid atrial fibrillation, with conversion to sinus rhythm spontaneously.

Past history is positive for CAD and hypertension. Patient is status post coronary artery bypass × 3. No chest pain or anginal symptoms have been noted.

Cardiac examination at present shows regular rate and rhythm; no gallops or murmurs are noted.

ASSESSMENT: Atrial fibrillation, status post left total mastectomy.

RECOMMENDATION: Treat conservatively with Coumadin at present. Monitor closely for signs of rhythm not converting spontaneously. Consideration would then have to be given to converting medically. Electrocardioversion is not recommended at this time.

76. 2/14/XX ANTHONY CASH, MD, CONSULTING PHYSICIAN

CHIEF COMPLAINT: Second-opinion surgery consultation *(inpatient)* regarding acute onset of no palpable pulses in lower extremities.

Mrs. Smith is a 68-year-old female with known history of CAD, status post coronary bypass in the 1970s. She recently underwent a total mastectomy 2/10/XX by Dr. Bond. Postoperatively, the patient has had an unremarkable course. Diet and activity were gradually increased. This morning she got up from bed about 4:30 and was weighed and had no problems. About 6:30 she suddenly experienced an acute onset of bilateral leg pain. The pain was excruciating. She was lying in bed when this first occurred. The surgical service was consulted about 7:30 this morning. By history from the patient, the pain gradually decreased. At the time of initial examination, she was complaining of a greater pain in her left thigh. She did state that her right leg had more of a numb feeling. She claimed that both legs were heavy feeling and that she would have to move every now and then to get relief from the pain.

Pertinent history reveals that the patient has been intermittently in atrial fibrillation. She has received two doses of Coumadin postoperatively for this atrial fibrillation.

Initial examination of the patient reveals a well-developed, well-nourished white female in no apparent distress. Heart: Regular rate and rhythm. Lungs are clear to auscultation bilaterally. Chest: The patient has a well-healing incision. There are no signs of infection, such as erythema or discharge. Abdomen: Positive bowel sounds, soft, nontender, nondistended. No rigidity on palpation. Examination of the pulses reveals the following: 2/4 in the radial, 2/4 in the carotid. No palpable pulses from the femoral on down. The patient does have dopplerable pulses in the femorals bilaterally. She has dopplerable left posterior tibial and no dopplerable right dorsalis pedis pulse. Neuro: Cranial nerves II–XII grossly intact.

IMPRESSION: Probable saddle embolus to the distal aorta.

PLAN: Patient in need of emergent embolectomy with possible aortofemoral reconstruction. Acute onset of bilateral leg pain and numbness. Embolism most likely from left atrium. Patient has been in and out of atrial fibrillation postoperatively. Discussed the risks, benefits, and complications of the procedure with the patient. The patient understands she will be cared for postoperatively in the surgical intensive care unit.

Thank you for this interesting consultation. We agree with your initial assessment and are happy to participate in the care of this nice lady.

77. 2/14/XX JACOB BOND, MD

PREOPERATIVE DIAGNOSIS: Saddle embolus, distal aorta.

POSTOPERATIVE DIAGNOSIS: Same.

PROCEDURE PERFORMED: Bilateral aortofemoral embolectomy via femoral artery approach, femoral embolectomy.

PROCEDURE: The patient was placed in the supine position and given a general anesthetic. She was prepped from her nipples to her toes. Following this, two bilateral groin incisions were made and dissection was carried down. The common femoral, profunda femoral, and superficial femoral arteries were identified on both sides and controlled with vessel loops. Following this, starting with the right side, a linear arteriotomy was made over the superficial femoral artery and profunda arteries. No. 3 Fogarty catheters were passed distally down the superficial femoral arteries and profunda arteries. No thrombus was recovered. They were then flushed with heparinized saline and controlled with vessel loops. Following this, no. 4 and no. 6 Fogarty catheters were sequentially placed up the common femoral artery toward the iliofemoral area. A lot of thrombus was removed, and good arterial inflow was established in the right leg. Before any arteriotomies had been made, the patient had been given 5000 units of IV heparin that had been given 5 minutes to circulate.

Following this, the arteriotomy on the right was closed with a running 5-0 Prolene suture. Before the arteriotomy was closed, it was back-flushed and fore-flushed. The clamps and vessel loops were all removed, and flow was restored to the right lower extremity. The patient had dopplerable posterior tibial pulses and palpable dorsalis pedis pulses at this point. Following this, a similar incision was made in the left lower extremity, and catheters were placed distally down the profunda and superficial femoral arteries, also flushing them sequentially with heparinized saline. No thrombus was removed from the distal arteries on the left; following this, no. 4 and no. 6 Fogarty catheters were placed sequentially toward the iliofemoral artery and more thrombotic material was removed, restoring good arterial inflow. The arteriotomy on the left was closed in a similar fashion with running 5-0 Prolene. All the clamps were removed. There were palpable dorsalis pedis and dopplerable posterior tibial pulses at this junction of the procedure. Following this, both wounds were irrigated free of clot and debris. They were closed with three layers of interrupted 3-0 Vicryl, and the skin was closed with staples. The patient tolerated the procedure well and went to the recovery room in good condition.

78. 2/17/XX ERIC ARNOLD, MD, CONSULTING PHYSICIAN

REASON FOR CONSULTATION: Pleural effusion.

Patient is a 68-year-old female who was initially admitted for a left breast biopsy. Pathology confirmed carcinoma, and patient proceeded to have left total mastectomy. Hospital course has been complicated by atrial fibrillation and saddle embolism, requiring embolectomy. Patient is now 4 days postop embolectomy and has developed persistent pleural effusion. Attempts at medical management have failed, and patient is developing respiratory failure. A pleuracentesis is accomplished, with 500 ml of blood-tinged fluid immediately aspirated. Patient appears to receive immediate relief. Patient will be closely monitored in intensive care unit for additional signs of respiratory failure.

79. 3/10/XX JACOB BOND, MD

Patient in for follow-up appointment, as status post mastectomy on 2/10/XX. Hospital course was complicated by atrial fibrillation and embolism, requiring embolectomy. Patient also developed pleural effusion requiring pleuracentesis. Patient has now been discharged from the hospital for 10 days. Other than some incisional pain, patient seems to be doing well. No major complaints: denies shortness of breath, nausea, loss of appetite, fever, or pain in extremities. Energy levels seem to be returning to normal. Incision sites are examined, with no erythema or infection noted. Sutures are removed. Patient is instructed not to lift, push, or pull objects and to return to activities slowly. Wound care is reviewed. Patient is instructed to follow-up in 2 weeks or sooner if complaints.

80. PULMONARY FUNCTION STUDY

This 49-year-old presents with dyspnea. He has previous cigarette smoking history.

COMPLETE PULMONARY FUNCTION STUDY: Forced vital capacity is 4.87 L, 112% of predicted. FEV1 is 4.02 L, 113% of predicted. FEV1 is 83%. FEF 25% to 75% is normal. There is no significant response to bronchodilators. Flow volume loop shows a well-preserved inspiratory limb.

Total lung capacity by plethysmography is 6.82 L, 111% predicted. RV/TLC ratio and airway resistance are normal. Corrected DLCO was 18.99, 70% of predicted.

IMPRESSION:

1. Normal expiratory flow rates.
2. Normal lung volumes.
3. Mild reduction of DLCO is noted.

The cause of decreased diffusion capacity is unclear in this patient. Possible causes could include heart disease, pulmonary embolism, anemia, obstructive sleep apnea. Clinical correlation is advised for cause of abnormal diffusion. There is no evidence of coexisting obstructive or restrictive pulmonary disease.
Note: The items to be coded listed below:

- Spirometry before and after bronchodilator
- Respiratory flow volume loop
- Functional residual capacity
- Carbon monoxide diffusing capacity
- Bronchodilator supply

81. OPERATIVE REPORT

PREOPERATIVE DIAGNOSIS: History of adenocarcinoma of the prostate.

POSTOPERATIVE DIAGNOSIS: History of adenocarcinoma of the prostate.

PROCEDURES PERFORMED:

1. Transrectal ultrasound performance with:
2. Volume study.
3. Needle localization.
4. Needle implantation.
5. Cystoscopy.

ANESTHESIA: General.

ESTIMATED BLOOD LOSS: Minimal.

PROCEDURE: Please see the preoperative note for indications of the procedure, as well as full informed consent. The patient underwent a general anesthetic and was put in the extended dorsal lithotomy position. The table was decanted or in Trendelenburg 5 degrees. He was prepped and draped in the usual fashion, which included a 14-French Foley catheter with 120 ml of sterile saline in his bladder. The testicles and scrotum had been taped back and away. We irrigated the rectum with sterile saline, performing

Brachytherapy (putting in the seeds)

a pseudo-enema. The patient underwent transrectal ultrasound placement. This was connected to the gantry. The placement of ultrasound and the grid work were set up so that the base of the prostate is noted at #1 on the grid work. The anterior most component at approximately 4.5–5, prostate extended from side-to-side from A to F.

Five-mm increment imaging slices were obtained, starting at the base of the prostate, carrying it back for a total of 3 cm to 30. Volume of the prostate is approximately 33 ml.

The outline of the prostate was drawn during the volume study. This information was given to the computer electronically so that a plan could be developed. Once the plan had been completed, the placement of the needles was performed in the usual fashion. The dose was delivered via 125 seeds after placement of the needles.

The total number of needles was 41 for 107 seeds (radioelements) placed with ultrasound guidance. The patient tolerated this well. At the conclusion, the patient was re-prepped and draped with the Foley catheter being removed and a cystoscopic evaluation was performed. There is no evidence of perforation of the urethra, bladder neck, or bladder. Urine within the bladder was clear. No seeds or spacers could be identified. An 18-French Foley catheter was then placed along with Triple antibiotic salve to the perineum and mesh panties. He tolerated the procedure well overall. Estimated blood loss minimal.

82. OPERATIVE REPORT

PREOPERATIVE DIAGNOSIS: History of a nodular mass, mid-prostate with urinary retention.

POSTOPERATIVE DIAGNOSIS: History of a nodular mass, mid-prostate with urinary retention; possible macronodular prostate.

PROCEDURE: Cystoscopy, transurethral resection of the prostate, one stage.

ANESTHESIA: Spinal.

ESTIMATED BLOOD LOSS: Approximately 100 ml.

FINDINGS: Benign prostatic hypertrophy type changes.

This is a 76-year-old gentleman who has a history as outlined in the preoperative note. Cystoscopically there is a large, red, macronodular area along the base of the prostate, which has been noted. The patient is having outlet obstructing symptoms. He has some decompensation in his urinary bladder but in discussion with the findings he wishes to go through the transurethral resection of prostate as outlined and discussed.

The patient underwent a spinal anesthetic, was put in the dorsolithotomy position, prepped, and draped in the usual fashion. Cystoscopic evaluation reveals the 1-cm nodule along the base of the prostate. This appears more macronodular but is not really prostatic or is very minimally prostatic. It could represent a deteriorating median lobe.

Resection of the prostate was started at the 12-o'clock position and was carried between 3 and 9 o'clock back to the plane of the verumontanum. The base tissue and the rest of the lateral walls were then resected. This was a pretty small prostate, around 20 ml of tissue. The area was separately resected.

At the conclusion of this procedure, the chips were irrigated out of the bladder. Final hemostasis was achieved. A 22-French three-way Foley catheter was inserted, inflated, and irrigated with slightly tinged irrigant returning. He was taken to the Recovery Room in satisfactory condition.

83. OPERATIVE REPORT

PREOPERATIVE DIAGNOSIS: History of left cryptorchid testicle.

POSTOPERATIVE DIAGNOSIS: Left ectopic testicle.

PROCEDURE PERFORMED: Left groin exploration with orchiopexy.

ANESTHESIA: General.

Please see the preoperative note for indications of the procedure as well as full informed consent. This 14-year-old was recognized on a sports physical as having a nonpalpable testicle. Through his younger years, it had been palpable.

The testicle on physical exam sat in the superficial inguinal canal next to the external ring. With him asleep, we went ahead and evaluated again and, again, the testicular cord was foreshortened, not allowing the testicle to get into the scrotum proper and sat slightly lateral as noted on the preoperative note.

He underwent a general anesthetic as noted previously and was prepped and draped in the usual fashion. A transverse incision was made halfway between the anterosuperior iliac spine and pubic tubercle at the presumed location of the internal ring. The external oblique aponeurosis was opened along the course of its fibers to the external ring. The inguinal canal was opened. The external ilioinguinal nerve was identified and preserved. The testicle could be identified outside the inguinal canal lateral to it in its own small covering. This was opened and the cord, with the testicle, could be freed up. We removed some of the adhesions along the cord, which allowed very satisfactory length to allow it to fit well into the inferior aspect of the left hemiscrotum.

inguinal approach

A separate incision was made in the left hemiscrotum. Subdartos pouch was formed using sharp and blunt dissection. The testicle was brought through in a medial tract performed by using blunt dissection with a hemostat. The testicle was brought down into the scrotum and out of the incision with ease. On the inferior pole of the testicle, a small 3-0 chromic was placed in the inferior most portion of the septum. The scrotal wall was then closed over the testicle with interrupted 3-0 chromic. Irrigation of the wound was performed. No active bleeding could be identified. The external oblique aponeurosis was closed utilizing 3-0 silk. Bupivacaine 0.25% without epinephrine was placed approximately 3 ml in the internal ring and 3 ml in the subcut. The subcut was closed with interrupted 3-0 chromic and 4-0 undyed Vicryl for subcuticular incision closure with Steri-Strips. He tolerated the procedure well.

84. TRANSURETHRAL NEEDLE ABLATION (TUNA) THERAPY

The procedure was performed in the usual fashion and multiple segments as noted.

Transrectal ultrasound was performed with the patient in the left lateral position. The ultrasound is performed in order to evaluate the prostate in detail, bladder neck, and seminal vesicles. Ultrasound shows a width of the prostate at 45 mm. The entire calculated volume of the prostate is approximately 40 cc's. Large amount of the bladder neck/median lobe is noted as prominent. No other findings are noted in the prostate.

A prostatic block was then performed. Using an 83, 18-gauge spinal needle, the area between the "angle" of the prostate to seminal vesicle laterally is identified. Needle is placed into position at that point under the rectum. 8 cc's of 2% Xylocaine are used to create the block.

The patient was then brought to the cystoscopic area. Further preparation includes viscous Xylocaine and liquid Xylocaine to the bladder. After a 15-minute wait, we proceeded with the procedure as follows.

The scope was advanced down into the urethra through the sphincter and prostatic urethra and into the bladder. A prominent bladder neck is noted. The length of the prostate is about 28 mm. The obstructing components are definitely the median lobe.

After introduction of the radiofrequency thermotherapy stylet, treatments were performed utilizing a suggested needle-length of 16 mm.

The treatments were performed 1 cm back from the bladder neck laterally. One cm back from that positioning, the next treatment halfway between the original and the verumontanum. This was performed bilaterally. All target temperatures were reached without difficulty. The fifth treatment zone was the median lobe. We retracted the needles to 12 mm to do this. The patient tolerated the procedure well. Foley catheter was placed at the conclusion of the procedure. Usual post procedure protocol to include antibiotics and pain relief medications.

85. OPERATIVE REPORT

PREOPERATIVE DIAGNOSIS: Glaucoma, severe stage, open angle, right eye.

POSTOPERATIVE DIAGNOSIS: Same.

OPERATION PERFORMED: Sequential cyclocryotherapy, right eye.

INDICATION: This 74-year-old white female has an out-of-control glaucoma in her right eye. She is pseudophakic and has been allergic to multiple drops and has had one sequential therapy before that worked quite well and then she stopped taking her drops. It is obvious that despite the cyclocryotherapy, she will need to continue on the Pilocarpine.

DESCRIPTION OF PROCEDURE: After the patient was placed on the OR table, she was given a retrobulbar anesthesia of Xylocaine 2% with 0.75% Marcaine and Wydase for a volume of 3.5 cc. After this, she was prepped and draped in the usual sterile fashion for ophthalmic surgery and a wire lid speculum was used to separate the lids of the right eye. 3.5 mm from the limbus was marked out with a marking pen in the superior temporal quadrant and the right inferior nasal quadrant of her eye. The cryoprobe was liquid nitrogen and nitrous oxide and was applied to −80 for a 5-second treatment in a freeze-thaw-freeze triple row of cryotherapy laid down in both the defined quadrants. There were no complications. Maxitrol ointment, Telfa, and two pads were applied and the patient sent to the Recovery Room.

86. OPERATIVE REPORT

PREOPERATIVE DIAGNOSES:

1. Blunt trauma with paint ball, right eye.
2. Hyphema, right eye, secondary to #1.
3. Recurrent hyphema, right eye, secondary to #1.
4. Corneal staining, right eye, secondary to #1.

5. Increased intraocular pressure, right eye, secondary to #1.
6. Dense cataract, right eye, secondary to #1.

POSTOPERATIVE DIAGNOSIS: Same.

PROCEDURE PERFORMED: Irrigation and aspiration of hyphema and blood clot anterior chamber, right eye.

ANESTHESIA: General endotracheal anesthesia.

INDICATION: This 14-year-old white male has had persistent problems since he was hit with a paint ball in his right eye 2 weeks ago. It has not resolved. It has continued to bleed and now it has formed a huge clot. Because of the increase in pain and obvious corneal staining, it was elected to irrigate the clot at this time. No guarantees were made to the mother for vision.

DESCRIPTION OF PROCEDURE: After the patient was prepped and draped in the usual sterile fashion for ophthalmic surgery under general endotracheal anesthesia, a wire lid speculum was used to separate the lids of the right eye. The Super knife was then used in the limbal area to make a 2-mm–wide incision at the 8-o'clock meridian, and the chamber was filled with BSS Plus. Using the Simcoe I&A apparatus, gentle suction, and a push-pull method, the clot was removed and the blood was irrigated. There was no damage done to the lens surface or to the iris and the pupil remained round. Healon was used to help dissolve the clot and make it easier for aspiration. At the end of the procedure, all the Healon and blood clot was removed and the pupil remained round. There was a dense cataract well on its way to hypermaturity already present, but no evidence of any vitreous or subluxation of the lens. The wound was closed with a 10-0 nylon suture, and the knot was buried. Healon was then placed over the cornea because the cornea showed some irregularity secondary to the paint ball explosion. Solu-Medrol was injected inferiorly Sub-Tenon's. Atropine 1% was placed in the eye and Maxitrol ointment and a Telfa pad, patch, and shield applied. The patient was sent to the Recovery Room. There were no complications.

87. OPERATIVE REPORT

PREOPERATIVE DIAGNOSES:

1. Cataract, right eye.
2. Pseudophakia, left eye.
3. Excess myopia, both eyes.
4. Diabetes mellitus.
5. Atrial fibrillation, controlled.
6. Hypothyroidism.
7. Pacemaker for history of bradycardia.

POSTOPERATIVE DIAGNOSIS: Same.

PROCEDURE PERFORMED: Extracapsular cataract extraction, right eye, with insertion of intraocular lens implant, right eye.

ANESTHESIA: MAC anesthesia.

INDICATION: This 86-year-old white female has had progressively decreasing vision in her right eye secondary to a nuclear sclerotic cataract that has reduced her vision to 20/400, which can be corrected to 20/100. She had successful cataract surgery in her left eye a year ago and has returned to 20/40 vision without glasses. She was counseled again as to the type of procedure, the need for medical clearance, anticoagulation regulation, and pacemaker regulation.

PROCEDURE: After the patient was placed on the OR table, she was given Nadbath and Van Lint anesthesia on a 25-gauge needle for a volume of 9 cc of Xylocaine 2% with 0.75% Marcaine and Wydase. The same mixture was administered on a blunt retrobulbar Atkinson needle for a volume of 4 cc without complications. After this, she was prepped and draped in the usual sterile fashion for ophthalmic surgery, and the Honan balloon was placed for four minutes by the clock at 35 mm Mercury. After this, the lid speculum was used to separate the lids of the right eye and a fornix-based flap was raised from 9 o'clock to 3 o'clock and the wet-field cautery was used. There was no excessive bleeding despite the use of the Coumadin. A 69-Beaver blade made a half-thickness O'Malley groove from 9:30 to 2:30 and the Super knife was used to enter the eye at 11 o'clock. The chamber was filled with Healon, and a dry, nonirrigating anterior capsulotomy was performed on a bent 25-gauge needle. The wound was extended with left and right corneal-cutting scissors, and three 8-0 Vicryls were post placed. Using a lens vectis, the nucleus was expressed without capsular rupture or iris prolapse. The post placed sutures were tied down and the Simcoe I&A apparatus was used to clean up excess cortex. It was noted that there was very weak zonular support and positive vitreous pressure. We elected at this point to fill the chamber with Healon, insert a lens glide, and a 14 diopter L122 UV lens was inserted. Miochol was used to bring down the pupil and eight 10-0 nylons were used to close the wound. A peripheral iridectomy was performed at 1 o'clock and there was no evidence of any vitreous. The Healon was left in the eye. The pupil was round and two 8-0 Vicryls closed the conjunctiva. Solu-Medrol was used sub-Tenon's inferiorly, and Pilopine gel, Maxitrol ointment, Telfa, two pads, and an eye shield were applied. There were no complications, and the heart rate was not out of ordinary since it was protected with a magnet.

88. OPERATIVE REPORT

PREOPERATIVE DIAGNOSES:

1. History of corneoscleral laceration, right eye.
2. History of retained sutures, right eye.

POSTOPERATIVE DIAGNOSIS: Same.

PROCEDURE PERFORMED: Removal of retained sutures, anterior cornea, right eye.

ANESTHESIA: General anesthesia.

INDICATIONS: This 17-year-old white male who suffered a severe injury to his eye with multiple lacerations of his right cornea has now recovered to the point that his vision is correctable with a contact lens to 20/25; however, there is a large amount of suture material, and it was elected to remove the sutures at this time.

PROCEDURE: After the patient was prepped and draped in the usual sterile fashion for ophthalmic surgery and he was under general anesthesia, the lid speculum was used to separate the lids of the right eye. Healon was placed over the sutures, a Super knife was used to cut them, and they were pulled with a combination of straight tiers and 0.12 forceps. One suture remained deeply buried and was left alone. None of the scleral sutures were removed. There were no complications and the chamber remained intact.

He was patched with TobraDex ointment without Telfa for 24 hours, and we will make arrangements to see him within the week.

89. OPERATIVE REPORT

PREOPERATIVE DIAGNOSIS: Splenic hematoma.

POSTOPERATIVE DIAGNOSIS: Same.

PROCEDURE PERFORMED: Splenectomy.

ANESTHESIA: General.

PROCEDURE: A surgical technique was used to remove the spleen due to splenic hematoma following trauma in football game, kicked. The patient was given general anesthesia. The anesthesiologist inserted a temporary tube into the patient's stomach to empty it. This helped to decompress the stomach and prevent postoperative nausea. A catheter was inserted into the bladder to drain the urine. Surgery was done with the patient lying flat on his back. Several small incisions were made into the abdomen. One was used for the laparoscope, which was attached to a camera that sent images to the video monitor. The other incisions were used to hold or manipulate tissue in the abdomen. Carbon dioxide gas is insufflated into the abdominal cavity to allow room to work and to allow visualizing the area. Parts of the spleen were freed from surrounding tissue. Blood vessels to the stomach and spleen were visualized, clipped with metal clips, and divided. Once the spleen was dissected free of its attachments in the abdominal cavity, it was placed in a special surgical plastic bag and removed through one of the small abdominal incisions. At the end of the surgery, carbon dioxide gas was removed. The small incisions were closed with suture, the skin cleaned, and the incisions covered with a small dressing. Patient tolerated the procedure well.

90. RECORD OF OPERATION

PREOPERATIVE DIAGNOSIS: Prostate cancer.

POSTOPERATIVE DIAGNOSIS: Same.

PROCEDURE PERFORMED: Cryoablation of prostate including suprapubic catheter insertion, transrectal ultrasound for prostate volume determination, placement of probes, and guidance of tissue ablation. Suprapubic catheter insertion.

CLINICAL NOTE: This gentleman has had prostate cancer. He has elected to proceed with cryoablation.

PROCEDURE NOTE: The patient was given a spinal anesthetic, prepped and draped in the lithotomy position. The Foley catheter placed into the bladder and transrectal ultrasound probe introduced. Prostate measurements and volumes were determined. Using the Cryoguide system, an 8 probe freeze was selected. Probes were placed under ultrasound guidance. Once all temperature monitors and Cryoprobes were placed the Foley catheter was withdrawn and patient then cystoscoped using the flexible instrument. This ensured the needles had not violated the urethra and the probes were in good position. A 12 French suprapubic catheter was then placed using a trocar technique under endoscopic and ultrasound guidance into the anterior wall of the bladder using a single pass technique. Once probe position was confirmed the urethral warming catheter was placed over a guide wire. A two cycle freeze was undertaken, please see the details. Temperature was recorded in the operative part of the chart. Ice bulb was monitored on ultrasound guidance. At the end of the procedure Cryoprobe was withdrawn. A Foley catheter was placed because of hematuria. CBI was started. Five minutes of pressure was applied to the perineum. Bacitracin ointment was applied to the perineum. The patient tolerated the procedure well and was transferred to the recovery room in good condition.

91. CLINIC PROCEDURE

PREOPERATIVE DIAGNOSIS: Left shoulder bursitis

POSTOPERATIVE DIAGNOSIS: Same

PROCEDURE PERFORMED: Left shoulder injection

PROCEDURE: After obtaining consent, the patient was brought to the Special Procedures area. His left shoulder area was cleaned with Betadine. 7 cc of lo lidocaine and 1 cc of Kenalog were injected in his left subacromial bursa without complications. The patient was slightly nauseated. His blood pressure was 168/107. Heart rate was 79/minute and regular.

I was planning on injecting his right shoulder, however, because of his symptoms I elected to withhold that at this time and do it at some other time.

92. REPORT OF OPERATION

PREOPERATIVE DIAGNOSIS: Left renal calculus.

POSTOPERATIVE DIAGNOSIS: Same.

PROCEDURE PERFORMED: Left ESWL *(extracorporeal shock wave lithotripsy).*

CLINICAL NOTE: This gentleman came in with renal colic, a stent was placed. He presents now for ESWL. The patient was given a general laryngeal mask anesthetic, prepped and draped in the supine position. Stone targeted and shock head engaged. A total of 2400 shocks at maximum KV and stone partial fragmentation and dissolution could be seen. The patient tolerated the procedure well and transferred to the recovery room in good condition. He will be seen in follow-up in two weeks' time for KUB.

93. REPORT OF OPERATION

PREOPERATIVE DIAGNOSIS: Acute renal failure, possible rejection, possible ischemic nephropathy.

POSTOPERATIVE DIAGNOSIS: Same.

PROCEDURE PERFORMED: Transplant kidney biopsy.

PROCEDURE: The transplant kidney in the right iliac fossa was visualized with ultrasound. The previous arteriovenous malformation was noted in the lower pole. We avoided that area as much as we could. At least three core biopsies were obtained after prepping the area in the usual fashion and injecting 1% Lidocaine. A post biopsy ultrasound showed no evidence of hematoma or new AVN. The patient had some pain after the procedure and was sent to the procedure area. She will be getting some intravenous morphine.

Hemoglobin will be done in six hours.

94. WALKING OXYGEN DESATURATION STUDY

ENTRANCE DIAGNOSIS: Dyspnea. He gave a board rating of 5 by the time he finished; it was 3 at the beginning and showed some discomfort or effort to do this. He was able to walk 6 minutes at a slow pace without stopping. He did have some wheezing, some coughing, and was able to go 300 feet, which for this age group is relatively poor exercise tolerance. The 02 sats never dropped below 92%.

This patient does not need oxygen therapy with this form of exercise.

95. CLINIC PROGRESS NOTE

SUBJECTIVE: This is a 42-year-old Caucasian female who presents to the clinic today to establish with me as her primary care provider. At this particular visit she is complaining of right hip pain. She also complains of a nagging dry cough and would like to find out what might possibly be causing that. Her right hip pain has been going on for about three months now, which is constant and is aggravated by standing up from sitting. She does not feel the pain as much when walking and she says that this pain sometimes radiates to the buttocks and all the way down to her heel area. She occasionally feels a tingling sensation at the lateral aspect of the thigh, particularly at night. She has been treating this with over-the-counter pain medication but that is not found to be helpful. In terms of her cough, she noticed that she usually gets this whenever she has heartburn.

PAST MEDICAL HISTORY is remarkable for:

1. Gastroesophageal reflux disease and has been taking medication for this but she cannot recall the name of that medication right now.
2. She also was found to have only one kidney and this was thought to be congenital.
3. Obesity.

PAST SURGICAL HISTORY is remarkable for a hysterectomy due to a bicornuate uterus.

SCREENINGS: She gets a Pap smear and mammogram every year. Last time was last year, which were normal.

ALLERGIES: She otherwise has no known drug allergies.

FAMILY MEDICAL HISTORY: Her father died at the age of 70 from a myocardial infarction. Mother is presently having high blood pressure and is taking medication for her heart. She also has high blood cholesterol. She is presently 67 years old. There is one brother who has spondylitis, and she has a total of three other sisters. One sister has a benign breast tumor.

PERSONAL AND SOCIAL HISTORY: She is married. She has been doing this job for about 11 years now. She denies alcohol use. She has a total of two children. One is 18 years old and one is 6 years old. She had a miscarriage and one stillbirth.

REVIEW OF SYSTEMS: Constitutional: Head and neck, chest and lungs, cardiovascular, gastrointestinal, genitourinary, and extremities are otherwise negative other than what is already mentioned above.

OBJECTIVE FINDINGS: Vital signs: Blood pressure is 110/70. Pulse rate of 88. Weight is 202 pounds. General survey: She is an obese middle-aged lady who is pleasant in no acute distress. Head and neck: Normocephalic and atraumatic. Pink conjunctivae. Pupils are equal, round, and reactive to light and accommodation. Extraocular movements are intact. Neck is supple. No jugular venous distention. No carotid bruit. No thyromegaly. No cervical lymphadenopathy. Chest and lungs: Symmetrical expansion. Clear breath sounds. No roles or wheezes. Cardiovascular: Normal rate and regular rhythm. No murmur and no gallop. Abdomen is obese, soft; normoactive bowel sounds; nontender. No organomegaly. Extremities: She has no edema, cyanosis, or clubbing. Palpable distal pulses. Straight-leg testing on both lower extremities is essentially negative. She has pain on internal rotation of the right hip joint. No pain on external rotation. On the left side internal and external rotation of the hip joints are negative.

ASSESSMENT/PLAN:

1. Hip pain, exact etiology is uncertain but this could be most likely secondary to degenerative joint disease of the hip versus mild trochanteric bursitis. Superficial femoral nerve syndrome is also a consideration but not very likely. Discussed management with Patient and we will just continue to observe for now. I advised her to give us a call when she develops progression of symptoms and referral to Orthopedics might be appropriate if that happens.
2. Cough, dry, probably related to heartburn symptoms.

Answers to Workbook Questions

CHAPTER 1: REIMBURSEMENT, HIPAA, AND COMPLIANCE

Theory

1. a. persons eligible for disability benefits from Social Security
   b. persons with permanent kidney failure
3. Social Security Administration
5. 80%
7. 12
9. OBRA
11. beneficiaries
13. Medicare Advantage
15. Administrative Simplification
17. National Provider
19. limiting
21. Internet Only
23. Staff
25. Program, All-Inclusive

CHAPTER 2: AN OVERVIEW OF ICD-10-CM

Theory

1. True
3. True
5. False
7. True
9. True

Practical

11. f
13. b
15. c
17. d
19. f
21. e

CHAPTER 3: ICD-10-CM OUTPATIENT CODING AND REPORTING GUIDELINES

Theory

1. False
3. False
5. True
7. False
9. False
11. True
13. True
15. False

Practical

17. Congestive heart failure, **I50.9**. The shortness of breath is a symptom of congestive heart failure and is not reported.

19. Hypertension with end stage renal disease, **I12.0**; end stage renal disease, **N18.6**. There is a combination code for hypertension with end stage renal disease. **I12.0** assumes a causal relationship in this scenario. Under code **I12.0** in the Tabular, a notation states "Use additional code to identify the stage of chronic kidney disease (**N18.5**, **N18.6**)."

21. Acute lower respiratory infection, **J22**. The Excludes2 note indicates both the infection and COPD may be coded, but the infection is the reason for the encounter.

23. Exposure to tuberculosis, **Z20.1**.

25. Abnormal perfusion study, **R94.39**; cardiovascular disease, **I25.10**. The purpose of the visit is the abnormal perfusion study; therefore, it is reported first, followed by the cardiovascular disease.

27. Contusion of the left cheek, **S00.83XA**; fist fight, **Y04.0XXA**. External cause codes are never reported as a first-listed diagnosis.

29. Encounter for insulin pump titration, **Z46.81**

31. Infant, liveborn, twin, born in hospital, **Z38.30**.

33. Abrasion of left upper arm, **S40.812A**.

35. Acute bronchitis, **J20.9**; COPD, **J44.0**; cigarette smoker, **F17.210**.

CHAPTER 4: USING ICD-10-CM

Theory

1. False
3. False
5. True
7. True
9. False
11. False
13. False
15. False

17. Heartburn, acid regurgitation, belching, hoarseness in the morning, reflux, pain in chest, trouble swallowing, choking feeling, dry cough

19. Swelling, pain, discoloration, disfiguration
21. Residual: Constrictive Pericarditis
    Cause: Tuberculosis infection

Practical

23. **J01.90** (Sinusitis, acute), **J32.9** (Sinusitis [chronic])
25. **J62.8** (Pneumoconiosis, dust, lime)
27. **J14** (Pneumonia, in, Hemophilus influenzae)
29. **I95.9** (Hypotension)
31. **K85.9** (Pancreatitis, acute), **K86.1** (Pancreatitis, chronic)
33. **E83.31, M90.80** (Rickets, vitamin-D-resistant)
35. **K70.11** (Ascites, due to, hepatitis, alcoholic), **F10.288** (Dependence, alcohol, with, specified disorder NEC)

CHAPTER 5: CHAPTER-SPECIFIC GUIDELINES (ICD-10-CM CHAPTERS 1-10)

Theory

1. True
3. True
5. False
7. True
9. True
11. True
13. True
15. True
17. False
19. True

Practical

21. **A41.9** (Sepsis [generalized]), **R65.20** (Sepsis, severe), **N17.9** (Failure, renal, acute), **J96.00** (Failure, respiration, respiratory, acute)
23. **E86.0** (Dehydration), **B19.10** (Hepatitis, B)
25. **J85.2** (Abscess, lung), **B95.62** (Infection, methicillin, resistant, Staphylococcus aureus)
27. **Z09** (Examination, follow-up [routine] [following] surgery), **Q54.9** (Hypospadias). Because this follow-up exam is part of the episode of care in which surgery corrected the hypospadias, the hypospadias is still coded as if it is an active disease. Once all treatment for the surgery is complete, a history of hypospadias would be reported instead.
29. **C80.0** (Neoplasm, disseminated, Malignant Primary), **R18.0** (Ascites, malignant)
31. **L03.116** (Cellulitis, lower limb), **E11.65** (Diabetes, type 2, with, hyperglycemia)
33. **O9A.111** (Pregnancy, complicated by, neoplasm, malignant), **C50.912** (Neoplasm, breast, Malignant Primary)
35. **C61** (Neoplasm, prostate, Malignant Primary), **D63.0** (Anemia, in, neoplastic disease)

37. **K56.60** (Obstruction, intestine), **I12.0** (Hypertension, kidney, with stage 5 chronic kidney disease), **N18.5** (Disease, kidney, chronic, hypertensive, stage 5)

39. **C79.31** (Neoplasm, brain NEC, Malignant Secondary), **Z85.3** (History, personal [of], malignant neoplasm, breast), **Z90.12** (Absence, breast(s) [acquired])

41. **D45** (Polycythemia, vera)

43. **T85.614A** (Complication, insulin pump, mechanical, breakdown), **T38.3X1A** (Substance, Insulin NEC, Poisoning, Accidental [Unspecified]), **E10.641** (Diabetes, type 1, with, hypoglycemia)

45. **C34.11** (Neoplasm, lung, upper lobe, Malignant Primary)

47. **I21.3** (Infarct, myocardium [acute], Q wave)

49. **F20.9** (Schizophrenic), **Z91.14** (Noncompliance, with, medication regimen NEC), **F91.8** (Disorder, conduct, specified NEC)

51. **B05.1** (Meningitis, in [due to], measles)

53. **A52.15** (Polyneuropathy, in [due to], syphilis [late]), **A52.77** (Syphilis, joint [late])

55. **G80.2** (Palsy, cerebral, hemiplegic, spastic)

57. **H81.09** (Meniere's disease, syndrome or vertigo)

59. **J81.0** (Edema, lung, acute), **I50.1** (Failure, ventricle, left), **Z99.11** (Dependence, on, ventilator)

CHAPTER 6: CHAPTER-SPECIFIC GUIDELINES (ICD-10-CM CHAPTERS 11-14)

Theory

1. True

3. True

5. False

7. False

9. True

Practical

11. **K03.2** (Erosion, dental [idiopathic] [occupational] [due to diet, drugs, or vomiting])

13. **N83.6** (Hemorrhage, fallopian tube)

15. **N76.4** (Cellulitis, genital organ NEC, female [external])

17. **N47.2** (Paraphimosis [congenital])

19. **N91.1** (Amenorrhea, secondary)

21. **M79.81** (Hematoma, nontraumatic, soft tissue)

23. **K51.412** (Polyp, polypus, colon, inflammatory, with, intestinal obstruction)

25. **L97.112** (Ulcer, lower limb, thigh, right, with, exposed fat layer)

27. **K40.41** (Hernia, inguinal [internal], with, gangrene, recurrent)

29. **N03.1** (Nephritis, nephritic [focal], chronic, with, focal and segmental glomerular lesions)

31. **L05.02** (Sinus, pilonidal [infected] [rectum], with abscess)

33. **M60.162** (Myositis, interstitial, lower leg)

35. **M32.13** (Lupus, erythematosus, systemic, with organ or system involvement, lung)

37. **M00.242** (Arthritis, streptococcal NEC, hand joint), **B95.1** (Streptococcus, group, B, as cause of disease classified elsewhere)

39. **M60.221** (Granuloma, foreign body [in soft tissue], upper arm)

41. **N61** (Abscess, areola [chronic])

Reports

43. Report 91: **M75.52** (Bursitis, shoulder)

45. Report 93: **T86.10** (Complication, transplant, kidney), **N17.9** (Failure, renal, acute)

CHAPTER 7: CHAPTER-SPECIFIC GUIDELINES (ICD-10-CM CHAPTERS 15-21)

Theory

1. True

3. True

5. True

7. True

9. False

11. False

13. True

15. True

17. anomaly

19. abnormal

21. third degree

23. 18

25. severity

Practical

27. **S40.812A** (Abrasion, arm [upper])

29. **T78.2XXA** (Shock, anaphylactic)

31. **O00.9** (Pregnancy, ectopic), **O08.0** (Peritonitis, following ectopic or molar pregnancy)

33. **Q55.64** (Concealed penis)

35. **O26.53** (Pregnancy, complicated by, hypotension)

37. **R13.0** (Aphagia)

39. **S93.402A** (Sprain, ankle)

41. **T23.201D** (Burn, hand[s], right, second degree)

43. **R80.1** (Proteinuria, persistent)

45. **S00.33XD** (Contusion, nose)

47. **Q99.2** (Syndrome, fragile X)

49. **O30.203** (Pregnancy, complicated by, multiple gestations, quadruplet)

51. **G25.1** (Tremor[s], drug induced), **T43.1X5A** (Table of Drugs and Chemicals, Substance, Monoamine oxidase inhibitor NEC, Poisoning Accidental [unintentional])

53. **S60.821A** (Blister, wrist)

55. **S42.001G** (Fracture, traumatic, clavicle)

57. **J80** (Distress, respiratory, adult), **R53.83** (Fatigue)

Reports

59. Report 94: **R06.00** (Dyspnea)

CHAPTER 8: AN OVERVIEW OF ICD-9-CM

Theory

1. f
3. a
5. h
7. j
9. d
11. b
13. a
15. f
17. c
19. a
21. g
23. d
25. True
27. True
29. reaction
31. obstruction
33. pregnancy
35. respiration
37. subcategory
39. category
41. subcategory
43. diagnosis code
45. procedure code
47. diagnosis code

Practical

49. Nephritis, Nephrotic Syndrome, and Nephrosis (580-589)

51. 580.0 Acute glomerulonephritis with lesion of proliferative glomerulonephritis

53. Essential

55. Essential

57. Essential

59. No, **770.0**

61. **002.0, 484.8** (in this order)

63. **075, 573.1** (in this order)

CHAPTER 9: ICD-9-CM OUTPATIENT CODING AND REPORTING GUIDELINES

Theory

1. True
3. False
5. False
7. False
9. True

Practical

11. **V18.19** (History [of], family, gout)
13. **V72.0** (Admission, for, vision examination)
15. **V73.4** (Screening (for), fever, yellow)
17. **V71.89** (Observation (for), suicide attempt, alleged)
19. **V04.1** (Vaccination, prophylactic, smallpox)
21. **V77.6** (Screening (for), cystic fibrosis)
23. **V06.4** (Vaccination, rubella, with measles and mumps)
25. **V59.3** (Donor, bone, marrow)
27. **V55.3** (Attention to, colostomy)

CHAPTER 10: USING ICD-9-CM

Theory

1. False
3. False
5. True
7. False
9. False

Practical

11. (any two) urgency, burning pain, urinary retention or inability to fully empty bladder, hematuria, pain lower abdomen, back or sides, chills, fever, nausea, and vomiting
13. Residual: severe intellectual disabilities, Code: **318.1** (Disabilities, intellectual, severe) Cause: encephalitis, viral, Code: **139.0** (Late effect[s] [of], encephalitis or encephalomyelitis, in infectious diseases, viral)
15. Residual Code: **733.00** (Osteoporosis) Cause Code: **138** (Late effect[s] [of], Poliomyelitis, acute)
17. **466.0** (Bronchitis, acute), **491.9** (Bronchitis, chronic)
19. **590.10** (Pyelonephritis, acute), **041.49** (Infection, *Escherichia coli*)
21. No code is assigned as there is no code for impending respiratory failure and no other information is given.
23. **482.2** (Pneumonia, *Hemophilus influenzae*)
25. **710.0** (Lupus, erythematosus, systemic), **581.81** (Nephritis, nephritic)

CHAPTER 11: CHAPTER-SPECIFIC GUIDELINES (ICD-9-CM CHAPTERS 1-8)

Practical

1. **110.4** (Infection, fungus NEC, foot)
3. **031.0** (Mycobacterium, mycobacterial (infection), atypical pulmonary)
5. **276.8** (Syndrome, hypokalemia)
7. **041.02** (Infection, streptococcal, Group B)
9. **279.03** (Deficiency, immunoglobulin, IgG)
11. **250.50** (Diabetes, retinopathy); **362.01** (Retinopathy, diabetic). Note: These codes need to appear in this order.
13. **266.2** (Deficiency, vitamin, B, specified type NEC)
15. **275.3** (Rickets, vitamin D-resistant)
17. **258.01** (Syndrome, Wermer's)
19. **296.7** (Disorder, bipolar, atypical)
21. **038.0** (Septicemia, streptococcal [anaerobic])
23. **295.32** (Schizophrenia, paranoid, chronic)
25. **305.1** (Tobacco, abuse)
27. **300.01** (Disorder, panic)
29. **362.83** (Edema, retina)
31. **366.22** (Cataract, traumatic, total)
33. **389.15** (Loss, hearing, sensorineural, unilateral)
35. **410.70** (Infarct, infarction, subendocardial)
37. **416.0** (Hypertension, pulmonary (artery), primary)
39. **427.0** (Tachycardia, paroxysmal, supraventricular)
41. **440.1** (Stenosis, renal artery)
43. **457.2** (Lymphangitis, chronic [any site])
45. **478.5** (Abscess, vocal cord)
47. **491.21** (Bronchitis, chronic, obstructive, with exacerbation [acute])
49. **414.01** (Arteriosclerosis, coronary [artery], native artery); **496** (Disease, lung, obstructive [chronic] [COPD])
51. **482.41** (Pneumonia, due to, *Staphylococcus aureus*)
53. **045.02** (Poliomyelitis, cerebral); **784.42** (Dysphonia)
55. **281.0** (Anemia, progressive, malignant)
57. **310.1** (Syndrome, organic personality)
59. **382.9** (Otitis, media)
61. **360.63** (Foreign body, lens, retained or old); **V90.89** (Foreign body, retained)
63. **008.47** (Diarrhea due to Paracolon bacillus, NEC)
65. **441.02** (Aneurysm, aorta, abdominal, dissecting)
67. **443.0** (Raynaud's, gangrene); **785.4** (Gangrene)
69. **451.11** (Thrombophlebitis, leg, deep (vessel), femoral vein)
71. **381.62** (Obstruction, Eustachian tube (complete) (partial) cartilaginous, intrinsic)
73. **793.11** (Nodules[s], lung, solitary)

Reports

75. Report 7: **214.8** (Lipoma, muscle)

77. Report 19: **513.0** (Abscess, lung)

79. Report 34: **455.0** (Hemorrhoids, internal); **455.3** (Hemorrhoids, external)

81. Report 42: **374.30** (Ptosis, eyelid); **368.46** (Hemianopia)

CHAPTER 12: CHAPTER-SPECIFIC GUIDELINES (ICD-9-CM CHAPTERS 9-17)

Practical

1. **601.0** (Prostatitis, acute); **041.00** (Infection, streptococcal NEC) in this order

3. **531.50** (Ulcer, stomach, with perforation [chronic])

5. **564.00** (Constipation)

7. **605** (Phimosis)

9. **626.0** (Amenorrhea)

11. **651.23** (Pregnancy, quadruplet NEC)

13. **710.0** (Lupus, erythematosus, systemic)

15. **698.8** (Itch, winter)

17. **556.9** (Colitis, ulcerative); **713.1** (Arthritis, due to or associated with, colitis, ulcerative) in this order

19. **726.73** (Spur, bone, calcaneal)

21. **730.06** (Osteomyelitis, acute or subacute, patella); **041.10** (Infection, staphylococcal)

23. **730.15** (Osteomyelitis, chronic or old, pelvic region and thigh)

25. **784.7** (Epistaxis)

27. **787.01** (Nausea, with vomiting)

29. **969.01** (Monoamine Oxidase Inhibitors, Poisoning); **785.1** (Palpitation); **E980.3** (Poisoning, Monoamine Oxidase Inhibitors, Undetermined)

31. **845.00** (Sprain, ankle)

33. **941.27** (Burn, forehead, second degree)

35. **935.2** (Foreign body, entering through orifice, stomach); **E915** (Foreign body, object or material, [entrance into (accidental)], stomach)

37. **896.0** (Amputation, traumatic, foot)

39. **887.2** (Amputation, traumatic, arm, at or above the elbow)

41. a. **564.2** (Syndrome, dumping)

    b. The "Excludes:" indicates that 997.4 does not include "postgastric surgery syndromes."

43. **965.01** (Table of Drugs and Chemicals, Heroin, Poisoning); **305.50** (Abuse, opioid, unspecified); **E850.0** (Table of Drugs and Chemicals, Heroin, Accident)

45. **792.1** (Blood, in, feces, occult)

47. **692.71** (Sunburn, first degree); **E926.2** (Sunburn)

49. **719.56** (Stiffness, joint, knee)

51. **759.0** (Splenomegaly, congenital); **780.61** (Fever)

53. **520.6** (Impaction, tooth)

55. **535.40** (Gastritis, allergic); **716.90** (Arthritis, site unspecified); **965.1** and **E935.3** (Table of Drugs and Chemicals, Aspirin, Therapeutic Use)

57. **601.1** (Prostatitis, chronic); **041.10** (Infection, Staphylococcal)

59. **600.00** (Hypertrophy, prostate, benign)

61. **642.41** (Pre-eclampsia); **656.31** (Pregnancy, management affected by, fetal distress); **V27.0** (Outcome of Delivery, single, liveborn)

63. **710.0**, **517.8** (Lupus, erythematosus, systemic, with lung involvement). Note: Must be coded in this order.

65. **716.15** (Arthritis, traumatic, pelvic region and thigh); **905.3** (Late effect, fracture, extremity, lower, neck of femur)

67. **780.09** (Unconscious, unconsciousness)

69. **576.8** (Jaundice, obstructive)

71. **789.64** (Tenderness, abdominal, left lower quadrant)

73. **914.6** (Injury, superficial, hand); **E920.8** (Cut, cutting by, splinters)

75. **965.61** (Ibuprofen, Poisoning); **E850.6** (Poisoning, Ibuprofen, Accident)

77. **907.0** (Late effect [of] injury, intracranial); **E989** (Late effect of, injury, undetermined whether accidentally or purposely inflicted)

79. **916.0** (Injury, superficial, leg)

81. **850.2** (Concussion, with, loss of consciousness, moderate)

83. **789.06** (Pain, epigastric)

Reports

85. Report 6: **709.2** (Scar)

87. Report 10: **952.04** (Injury, spinal [cord], cervical [C1–C4], with posterior cord syndrome); **E815.0** (Collision, motor vehicle, and other object [tree])

89. Report 12: **707.05** (Ulcer, pressure, ischial), **707.24** (Ulcer, pressure, necrosis). Note: The Tabular states to use additional code to identify pressure ulcer stage (707.20-707.25)

91. Report 14: **729.1** (Myositis), **V46.11** (Status, ventilation)

93. Report 28: **659.71** (Delivery, complicated (by), fetal heart rate or rhythm); **660.41** (Delivery, complicated (by), dystocia, shoulder girdle); **664.11** (Delivery, complicated (by), laceration, perineum, second degree)

95. Report 32: **532.70** (Ulcer, duodenum, chronic)

97. Report 35: **536.3** (Paresis, stomach)

99. Report 38: **788.30** (Incontinence)

101. Report 43: **722.10** (Displacement, displaced, intervertebral disc, lumbar)

CHAPTER 13: INTRODUCTION TO THE CPT AND LEVEL II NATIONAL CODES (HCPCS)

Theory

1–4. any of the following: service or procedure, anatomic site, condition or disease, synonym, eponym, abbreviation

5. d

7. b
9. Radiology
11. American Medical Association, or AMA
13. stand-alone code
15. CPT codes and/or HCPCS codes
17. 1966
19. Health Insurance Portability and Accountability Act, or HIPAA
21. g
23. f
25. a
27. c

Practical

Radiology
29. 77299

Pathology and Laboratory
31. 88399

Medicine
33. 95199
35. 90999

CHAPTER 14: MODIFIERS

Theory
1. A
3. preoperative services/management or preop
5. no

Practical
7. -50
   ICD-10-CM: **M71.21** (Cyst, Baker's), **M71.22** (Cyst, Baker's)
   ICD-9-CM: **727.51** (Cyst, Baker's)
9. -53
   ICD-10-CM: **M17.9** (Osteoarthritis, knee), **I95.81** (Hypotension, iatrogenic)
   ICD-9-CM: **715.96** (Osteoarthritis, lower leg), **458.29** (Hypotension, iatrogenic)
11. -32
   ICD-10-CM: **K50.10** (Enteritis, regional, large intestine)
   ICD-9-CM: **555.1** (Enteritis, regional, intestine, large)
13. -32
   ICD-10-CM: **Z02.6** (Examination, medical, insurance purpose)
   ICD-9-CM: **V70.3** (Examination, medical, insurance certification)
15. -76

17. -99

19. -55

21. -FA

CHAPTER 15: EVALUATION AND MANAGEMENT (E/M) SERVICES

Theory

1. c

3. a

5. e

7. b

9. high

11. low

13. elements

15. moderate severity

17. self-limited/minor severity

19. contributory

21. medical record

23. subjective

25. consultation, attending

27. concurrent

29. review of systems

Practical

Office or Other Outpatient Services and Hospital Inpatient Services

31. a. minimal, minimal/none

    b. minimal

    c. straightforward

    d. **99201**

33. **99219** (Evaluation and Management, Hospital Services, Observation Care)

35. **99223** (Hospital Services, Inpatient Services, Initial Hospital Care)

    ICD-10-CM: **I21.19** (Infarct, myocardium), **I25.10** (Arteriosclerosis, coronary [artery]), **Z98.61** (Status, angioplasty, coronary artery)

    ICD-9-CM: **410.41** (Infarct, myocardial, inferior wall), **414.01** (Arteriosclerosis, coronary [artery]), **V45.82** (Status, percutaneous transluminal angioplasty)

37. **99231** (Hospital Services, Inpatient Services, Subsequent Hospital Care)

    ICD-10-CM: **J15.9** (Pneumonia, bacterial)

    ICD-9-CM: **482.9** (Pneumonia, bacterial)

Consultation Services

39. **99243** (Consultation, Office and/or Other Outpatient)

    ICD-10-CM: **R10.2** (Pain, pelvic [female]), **N94.1** (Dyspareunia [female])

    ICD-9-CM: **625.9** (Pain, pelvic [female], **625.0** (dyspareunia [female])

Note: All three key components must be met for the service to qualify for the higher level code. In this case, only the MDM complexity was of a higher level, requiring the choice of the lower level code.

41. **99253** (New Patient, Inpatient Consultations)

43. **99232** (Hospital Inpatient Services, Subsequent Hospital Care)

    ICD-10-CM: **R21** (Rash)

    ICD-9-CM: **782.1** (Rash)

    Note that adverse effect from a drug would not be reported as the physician is looking for another cause.

45. **99231** (Hospital Inpatient Services, Subsequent Hospital Care)

    ICD-10-CM: **G44.209** (Headache, tension)

    ICD-9-CM: **307.81** (Headache, tension)

47. **99241** (Consultation, Office and/or Other Outpatient, New or Established Patient)

    ICD-10-CM: **K41.91** (Hernia, femoral, recurrent)

    ICD-9-CM: **553.01** (Hernia, femoral, unilateral, recurrent)

49. **99245-32** (Consultation, Office and/or Other Outpatient, New or Established Patient)

    ICD-10-CM: **M51.06** (Disorder, disc, with myelopathy, lumbar region)

    ICD-9-CM: **722.73** (Myelopathy, due to or with, intervertebral disc disorder, lumbar, lumbosacral)

Emergency Department Services, Nursing Facility, Domiciliary, and Home Services

51. **99282** (Emergency Department Services)

    ICD-10-CM: **S52.539A** (Colles, fracture), **W21.89XA** (External Cause Index, Striking against, other sports equipment), **Y93.64** (External Cause Index, Activity, baseball)

    ICD-9-CM: **813.41** (Colles' fracture [closed]), **E917.0** (Index to External Causes, Striking against or struck accidentally by others, in sports without subsequent fall), **E007.3** (Index to External Causes, Activity, involving other sports, baseball/softball)

53. **99342** (Home Services, New Patient)

    ICD-10-CM: **R60.0** (Edema, legs)

    ICD-9-CM: **782.3** (Edema, legs)

    Note that the leg pain is not reported because the medical documentation indicated that the pain was due to the edema.

55. **99309** (Nursing Facility Services, Subsequent Care)

    ICD-10-CM: **R41.0** (Confusion), **R42** (Dizziness), **I69.30** (Sequelae, infarction, cerebral)

    ICD-9-CM: **298.9** (Confusion), **780.4** (Dizziness), **438.9** (Late effect(s), cerebrovascular disease)

57. **99324** (Domiciliary Services, New Patient)

Prolonged Services and Preventive Medicine Services

59. **99205** for the office visit (Office and/or Other Outpatient Services, New Patient) and **99354** and **99355** for Prolonged Services (Prolonged Services)

Services from Throughout the E/M Section

61. **99205** (Office and/or Other Outpatient Services, Office Visit, New Patient)

63. **99234** (Discharge Services, Observation Care)

    ICD-10-CM: **T39.95XA** (Table of Drugs and Chemicals, Analgesic, Adverse Effect), **L29.8** (Pruritus, specified NEC), **R06.02** (Short, breath)

    ICD-9-CM: **698.9** (Pruritus), **786.05** (Short, breath), **E935.9** (Table of Drugs and Chemicals, Analgesics, External Cause, Therapeutic)

65. **99251** (Consultation, Inpatient)

67. **99291** (Critical Care Services, Evaluation and Management), **99292** × 3 (Critical Care Services, Evaluation and Management)

    ICD-10-CM: **J96.90** (Failure, respiratory), **I50.9** (Failure, heart), **J44.1** (Disease, pulmonary chronic obstructive, exacerbation, [acute]), **Z99.11** (Dependence, on, ventilator)

    ICD-9-CM: **518.81** (Respiratory, failure, acute), **428.0** (Failure, heart), **491.21** (Disease, pulmonary, with, exacerbation NEC [acute]), **V46.11** (Status, ventilator)

Reports

69. Report 1: **99283** (Evaluation and Management, Emergency Department)

    ICD-10-CM: **O23.43** (Infection, urinary, complicating pregnancy), **N39.0** (Infection, urinary [tract]), **R60.0** (Edema, legs)

    ICD-9-CM: **646.63** (Infection, urinary, complicating pregnancy), **599.0** (Infection, urinary [tract]), **782.3** (Edema, legs)

71. Report 3: **99212** (Evaluation and Management, Office and Other Outpatient)

    ICD-10-CM: **S93.401A** (Sprain, ankle)

    ICD-9-CM: **845.00** (Sprain, ankle)

73. Report 5: **99232** (Evaluation and Management, Hospital)

CHAPTER 16: ANESTHESIA

Theory

1. moderate sedation or conscious sedation

3. base unit

5. preoperative services

7. conversion

Practical

9. P4 (A patient with severe systemic disease that is a constant threat to life)

11. P3 (A patient with severe systemic disease)

13. P2 (A patient with mild systemic disease)

15. **01382** (Anesthesia, Knee)

17. **00144** (Anesthesia, Corneal Transplant)

19. **00124** (Anesthesia, Otoscopy)

21. **01920-P2** (Anesthesia, Cardiac Catheterization)

23. ICD-10-CM: **K57.33** (Diverticulitis, intestine, large, with, bleeding)

    ICD-9-CM: **562.13** (Diverticulitis, with hemorrhage)

25. ICD-10-CM: **E05.01** (Hyperthyroidism, with goiter)
ICD-9-CM: **242.01** (Goiter, toxic)

Reports

27. Report 7: **00400** (Anesthesia, Arm)
29. Report 44: **00140** (Anesthesia, Eye)

CHAPTER 17: SURGERY GUIDELINES AND GENERAL SURGERY

Theory

1. Female Genital
3. categories
5. unlisted
7. major
9. yes
11. local
13. general
15. 99070
17. same
19. dehiscence

Practical

21. 10021-69990
23. Operating
25. 42400
27. therapeutic
29. 40799

CHAPTER 18: INTEGUMENTARY SYSTEM

Theory

Integumentary System Terminology

1. b
3. i
5. a
7. f
9. c
11. a
13. i
15. c
17. e
19. f
21. d

Practical

23. **12032** (Repair, Wound, Intermediate), **99070** (Special Services, Supply of Materials)

    ICD-10-CM: **S41.101A** (Wound, open, arm, [upper])

    ICD-9-CM: **884.0** (Wound, open, arm)

    Note: You do not report an E/M code because this is an established patient and the treatment constitutes the main service provided to the patient.

25. **19081-LT** (Breast, Biopsy, Placement, with stereotactic guidance), **99070** (Special Services, Supply of Materials)

    ICD-10-CM: **D48.62** (Neoplasm, breast, Uncertain Behavior)

    ICD-9-CM: **238.3** (Neoplasm, breast, Uncertain Behavior)

    Note: You do not report an E/M code because this is an established patient and the treatment constitutes the main service provided to the patient.

27. **11451** (Hidradenitis, Excision)

    ICD-10-CM: **L73.2** (Hidradenitis)

    ICD-9-CM: **705.83** (Hidradenitis)

29. **11971** (Removal, Tissue Expanders, Skin)

31. **11976** (Removal, Contraceptive Capsules)

    ICD-10-CM: **Z30.432** (Contraception, device, removal)

    ICD-9-CM: **V25.12** (Removal, device, contraceptive)

33. **11444** (Excision, Skin, Lesion, Benign) for 4 cm face lesion, **11423-51** (Excision, Skin, Lesion, Benign) for 3 cm neck lesion

    ICD-10-CM: **D23.30** (Neoplasm, skin, face, benign), **D23.4** (Neoplasm, skin, neck, Benign)

    ICD-9-CM: **216.3** (Neoplasm, skin, face, Benign), **216.4** (Neoplasm, skin, neck, Benign)

35. **17000** (Destruction, Lesion, Facial), **17003 ¥ 2** (Destruction, Lesion, Facial)

    ICD-10-CM: **L57.0** (Keratosis, actinic)

    ICD-9-CM: **702.0** (Keratosis, actinic)

37. **12035** (Wound, Repair, Intermediate); **11042-51** (Debridement, Subcutaneous Tissue)

    ICD-10-CM: **S81.801A** (Wound, open, leg), **W09.1XXA** (External Cause Index, Fall, from, off, playground equipment, swing), **W27.1XXA** (External Cause Index, Contact with, garden fork), **Y92.830** (External Cause Index, Place of occurrence, park [public])

    ICD-9-CM: **891.0** (Wound, open, leg), **E884.0** (Index to External Causes, Fall, from, off, playground equipment), **E920.4** (Index to External Causes, Contact with, garden, fork), **E004.9** (Index to External Causes, Climbing), **E849.4** (Index to External Causes, Accident, occurring, park)

39. **17110** (Destruction, Warts, Flat)

    ICD-10-CM: **B07.8** (Wart, Flat)

    ICD-9-CM: **078.19** (Wart)

41. **11000, 11001** (Debridement, Skin, Eczematous)

ICD-10-CM: **L30.9** (Eczema)

ICD-9-CM: **692.9** (Eczema)

43. **16000** (Burns, Initial Treatment)

ICD-10-CM: **T23.169A** (Burn, hand, back, first degree, unspecified hand), **T31.0** (Burn, extent, less than 10 percent), **X16.XXXA** (External Cause Index, Burning, steam, pipe), **Y92.009** (External Cause Index, Place of occurrence, residence)

ICD-9-CM: **944.16** (Burn, hand, back, first degree), **948.00** (Burn, extent, less than 10 percent); **E924.8** (Index to External Causes, Burning, steam, pipe), **E849.0** (Index to External Causes, Accident, occurring, home, private)

45. **19020** (Mastotomy)

ICD-10-CM: **N61** (Abscess, breast)

ICD-9-CM: **611.0** (Abscess, breast)

Reports

47. Report 7: **21554** (Excision, Tumor, Thorax)

ICD-10-CM: **D17.39** (Lipoma, site, skin)

ICD-9-CM: **214.8** (Lipoma)

Note: 11406 because the report indicates "dissected free of the muscle."

49. Report 9: **19120-RT** (Excision, Breast, Lesion)

ICD-10-CM: **C50.111** (Neoplasm, breast, central portion, Malignant Primary)

ICD-9-CM: **174.1** (Neoplasm, breast, central portion, Malignant, Primary)

51. Report 12: **15940** (Ulcer, Pressure)

ICD-10-CM: **L89.224** (Ulcer, pressure, hip)

ICD-9-CM: **707.04** (Ulcer, pressure, hip), **707.24** (Ulcer, pressure, stage, 4)

Note: Modifier -22 may be added to 15940 due to the extensive size of the ulcer.

CHAPTER 19: MUSCULOSKELETAL SYSTEM

Theory

Musculoskeletal Terminology

1. d
3. j
5. b
7. c
9. h
11. g

Answer the Following

13. aspiration of a joint
15. fascia lata graft

17. arthroscopy

19. No, the removal is part of the cast service

21. The primary difference is extent. The codes in the musculoskeletal system subsection are of biopsies of deep subcutaneous tissue, muscle and/or bone, whereas the codes in the integumentary system subsection are for skin and subcutaneous tissue.

Practical

23. **29075** (Cast, Short Arm)

    ICD-10-CM: **Z46.89** (Admission, for, orthopedic [cast]), **S52.119D** (Fracture, forearm)

    ICD-9-CM: **V53.7** (Admission [Encounter], for, fitting of, orthopedic [cast]), **V54.12** (Aftercare, fracture, traumatic, arm, lower)

25. **28406** (Fracture, Calcaneus, with Manipulation)

    ICD-10-CM: **S92.009A** (Fracture, tarsal, calcaneus)

    ICD-9-CM: **825.0** (Fracture, calcaneus [closed])

27. **26700** (Metacarpophalangeal Joint, Dislocation, Closed Treatment)

    ICD-10-CM: **S63.269A** (Dislocation, finger)

    ICD-9-CM: **834.01** (Dislocation, finger, metacarpal, distal end)

29. **27520** (Fracture, Patella, Closed Treatment, without Manipulation)

    ICD-10-CM: **S82.009A** (Fracture, patella)

    ICD-9-CM: **822.0** (Fracture, knee cap, closed)

31. **27570** (Manipulation, Knee)

    ICD-10-CM: **S83.116A** (Dislocation, knee, proximal tibia, anterior)

    ICD-9-CM: **836.61** (Dislocation, tibia, proximal, anterior, open)

33. **21343** (Sinuses, Frontal, Fracture, Open Treatment)

35. **20615** (Aspiration, Cyst, Bone)

37. **20822** (Replantation, Digit)

39. **20526** (Injection, Carpal Tunnel, Therapeutic)

    ICD-10-CM: **G56.00** (Syndrome, carpal tunnel)

    ICD-9-CM: **354.0** (Carpal tunnel syndrome)

41. **20665** (Removal, Halo)

43. **21450** (Fracture, Mandible, Closed Treatment, without Manipulation)

45. **29750** (Cast, Wedging)

47. **29520** (Strapping, Hip)

49. **29200** (Strapping, Thorax)

51. **29049** (Cast, Shoulder)

53. **29860** (Arthroscopy, Diagnostic, Hip)

55. **29877** (Arthroscopy, Surgical, Knee)

57. **29848** (Ligament, Release, Transverse Carpal)

59. **21032** (Excision, Maxillary, Torus Palatinus)

Reports

61. Report 13: **20610-LT** (Injection, Joint)

    ICD-10-CM: **M75.102** (Syndrome, rotator cuff, shoulder)

    ICD-9-CM: **726.10** (Syndrome, rotator cuff, shoulder)

63. Report 15: **25606-LT** (Fracture, Radius, Distal)

    ICD-10-CM: **S52.572A** (Fracture, radius, lower end, intraarticular), **W10.9XXA** (Fall, from, unspecified, stairs and steps, initial encounter)

    ICD-9-CM: **813.42** (Fracture, radius, lower end, intraarticular), **E880.9** (Fall, from, off, stairs, steps)

65. Report 17: **27244** or **27244-RT** (Fracture, Femur, Intertrochanteric, Plate/Screw Implant)

    ICD-10-CM: **S72.21XA** (Fracture, femur, upper end, subtrochanteric)

    ICD-9-CM: **820.21** (Fracture, femur [closed], neck, intertrochanteric); **820.22** (Fracture, femur [closed], subtrochanteric)

CHAPTER 20: RESPIRATORY SYSTEM

Theory

Respiratory Terminology

1. d
3. k
5. b
7. c
9. f
11. m
13. a
15. e

Answer the Following

17. nasal button
19. septoplasty
21. posterior
23. transtracheal and cricothyroid
25. 50

Practical

27. **31267** (Antrostomy, Sinus, Maxillary)
29. **31628-RT** (Bronchoscopy, Biopsy), **31632-RT** (Bronchoscopy, Biopsy). Note: Code 31628 is for a single lobe and two lobes were biopsied. Code 31632 is an add-on code reporting the biopsy of the additional lobe.
31. **31575** (Laryngoscopy, Fiberoptic)
33. **30801** (Ablation, Turbinate Mucosa). Note: Code specified unilateral or bilateral.
35. **30115** and **30115-50** (Excision, Nose, Polyp)
37. **31536** (Laryngoscopy, Direct)
39. **31400** (Arytenoidectomy)
41. **31720** (Aspiration, Trachea, Nasotracheal)
43. **31830** (Revision, Tracheostomy, Scar)
45. **32658** (Thoracoscopy, Surgical, with Wedge Resection of Lung)
47. **32800** (Hernia Repair, Lung)

49. **30930** (Fracture, Nasal Turbinate, Therapeutic)

51. **31613** (Tracheostoma, Revision)

    ICD-10-CM: **J95.02** (Tracheostomy, complication, infection), **L03.221** (Cellulitis, neck)

    ICD-9-CM: **519.01** (Tracheostomy [complication], infection), **682.1** (Cellulitis of neck)

53. **32440** (Pneumonectomy)

    ICD-10-CM: **J61** (Asbestosis [occupational])

    ICD-9-CM: **501** (Asbestosis [occupational])

55. **32900** (Resection, Ribs)

    ICD-10-CM: **Q76.6** (Deformity, rib, congenital)

    ICD-9-CM: **756.3** (Deformity, rib, congenital)

57. **32560** (Pleurodesis)

    ICD-10-CM: **C56.9** (Neoplasm, ovary, Malignant Primary), **J91.0** (Effusion, pleura, malignant)

    ICD-9-CM: **183.0** (Neoplasm, ovary, Malignant Primary), **511.81** (Effusion, pleura, malignant)

Reports

59. Report 19: **32480-LT** (Lobectomy, Lung)

    ICD-10-CM: **J85.2** (Abscess, lung)

    ICD-9-CM: **513.0** (Abscess, lung)

61. Report 23: **32554** (Thoracentesis)

    ICD-10-CM: **J90** (Effusion, pleura)

    ICD-9-CM: **511.9** (Effusion, pleural)

CHAPTER 21: CARDIOVASCULAR SYSTEM

Theory

Cardiovascular Terminology

1. e
3. b
5. d
7. a
9. i
11. f
13. j
15. d
17. i
19. h
21. n
23. b
25. l

Answer the Following

27. internally or externally, or intracardiac or external

29. epicardial and transvenous

31. no, suture removal is bundled into the pacemaker procedure
33. 24
35. patient-activated event recorder
37. reversible
39. embolus

Practical

41. **33403** (Valvuloplasty, Aortic Valve)
43. **33464** (Valvuloplasty, Tricuspid Valve)
45. **93000** (Electrocardiography, Evaluation)
47. **92920** (Angioplasty, Coronary Artery, Percutaneous Transluminal)
49. **93010** (Electrocardiography, Evaluation)
51. **37609** (Ligation, Artery, Temporal)
53. **35452** (Angioplasty, Aorta, Intraoperative)
55. **33513** (Bypass Graft, Coronary Artery, Venous Graft)
    ICD-10-CM: **I24.8** (Insufficiency, coronary)
    ICD-9-CM: **411.89** (Disease, heart, ischemic acute, without myocardial infarction)
57. **33967** (Balloon Assisted Device, Aorta)
    ICD-10-CM: **I21.3** (Infarction, myocardium, myocardial [acute]), **R57.0** (Shock, cardiogenic)
    ICD-9-CM: **410.91** (Infarction myocardium myocardial), **785.51** (Shock, cardiogenic)
59. **33641** (Heart, Repair, Atrial Septum)
    ICD-10-CM: **Q21.1** (Defect, septal, congenital [atrial])
    ICD-9-CM: **745.5** (Defect, atrial septal, congenital)
61. **33533** (Bypass Graft, Coronary Artery, Arterial), **33517** (Coronary Artery Bypass Graft, Arterial-Venous), **33530** (Reoperation, Coronary Artery Bypass, Valve Procedure)
    ICD-10-CM: **I25.10** (Arteriosclerosis, coronary, artery)
    ICD-9-CM: **414.01** (Arteriosclerosis, coronary, artery, native artery)

Reports

63. Report 26: **33533** (Coronary Artery Bypass Graft [CABG], Arterial)
    ICD-10-CM: **I25.10** (Arteriosclerosis, coronary, artery), **I51.9** (Dysfunction, ventricular)
    ICD-9-CM: **414.01** (Arteriosclerosis, coronary, artery, native artery), **429.9** (Dysfunction, ventricular)

CHAPTER 22: HEMIC, LYMPHATIC, MEDIASTINUM, AND DIAPHRAGM

Theory

Hemic and Lymphatic Terminology

1. k
3. e
5. g
7. d

9. i

11. c

13. f

15. b

17. h

19. c

Mediastinum and Diaphragm Terminology

21. m

23. j

25. d

27. l

29. k

31. g

33. b

Practical

35. **38720** (Lymphadenectomy, Radical, Cervical)

    ICD-10-CM: **C77.0** (Neoplasm, lymph, gland, cervical, Malignant, Secondary), **C50.012** (Neoplasm, breast, nipple, Malignant Primary)

    ICD-9-CM: **196.0** (Neoplasm, lymph, gland, cervical, Malignant, Secondary); **174.0** (Neoplasm, breast, nipple, Malignant, Primary)

    Note: The lymph gland neoplasm is first-listed because it was the reason for the procedure.

37. **38241** (Bone Marrow, T-Cell Transplantation)

    ICD-10-CM: **C92.00** (Leukemia, myelogenous)

    ICD-9-CM: **205.00** (Leukemia, myelogenous). Fifth digit "0" is added to indicate the leukemia is not in remission.

39. **38230** (Harvesting, Bone Marrow)

    ICD-10-CM: **Z52.3** (Donor, bone, marrow)

    ICD-9-CM: **V59.3** (Donor, bone, marrow)

41. **39200** (Resection, Cyst, Mediastinal)

43. **38209** (Transplantation, Stem Cells, Washing)

45. **78195-26** (Nuclear Medicine, Lymph Nodes), **38792-59** (Lymphadenectomy, Injection), **38530** (Excision, Lymph Nodes)

CHAPTER 23: DIGESTIVE SYSTEM

Theory

Digestive Terminology

1. b

3. f

5. g

7. a

9. i

11. i

13. e

15. h

17. a

Practical

19. **43194** (Endoscopy, Esophagus, Removal, Foreign Body)

21. **43401** (Esophagus, Repair, Varices)

23. **44345** (Colostomy, External Fistulization, Revision)

25. **42104** (Excision, Lesion, Palate)

27. **42831** (Adenoids, Excision)

29. **49521** (Repair, Hernia, Inguinal)

31. **40650** (Repair, Lip)

33. **42507** (Parotid Duct, Diversion)

35. **43605** (Biopsy, Stomach)

37. **44604** (Suture, Intestines, Large, Wound)

39. **49320** (Laparoscopy, Diagnostic)

41. **99284-25** (Evaluation and Management, Emergency Department), **43752** (Tube Placement, Nasogastric Tube)

    ICD-10-CM: **K92.0** (Hematemesis), **R18.8** (Ascites [abdominal]), **D62** (Anemia, due to, blood loss, acute)

    ICD-9-CM: **578.0** (Hematemesis), **789.59** (Ascites), **285.1** (Anemia, due to, blood loss, acute)

Reports

43. Report 31: **45384** (Colonoscopy, Removal, Polyp)

    ICD-10-CM: **K63.5** (Polyp, colon)

    ICD-9-CM: **211.3** (Neoplasm, intestine, colon, Benign)

    Note: The entry listed under "Neoplasm, intestine, cecum, Benign" indicates 211.3, the same code as for the benign polyp of the colon and the code is only reported once.

45. Report 33: **44143** (Hartmann Procedure, Open), **43500-51** (Gastrotomy), **43830** (Gastrostomy, temporary)

    ICD-10-CM: **N49.3** (Disease, Fournier's); **T18.2XXA** (Foreign body, entering through orifice, stomach)

    ICD-9-CM: **608.83** (Fournier's disease, idiopathic gangrene), **935.2** (Foreign body, entering through, orifice, stomach)

47. Report 35: **43752** (Orogastric Tube Placement)

    ICD-10-CM: **K31.84** (Gastroparesis)

    ICD-9-CM: **536.3** (Gastroparesis)

CHAPTER 24: URINARY AND MALE GENITAL SYSTEMS

Theory

Urinary System Terminology

1. d

3. g

5. f

7. k

9. c

11. l

13. i

15. a

17. d

19. f

21. b

23. h

Male Genital Terminology

25. c

27. e

29. b

31. d

33. e

35. f

37. i

39. c

41. c

43. a

45. f

47. a

49. d

51. e

53. a

55. d

57. c

Practical

59. **50390** (Aspiration, Cyst, Kidney)

    ICD-10-CM: **N28.1** (Cyst, kidney, solitary, acquired)

    ICD-9-CM: **593.2** (Cyst, kidney, solitary)

61. **52450** (Incision, Prostate, Transurethral)

    ICD-10-CM: **N41.1** (Prostatitis, hypertrophic)

    ICD-9-CM: **600.00** (Prostatitis, hypertrophic)

63. **54650-50** (Orchiopexy, Abdominal Approach)

    ICD-10-CM: **Q53.21** (Nondescent, testicles, bilateral, abdominal)

    ICD-9-CM: **752.51** (Undescended, testis)

65. **50520** (Fistula, Kidney)

67. **53215** (Urethrectomy, Total, Male)

69. **53270** (Skene's Gland, Excision)

71. **55400** (Vasovasorrhaphy)

73. **54600** (Repair, Testis, Torsion)

75. **54056** (Destruction, Lesion, Penis, Cryosurgery)

77. **55100** (Abscess, Scrotum, Incision and Drainage)

Reports

79. Report 36: **52332-50** or **52332-RT** and **52332-LT** (Cystourethroscopy, Insertion, Indwelling Ureteral Stent)

81. Report 38: **53445** (Insertion, Prosthesis, Urethral Sphincter)

ICD-10-CM: **R32** (Incontinence), **Z85.46** (History, personal, malignant neoplasm, prostate)

ICD-9-CM: **788.30** (Incontinence), **V10.46** (History, personal, malignant neoplasm, prostate)

83. Report 82: **52630** (Transurethral Procedure, Prostate, Resection)

85. Report 84: **53852** (Transurethral Procedure, Prostate, Thermotherapy, Radiofrequency), **76872** (Ultrasound, rectal)

CHAPTER 25: REPRODUCTIVE, INTERSEX SURGERY, FEMALE GENITAL SYSTEM, AND MATERNITY CARE AND DELIVERY

Theory
Female Genital Terminology

1. d
3. h
5. b
7. m
9. c
11. j
13. f

Maternity Care and Delivery Terminology

15. e
17. g
19. f
21. j
23. l
25. o
27. i
29. n
31. introitus
33. colpocentesis
35. False
37. colposcope
39. loop electrode excision procedure
41. hysterectomy
43. Radiology
45. Oviduct/Ovary
47. trimesters
49. estimated date (of) delivery
51. E/M

Practical

53. **57400** (Dilation, Vagina)

55. **56441** (Adhesions, Labial, Lysis)

57. **58558** (Hysteroscopy, Surgical with Biopsy)

59. **58920** (Ovary, Wedge Resection)

61. **58800** (Cyst, Ovarian, Incision and Drainage)

63. **59514** (Cesarean Delivery, Delivery Only)

65. **59020** (Fetal Contraction Stress Test)

67. **56440** (Marsupialization, Bartholin's Gland, Cyst)

69. **57065** (Destruction, Lesion, Vagina, Extensive)

Reports

71. Report 28: **59409** (Vaginal Delivery, Delivery Only)

ICD-10-CM: **O76** (Delivery, complicated by, fetal, heart rate or rhythm), **O66.0** (Delivery, complicated. by, obstruction, due to, dystocia, shoulder), **O70.1** (Delivery, complicated, by, laceration, perineum, second degree), **Z37.0** (Outcome of delivery, single liveborn).

ICD-9-CM: **669.51** (Delivery, vacuum extractor), **659.71** (Delivery, fetal, heart rate or rhythm), **652.81** (Delivery, complicated, shoulder, presentation), **664.11** (Delivery, complicated, laceration, perineum, second degree, delivered), **V27.0** (Outcome of delivery, single liveborn)

Note: You report the delivery only because by reading this note you have no idea if the delivering physician was her regular obstetrician before and after delivery care.

73. Report 30: **59000** (Amniocentesis)

ICD-10-CM: **O09.293** (Pregnancy, complicated by, poor obstetric history), **Z36** (Screening (for), antenal (of mother)), **Z87.448** (History, personal, disorder, urinary system, specified NEC)

ICD-9-CM: **V23.49** (History of, obstetrical disorder, affecting management of current, pregnancy), **V28.2** (Screening (for) antenal, of mother, based on amniocentesis), **V13.09** (History, personal, disorder, urinary system, specified NEC)

CHAPTER 26: ENDOCRINE AND NERVOUS SYSTEMS

Theory

Endocrine System Terminology

1. c

3. f

5. d

7. g

9. h

11. b

Nervous System Terminology

13. g
15. h
17. b
19. d

Practical

21. **60000** (Thyroid Gland, Cyst, Incision and Drainage)
23. **64840** (Suture, Nerve)
25. **64831** (Repair, Nerve, Suture), **69990** (Operating Microscope)
27. **62311** (Injection, Spinal Cord, Anesthetic)
29. **61619** (Skull Base Surgery, Dura, Repair of Cerebrospinal Fluid Leak)
31. **63030** (Hemilaminectomy), **63035** (Hemilaminectomy)

Reports

33. Report 43: **63030-RT** (Hemilaminectomy)

   ICD-10-CM: **M51.16** (Displacement, intervertebral disc, lumbar, with neuritis, radiculitis, sciatica, or other pain)

   ICD-9-CM: **722.10** (Displacement, intervertebral disc, [with neuritis, radiculitis, sciatica, or other pain], lumbar)

CHAPTER 27: EYE, OCULAR ADNEXA, AUDITORY, AND OPERATING MICROSCOPE

Theory

Eye and Ocular Adnexa Terminology

1. a
3. b
5. c
7. d
9. i
11. g
13. k
15. f
17. d
19. h
21. j

Auditory System Terminology

23. g
25. n
27. h
29. i
31. k
33. a
35. c
37. l

Practical

39. **67570-RT** (Decompression, Optic Nerve)

41. **69620-LT** (Myringoplasty)

43. **69661** (Stapedectomy, with Footplate Drill Out)

Reports

45. Report 85: **66720-RT** (Glaucoma, Cryotherapy)

    ICD-10-CM: **H40.10X3** (Glaucoma, open-angle)

    ICD-9-CM: **365.10** (Glaucoma, open-angle); **365.73** (Glaucoma, severe stage)

47. Report 87: **66984-RT** (Cataract, Removal, Extraction, Extracapsular)

CHAPTER 28: RADIOLOGY

Theory

1. c
3. b
5. a
7. b
9. f
11. a
13. e
15. i
17. h
19. j
21. c

Practical

23. **78499** (Nuclear Medicine, Heart, Unlisted Services and Procedures)

25. -26

27. **75705** (Angiography, Spinal Artery)

29. **70130** (X-Ray, Mastoids)

31. **70542** (Magnetic Resonance Imaging [MRI], Neck)

33. **73510** (X-Ray, Hip)

35. **76098** (X-Ray, Specimen/Surgical)

37. **99219** for initial observation care (Evaluation and Management, Hospital Services, Observation Care); **70450** for CT Scan without mention of contrast (CT Scan, without Contrast), **76516** for A-scan (Ultrasound, Eye, Biometry); **77261** for therapeutic radiation (Radiation Therapy Planning); **77402** for radiation delivery of single treatment area (Radiation Therapy, Treatment Delivery, Single); **77427** for weekly radiology therapy management (Radiation Therapy, Treatment Delivery, Weekly)

39. **76604** (Ultrasound, Chest); **71550** for the MRI (Magnetic Resonance Imaging, Chest); **33020** for the pericardiotomy (Pericardiotomy, Removal, Clot)

41. **73092** (X-Ray, Arm, Upper)

43. **77002** (Fluoroscopy, Needle Biopsy)

45. **76872** (Ultrasound, Rectal)
47. **72240** (Myelography, Spine, Cervical)
49. **70140** (X-Ray, Facial Bones)
51. **74010** (X-Ray, Abdomen)
53. **75870** (Venography, Sagittal Sinus)
    ICD-10-CM: **G08** (Thrombosis, sinus, intracranial)
    ICD-9-CM: **325** (Thrombosis, sinus, intracranial)
55. **75945** (Ultrasound, Non-Coronary, Intravascular)
    ICD-10-CM: **I70.1** (Stenosis, artery, renal)
    ICD-9-CM: **440.1** (Stenosis, artery, renal)

Reports

57. Report 45: **71010** (X-Ray, Chest)
    ICD-10-CM: **R07.9** (Pain, chest)
    ICD-9-CM: **786.50** (Pain, chest)
59. Report 47: **70480-26** (CT Scan, without Contrast, Orbit)
    ICD-10-CM: **H57.12** (Pain, eye)
    ICD-9-CM: **379.91** (Pain[s], ocular)
61. Report 49: **74000-26** (X-Ray, Abdomen)
    ICD-10-CM: **E46** (Malnutrition)
    ICD-9-CM: **263.9** (Malnutrition)
63. Report 51: **74160-26** (CT, with Contrast, Abdomen)
    ICD-10-CM: **R94.5** (Findings, abnormal, inconclusive, function study, liver)
    ICD-9-CM: **794.8** (Findings, abnormal, function study, liver)
65. Report 53: **78451-26** (Myocardial, Perfusion Imaging)
    ICD-10-CM: **R07.9** (Pain[s], chest), **R06.02** (Shortness, breath)
    ICD-9-CM: **786.50** (Pain, chest), **786.05** (Shortness, breath)

CHAPTER 29: PATHOLOGY/LABORATORY

Theory

1. Surgery
3. presence, amount or amount, presence
5. section
7. one

Practical

9. **84520** (Urea Nitrogen, Quantitative), **84295** (Sodium), **84132** (Potassium), **82565** (Creatinine, Blood), **84550** (Uric Acid, Blood)
   ICD-10-CM: **E86.0** (Dehydration), **M25.50** (Pain, joint), **R50.9** (Fever)
   ICD-9-CM: **276.51** (Dehydration), **719.40** (Pain, joint), **780.60** (Fever)
   Note: The Blood Urea Nitrogen (BUN) is part of the blood chemistry for this patient, and there are two codes for blood as the source of the sample—84520 and 84525. Although there are other CPT codes to

identify urea nitrogen, the source of the sample for those codes is the urine (84540, 84545).

11. **80076** (Blood Tests, Panels, Hepatic Function), **80061** (Blood Tests, Panels, Lipid Panel)

 ICD-10-CM: **E78.5** (Hyperlipidemia)

 ICD-9-CM: **272.4** (Hyperlipidemia)

13. **80162** (Digoxin, Assay)

 ICD-10-CM: **I48.2** (Fibrillation, atrial)

 ICD-9-CM: **427.31** (Fibrillation, atrial)

Reports

15. Report 55: **88305** Urinary Bladder (Pathology, Surgical, Gross and Micro Exam, Level IV)

 ICD-10-CM: **D09.0** (Neoplasm, bladder, Malignant Ca in-situ)

 ICD-9-CM: **233.7** (Neoplasm, bladder, Malignant, Ca in situ)

17. Report 57: **88304** Intervertebral Disc (Pathology, Surgical, Gross and Micro Exam, Level III)

 ICD-10-CM: **M51.26** (Displacement, intervertebral disc, lumbar region)

 ICD-9-CM: **722.10** (Displacement, intervertebral disc, lumbar, lumbosacral)

19. Report 59: **88305** Muscle (Pathology, Surgical, Gross and Micro Exam, Level IV)

 ICD-10-CM: **D17.1** (Lipoma)

 ICD-9-CM: **728.2** (Atrophy, muscle, muscular)

21. Report 61: **88304** Skin Cyst (Pathology, Surgical, Gross and Micro Exam, Level III)

 ICD-10-CM: **L72.9** (Cyst, skin)

 ICD-9-CM: **706.2** (Cyst, skin)

23. Report 63: **88307** Liver (Pathology, Surgical, Gross and Micro Exam, Level V)

 ICD-10-CM: **E66.01** (Obesity, morbid), **K76.0** (Fatty, liver)

 ICD-9-CM: **278.01** (Obesity, morbid); **571.8** (Fatty, liver)

25. Report 65: **88309** Lung Lobe (Pathology, Surgical, Gross and Micro Exam, Level VI)

 ICD-10-CM: **J85.2** (Abscess, lung)

 ICD-9-CM: **513.0** (Abscess, lung)

27. Report 67: **88104** (Cytopathology, Fluids, Washings, Brushings)

 ICD-10-CM: **J90** (Effusion, pleura)

 ICD-9-CM: **511.9** (Effusion, pleura)

CHAPTER 30: MEDICINE

Theory

1. m

3. h

5. n

7. i

9. g

11. l

13. a

15. g

17. f

19. a

21. c

23. hearing test

25. stimulation of the cochlea to measure electrical activity

27. studying the capillaries of the eyes

29. a device for detecting color blindness

31. cornea and sclera together forming one organ

33. the thick outer coat of the eye, mostly white and opaque

Practical

35. **95052** × 2 (Allergy Tests, Patch, Photo Patch)

37. **92341** (Spectacle Services, Fitting, Spectacles)

39. **92534** (Nystagmus Tests, Optokinetic)

41. **91034** (Esophagus, Acid Reflux Tests)

43. **90880** (Hypnotherapy)

45. **92626** (Rehabilitation, Auditory, Status Evaluation)

47. **90940** (Hemodialysis, Blood Flow Study)

49. **93503** (Catheterization, Cardiac, Flow Directed)

51. **94003** (Ventilation Assist)

    ICD-10-CM: **J96.00** (Failure, respiration, respiratory, acute)

    ICD-9-CM: **518.81** (Failure, respiration, respiratory, acute)

53. **99144** (Sedation, Moderate)

55. **90471** (Administration, Immunization, One Vaccine/Toxoid), **90472** (Administration, Immunization, each additional Vaccine/Toxoid)

57. ICD-10-CM: **I21.19** (Infarct, myocardium), **I23.1** (Defect, atrium, acquired)

    ICD-9-CM: **410.21** (Infarct, myocardium), **429.71** (Defect, atrial septal, acquired)

Reports

59. Report 68: **99203** (Office and/or Other Outpatient Services, New Patient)

    ICD-10-CM: **I25.10** (Arteriosclerosis, coronary), **I10** (Hypertension), **N63** (Mass, breast), **Z95.1** (Status, coronary artery bypass), **Z79.890** (Long-term, hormone replacement), **Z82.49** (History, family, cardiovascular disease), **Z80.3** (History, family, malignant neoplasm, breast)

    ICD-9-CM: **414.01** (Arteriosclerosis, coronary, native artery), **401.9** (Hypertension, Unspecified), **611.72** (Mass, breast), **V45.81** (Status, coronary artery bypass), **V49.81** (Status, postmenopausal), **V17.49** (History, family, cardiovascular disease), **V16.3** (History, family, malignant neoplasm, breast)

61. Report 70: **99241** (Consultation, Office and/or Other Outpatient)

63. Report 72: **none,** as the admission is part of the surgical package

65. Report 74: **19307-LT** (Mastectomy, Modified Radical)

   ICD-10-CM: **C50.912** (Neoplasm, breast, Malignant Primary)

   ICD-9-CM: **174.9** (Neoplasm, breast, Malignant, Primary)

67. Report 76: **99252-57** (Consultation, Inpatient) modifier -57 indicates the decision for major surgery

   ICD-10-CM: **I97.89** (Complication, circulatory, system, post procedural), **M79.606** (Pain, leg)

   ICD-9-CM: **997.79** (Complication, vascular, postoperative, other vessels) for postoperative vascular complications, **729.5** (Pain, leg)

69. Report 78: **32554** (Thoracentesis)

   ICD-10-CM: **J90** (Effusion, pleural)

   ICD-9-CM: **511.9** (Effusion, pleura). Note that the report indicated the patient was developing respiratory failure; if the failure was confirmed, the diagnosis would be reported with **518.81** (Respiratory, failure).

   Note: The report indicated the patient was developing respiratory failure; if the failure was confirmed, the diagnosis would be reported with **J96.00** (Failure, respiration, respiratory, acute).

71. Report 80: **94060** (Spirometry), **94729** (Pulmonology, Diagnostic, Carbon Monoxide Diffusion Capacity), **99070** (Supplies, Materials) for the bronchodilator

CHAPTER 31: INPATIENT CODING

Theory

1. Inpatient

3. Outpatient

5. False

7. False

9. a

11. b

13. c

15. c

Sequencing Exercises

Cases of Principal Diagnosis and Other Diagnoses

17. Principal diagnosis: cellulitis ankle or leg

   Other diagnoses: none

19. Principal diagnosis: colon cancer, primary malignancy

   Other diagnoses: bone cancer, secondary

21. Principal diagnosis: menorrhagia

   Other diagnoses: acute, bronchitis, canceled surgery

23. Principal diagnosis: bronchitis with exacerbation [acute]

   Other diagnoses: none

Principal Diagnosis

25. **ICD-10-CM: Principal diagnosis and code:** Right orbital fracture, **S02.3XXA** (Fracture, traumatic, orbit, floor [blowout])

    Other diagnoses and codes:

    Right zygoma fracture **S02.44XA** (Fracture, traumatic, zygoma)

    Abrasion to head **S00.81XA** (Abrasion, forehead), S00.01XA (Abrasion, scalp)

    Assault by striking **Y00.XXXA** (External cause Code, Assault, weapon, blunt)

    Procedure: 0NRP0JZ implant (Replacement, Orbit, Right)

    ICD-9-CM: **Principal diagnosis and code: 802.6** (Fracture orbit, floor)

    Other diagnoses and codes:

    802.4 (Fracture, zygoma), **910.0** (Injury, superficial, head), **E968.2** (Index to external causes, Assault, weapon, blunt)

    Procedure: 76.92 implant (Implant, facial bone, synthetic)

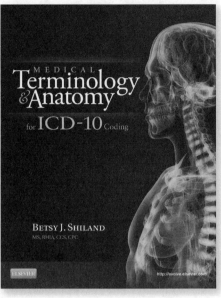
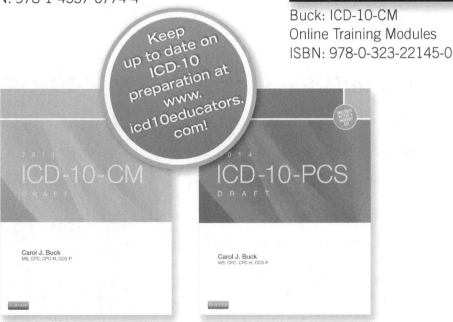

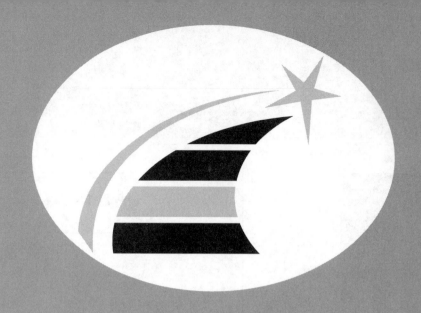

Step 2: Practice

"Before everything else, getting ready is the secret of success."

— Henry Ford

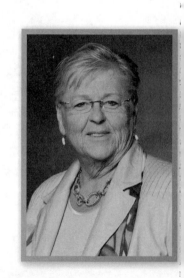

Thank you for pursuing excellence in your coding education! As coding becomes a more complex and specialized career, it is extremely important that we coders stay at the top of our coding game. That's why, as a lifelong coder and educator, I know that tools for more advanced learning and practice are crucial for today's top coders. ***Thank you for being committed to being one of the best and rising to the top in your career.***

— Carol J. Buck, MS, CPC, CPC-H, CCS-P

Track your progress!

See the checklist in the back of this book
to learn more about your next step toward coding success!

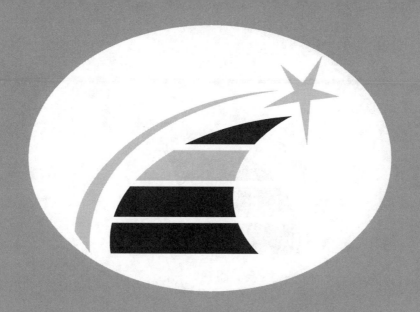

Step 3: Certify

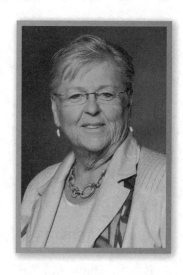

Congratulations on reaching the certification step in your career! As you know, certified coders are in top demand in today's marketplace. That's why, as a lifelong coder and educator, I have dedicated myself to providing the most up-to-date, comprehensive, and user-friendly certification review books on the market. I update these books every year so that you will have the best tools possible when studying for your certification exam.

It's time to hit the books. ***You can do it! I know you can!***

— Carol J. Buck, MS, CPC, CPC-H, CCS-P

Track your progress!

See the checklist in the back of this book
to learn more about your next step toward coding success!

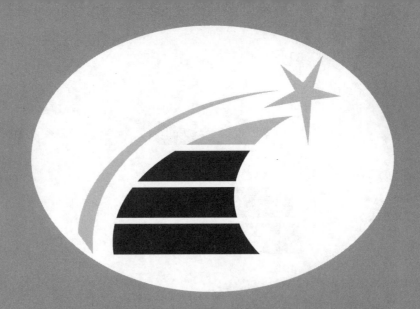

Step 4:
Professional Resources

"Nothing is particularly hard if you divide it into small jobs."

— Henry Ford

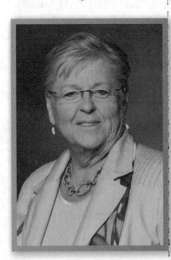

As you reach higher and more specialized levels of coding, I want to applaud you for taking this step in your career. You won't be disappointed. Specialized coders are like rare gems—**they are harder to find and greatly valued** in the profession.

— Carol J. Buck, MS, CPC, CPC-H, CCS-P

Track your progress!

See the checklist in the back of this book
to learn more about your steps toward coding success!

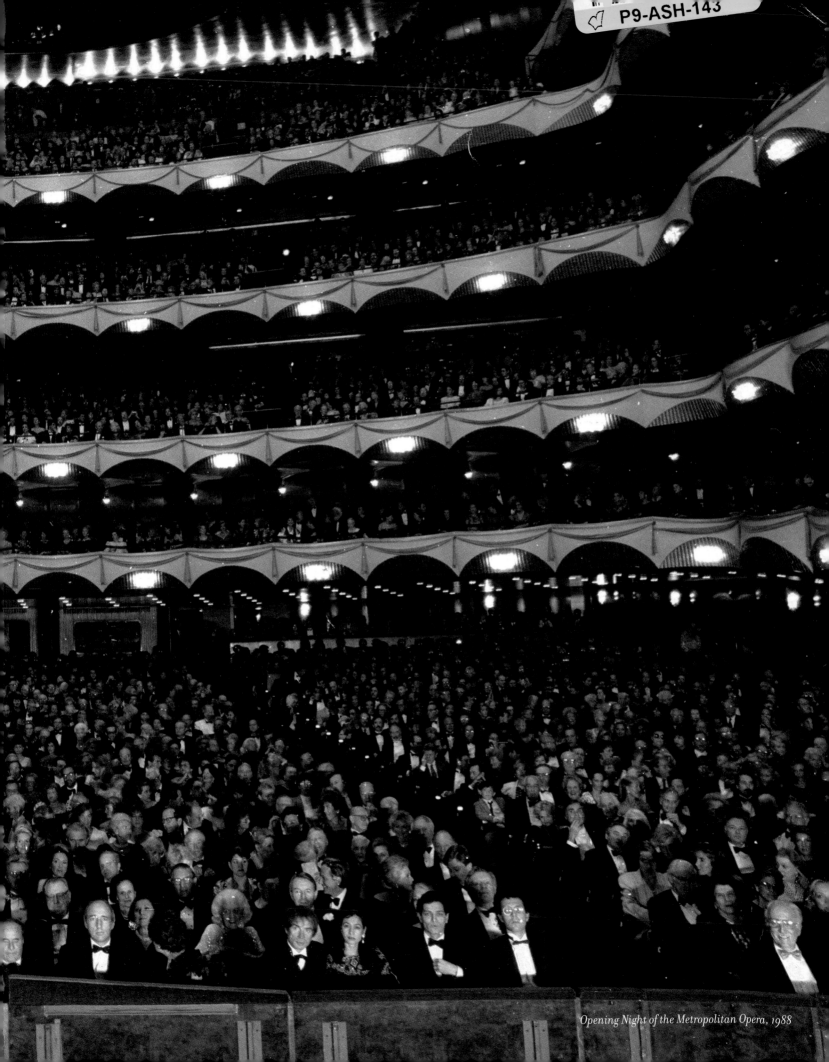

Opening Night of the Metropolitan Opera, 1988

James Levine

40 YEARS at The Metropolitan Opera

James Levine

40 YEARS at The Metropolitan Opera

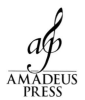

AMADEUS
PRESS

AN IMPRINT OF HAL LEONARD CORPORATION

Published in 2011 by Amadeus Press
An Imprint of Hal Leonard Corporation
7777 West Bluemound Road
Milwaukee, WI 53213

Trade Book Division Editorial Offices
33 Plymouth St., Montclair, NJ 07042

www.amadeuspress.com

Editorial Director
Elena Park

Senior Editor
Ellen Keel

Associate Editor
Casey Elsass

Contributing Editors
Katrine Ames, Matt Dobkin

Design
AdamsMorioka, Inc.

Managing Editor
Hilary Ley

Met Archivist
Robert Tuggle

Special thanks to the friends and colleagues of Maestro Levine who contributed to the book.
Additional thanks to Amadeus Press, Research Editor Michael Griebel, Editorial Coordinator
Matthew Principe, and Photo Researcher Jonathan Tichler, as well as Philipp Brieler,
Jonathan Friend, Matthew Galek, Mary Jo Heath, Ken Hunt, Kit Morrison, and Rose Schwartz.

Printed in the United States of America

Library of Congress Cataloging-in-Publication Data

James Levine : 40 years at the Metropolitan Opera.
   p. cm.
Includes discography and index.
ISBN 978-1-57467-196-4
1. Levine, James, 1943- 2. Metropolitan Opera (New York, N.Y.)—History.
ML422.L67J35 2011
782.1092—dc22
[B]   2011007606

For me, Jim was the first "love conductor," versus
the old-time "fear conductors." I'm old enough to
have worked with Karajan, Böhm, Bernstein, Solti,
Leinsdorf, Reiner... They were great conductors,
but when you looked down at the pit, you were a little
afraid. With Jim you have huge respect—and love.
   —*Sherrill Milnes*

He's unbelievably generous with his gift. He creates
a space filled with love of what he's doing, as if he
would rather be doing that than anything in the world,
and he makes you part of it.
   —*Frederica von Stade*

Contents

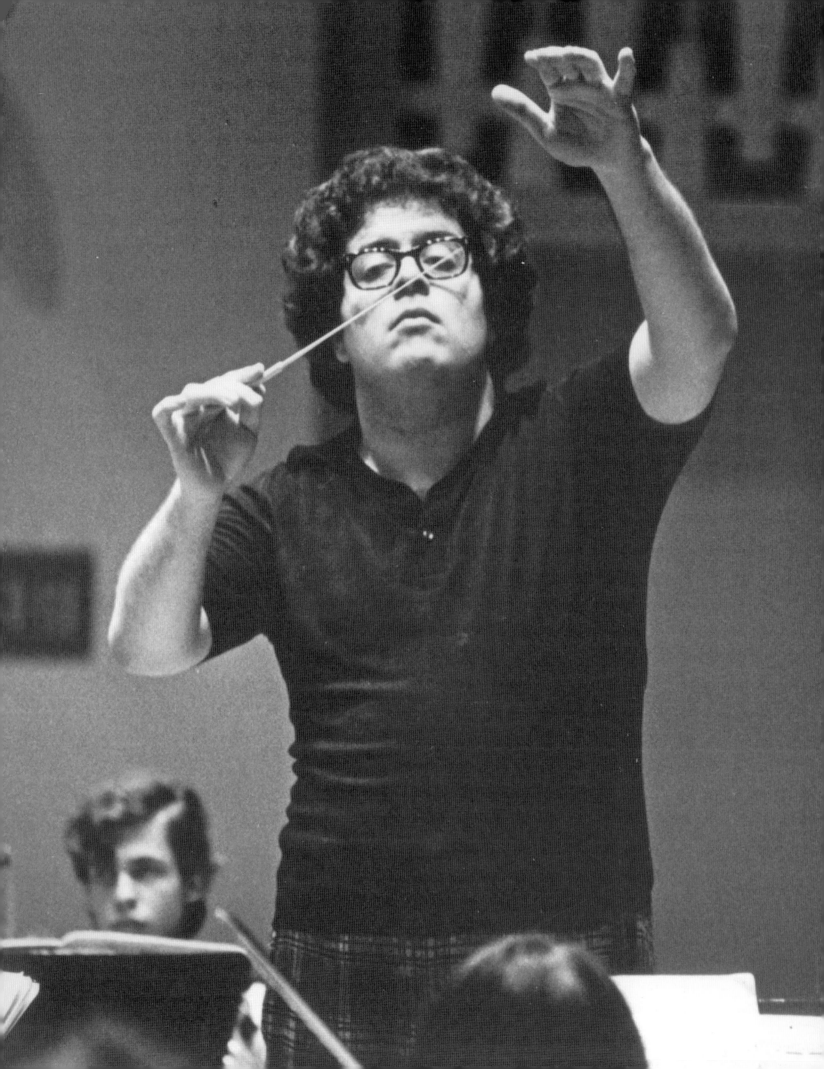

Foreword

PETER GELB

General Manager, Metropolitan Opera

This book is filled with loving and informed commentary about one of the most beloved and legendary conductors of all time. It is also full of James Levine's own frank commentary, providing a revealing glimpse into his unparalleled 40-year run at the Met.

In 1971, when Jim made his noteworthy debut at the Met, I was working there as a part-time usher, still in my teens. But it wasn't until some years later, when I worked with Jim on some television projects, that I was first exposed to his masterful approach with singers and orchestras. Jim didn't merely conduct everything extraordinarily; he was also a genius at human relations—flattering, cajoling, and ultimately inspiring his forces to greater heights.

In the 1980s, I approached Jim with the idea of a special concert program of spirituals, starring Kathleen Battle and Jessye Norman. They were two of the greatest soprano stars of the Met—but not necessarily considered to be a compatible pairing. I immediately realized that only Jim and his finely honed persuasive skills could manage this high-wattage duo. As he guided them through the rehearsals, carefully balancing solos and duets, he was an effervescent and soothing force. With tensions running a little high, Jim would choose to reinforce only the positive aspects of the rehearsals. "That really tickles me," he told them both. How could any diva not behave after a compliment like that?

For 40 years, Jim has been enveloping singers and instrumentalists with his energetic, but tender approach. So, it's really no surprise that this book contains so many warm accounts from his many admirers. Of course, not everyone who has been exposed to the Levine treatment is immediately enthralled. About 25 years ago, I remember one slightly suspicious member of the Vienna Philharmonic saying to me, "Why is he so nice to us?" At the time, I didn't quite know how to respond. Today, I would surely say, "To make you play better."

Musician with a Conscience

MARTIN BERNHEIMER

James Levine isn't like most conductors.

He doesn't do a lot of deep emoting on the podium. He doesn't go in for conspicuous perspiration. If he does a lot of sweating, he does it in rehearsals. He's not a frantic dancer or a daring acrobat. He doesn't exert a lot of picturesque energy stomping or flailing or leaping. He doesn't choreograph showy cues when his players don't need them. He simply lavishes his attention on the people working in front of him, not on the people sitting behind him.

He doesn't live on jet planes, flitting from city to city to city in short-term quest of hit-and-run adventure. He doesn't place his own ego before that of the composer. He doesn't concentrate on a short list of hum-along hits for clap-happy audiences. He takes chances in matters of repertory—an astonishingly diverse repertory—but not in matters of interpretation.

He likes to rehearse and polish. He likes to watch things grow. A virtuoso technician and a stubborn perfectionist, he shows a healthy respect for tradition. But he certainly isn't paralyzed by that respect.

Essentially, he's a musician blessed with a conscience. Even when confronting old war-horses, he enjoys the saving graces of flair and imagination. His sense of proportion invariably precludes breaching any bonds of taste.

Levine savors the stability and intimacy of long-term relationships—40 years so far at the Met, 23 summers with the Chicago Symphony at Ravinia, 18 festivals in Salzburg, 15 in Bayreuth. His early experience as assistant to George Szell in Cleveland no doubt taught him the interpretive virtues of discipline and economy. His dedication to the world of opera has taught him the value of lyricism, a quest for the graceful vocal line even when it happens to be sung by instruments in a symphonic context.

He works on a broad dynamic scale, and in flights of romantic generosity tends to favor slow tempos. The tempos never seem sluggish, just spacious. This conductor knows how to explore meaningful detail, how to maintain linear tension, how to keep the rhythmic pulse vital and the textures clear. This conductor is sensitive to subtle shifts in mood and color. With James Levine a leisurely pace leads to contemplation, and to grandeur.

Pulitzer Prize-winning critic Martin Bernheimer covers music in New York for the Financial Times *and* Opera *magazine. A version of this essay originally appeared in a program for the Verbier Festival.*

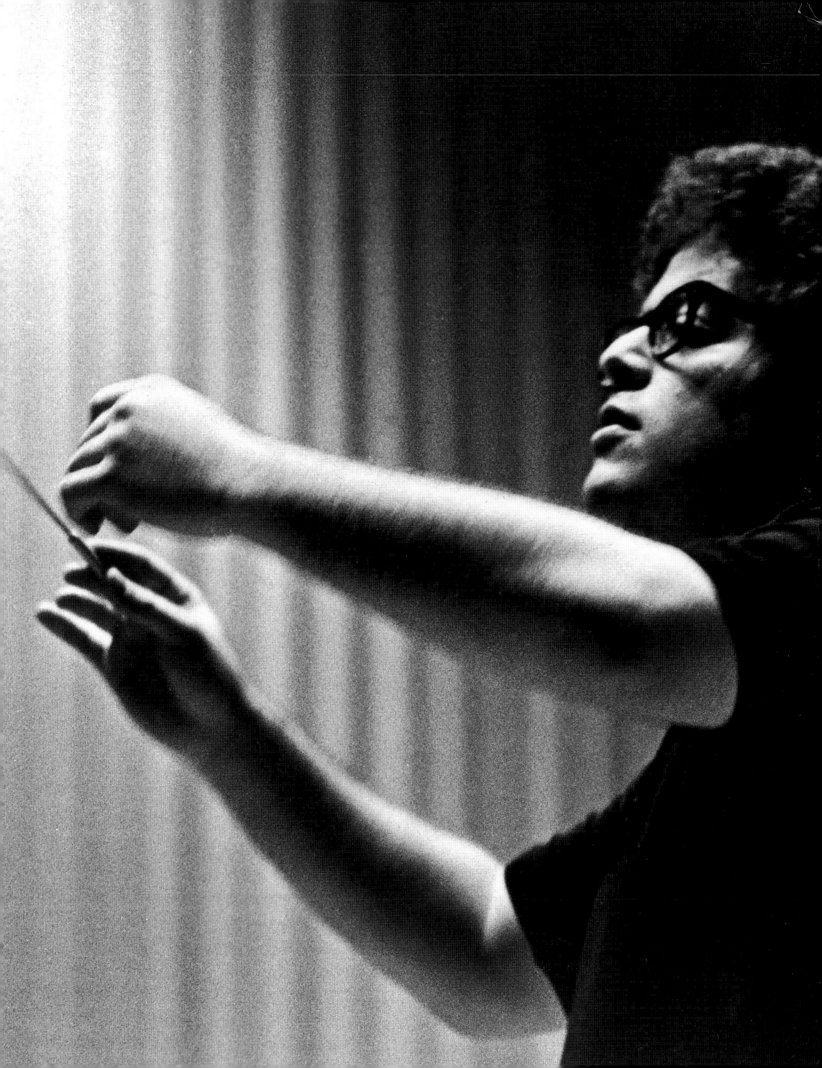

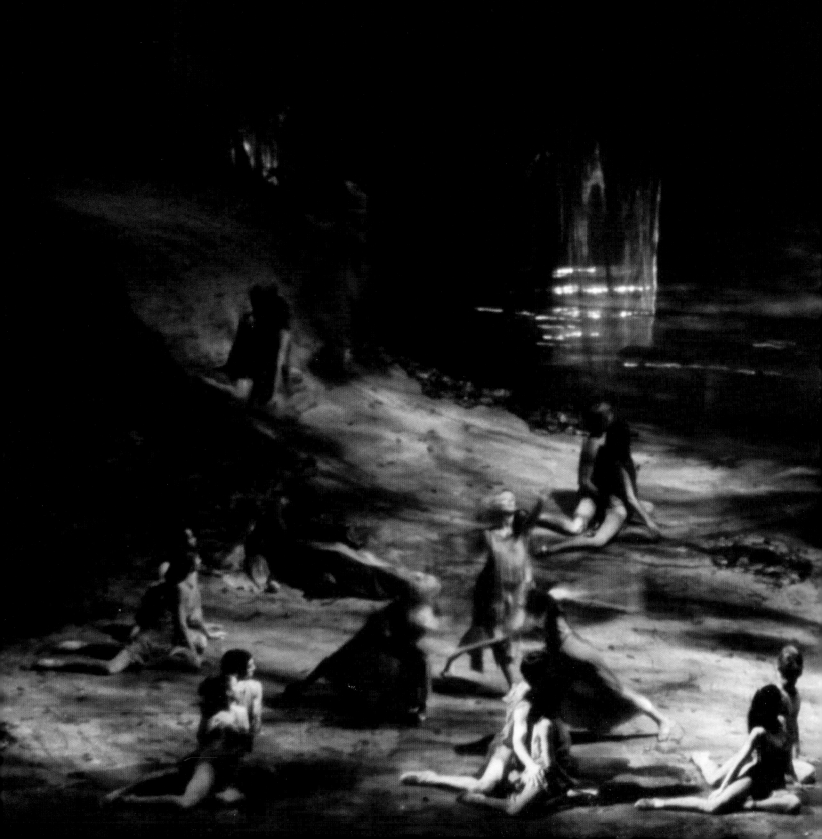

1970–1980

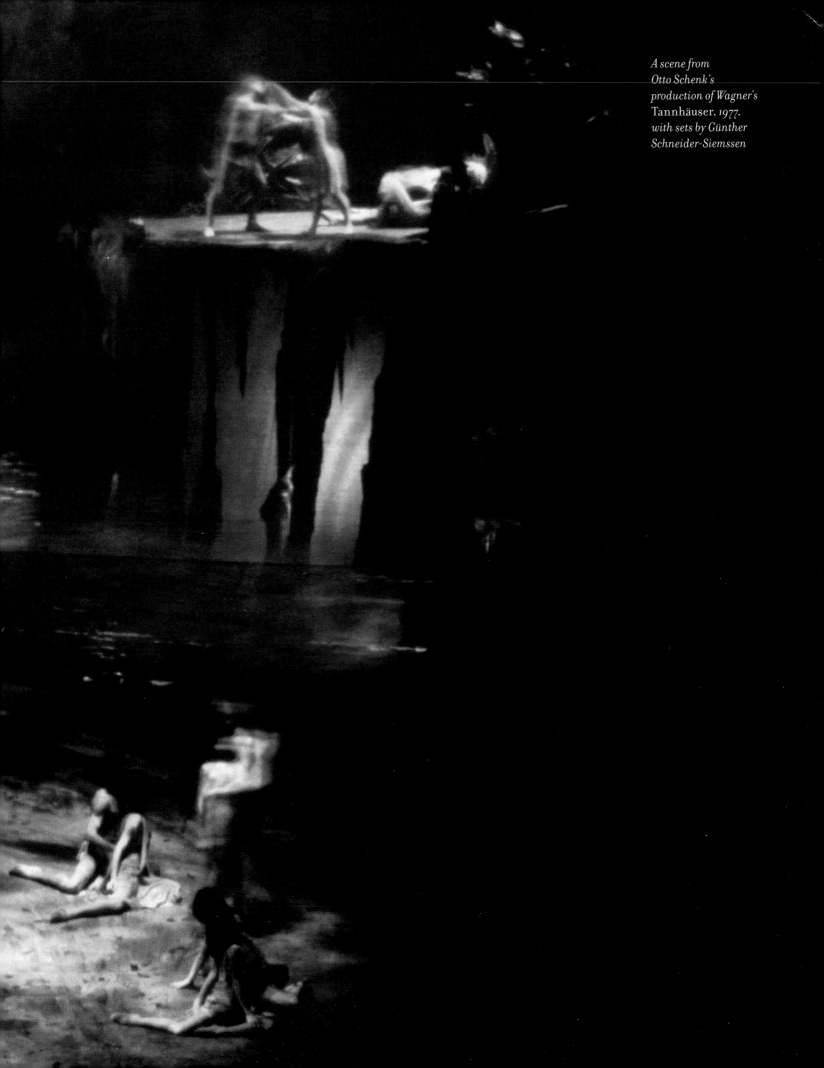

A scene from Otto Schenk's production of Wagner's Tannhäuser, *1977, with sets by Günther Schneider-Siemssen*

A Guiding Hand

HARVEY SACHS

When I was 20 years old I had a summer job in the publications office of The Cleveland Orchestra. George Szell was then Music Director and undisputed generalissimo of my home town's great local ensemble; he was supremely knowledgeable but also supremely tough and demanding in all matters musical. Paying compliments was definitely not his forte. But I remember staff people mentioning with amazement that Szell had been heard to express high hopes for one of his young assistant conductors—a certain James Levine—whom he considered to be exceptionally gifted.

One day, a curly-haired young man came into the office, introduced himself as Jimmy Levine, and told me that he sometimes listened to a radio program that I hosted on a local FM station; the program was dedicated to the recordings of Arturo Toscanini, and Jimmy said that he was a great admirer of the Maestro. He knew a lot about historic performers and different approaches to musical interpretation, and it was immediately clear that he was a musician who wanted not only to get the notes right and perform them convincingly— he wanted to dig beneath the surface, to figure out why it made more sense to do a piece at a certain tempo rather than another, to break or not to break a melodic line at a certain point, to accentuate a certain harmonic shift or let it speak for itself. Jimmy was voluble, enthusiastic, and impressive—even before I had heard him conduct a note.

That was back in 1966. Szell died in 1970, and within a very few years the high hopes he had expressed for his young assistant had been fulfilled. In the decades that followed those hopes were fulfilled many times over: James Levine has worked all over the world with the greatest orchestras and singers—and most significant of all, he has been the Metropolitan Opera's moving force for most of his life.

As a teenager, I had listened to Toscanini's impassioned yet disciplined recordings day after day and to Szell's meticulously prepared Cleveland Orchestra week after week, and I used to find the Met's Saturday afternoon radio broadcasts puzzling. Of course there were outstanding singers, but the ensemble as a whole seemed to lack direction and distinction. The orchestra was often ragged, even when renowned conductors were at the helm; coordination between stage and pit seemed frayed; and—when outstanding conductors were not at the helm—each singer seemed to do more or less what he or she felt like doing at any given moment without necessarily paying much attention to what colleagues were doing. I probably couldn't have expressed the problem at the time, but what was missing was the guiding hand of a conductor who possessed both artistic vision and the ability to work steadily at improving and coordinating each of the ensemble's musical components. Mahler and Toscanini had no doubt achieved such standards and enforced unifying musical-dramatic concepts during their relatively short conductorships at the Met a hundred years ago, but they were able to use terror tactics that had become unacceptable by the 1960s. Also, at the turn of the last century most of the members of major American orchestras had been born and trained in Europe and were accustomed to the iron discipline that prevailed there at the time and that American-trained musicians today would not tolerate. In this country and in our day, an orchestra with excellent personnel plus internal pride and esprit de corps can achieve anything, but a demoralized or fragmented orchestra will never rise above average, no matter how good its individual elements may be.

Levine's early Met appearances, beginning with his 1971 debut, coincided with a series of administrative changes, both planned and accidental, within the company, and those changes made the need for fresh thinking and first-rate music-making all the more imperative. He was the right man in the right place at the right time. Appointed Principal Conductor in 1973, at the age of 30, and Music Director three years later, he brought to his tasks a winning combination of qualities: tremendous talent, knowledge, and curiosity; considerable experience (he had already worked with most of the major American

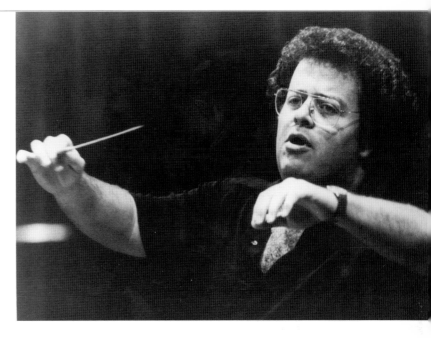

orchestras and several major opera ensembles here and abroad); awareness of and respect for what was then the company's nearly century-long history and for its remarkable accomplishments; a naturally outgoing personality; and a truly collaborative spirit. When the going gets rough—as inevitably happens at times within such a gigantic operation as the Met—Levine is perfectly capable of laying down the law, but he would much rather coach and convince than demand or dictate.

With the combination of enjoyment, patience, and insistence that are the hallmarks of his approach to music-making, Levine began to hone the ensemble, and within a very few years the results were evident to anyone who had a good pair of ears. Today, there is no other opera ensemble in the world that can compare to the Met in both the quantity and the quality of the work it produces. Nearly 2,500 performances after his debut, Levine is still at the helm of this fantastic mechanism, putting the finest craftsmanship at the service of high art day after day and year after year. Other conductors who work at the Met are astonished by the standards that have been achieved.

Yet despite all the admiration and love that flow in his direction, Levine's frankness on the subject of the limits of a conductor's power is refreshing. "You rehearse a piece, you try to reach a point where you're doing what you think you should be doing with it," he says, "and then, when you perform it before a full house, you try to do the same thing, as closely as possible. But once rehearsals are over, conductors are not protagonists. They're on hand to guide, organize, and even inspire the people who are making the sounds, but they themselves are not making those sounds." This is not false modesty: this is an honest and correct job description for conductors—gifted and serious conductors, at any rate.

There is always a potential conflict between a composer's wishes and a performer's musical sensibility and approach to interpretation. Most composers want their works to be performed according to their intentions, without extraneous ideas injected—but not slavishly or spinelessly by performers who lack strong intelligence and personality. One artist's work may be conscientious but bland; another's may be flavorful but wrong-headed. The problem is how to reach an ideal mixture of conscientiousness and imagination, with a great deal of conviction to support both. This is the balance that James Levine has been seeking and finding throughout his artistic life. Walter Levin, first violin of the legendary LaSalle String Quartet, which was in residence at the University of Cincinnati when young Jimmy was growing up in the city, has told of the explosive talent and endless curiosity of the budding, 11-year-old musician whom he took under his wing in the mid-1950s. Fortunately, the brilliance has never dimmed, nor has the two-pronged desire to explore new musical horizons and to dig deeper and deeper into familiar works.

James Levine's contribution to the Metropolitan Opera, to the musical life of New York City and beyond, and to the art of musical performance cannot be overestimated. His 40th Met anniversary gives all of us who have benefited from his work an opportunity to tell him how grateful we are and to give him our very best—and not entirely unselfish—wishes for the future.

Harvey Sachs's most recent book is The Ninth: Beethoven and the World in 1824 *(Random House, 2010). The biographer of Arturo Toscanini and Arthur Rubinstein, he is on the faculty of the Curtis Institute of Music.*

Milton Babbitt, composer: I first heard of this pudgy little boy of 13 when he was at the Marlboro Festival for chamber music, running around with a piano part of the Schubert Quintet looking for someone to play it with him. My next awareness of him was in the mid '60s, when George Szell turned over The Cleveland Orchestra to Gunther Schuller for a program of contemporary music, and Gunther chose to conduct my *Relata I.* When I arrived at the first rehearsal, I found that little boy was now the pianist and assistant conductor for the orchestra. The rehearsals were not easy, but they were smoothed somewhat by the ability of this pianist to play every part, at the correct transposition, of course. The next big occasion was the result of my receiving a call from Herman Krawitz, then assistant manager of the Metropolitan Opera. He had asked me at an earlier time for the names of any young musicians who had impressed me. My list included Jimmy, but nothing came of it until Herman called and asked if I knew whether Jimmy knew *Tosca.* I couldn't be certain, but I told Herman that knowing the range of Jimmy's knowledge of the repertory he probably did. He did. The rest is music history.

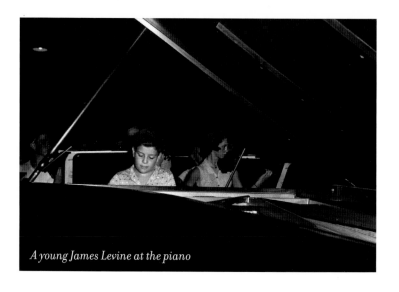

A young James Levine at the piano

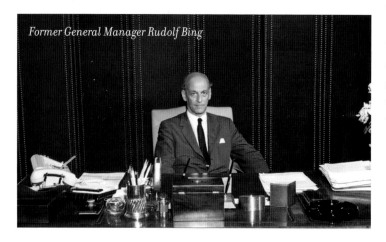

Former General Manager Rudolf Bing

James Levine: When I got the invitation, my strongest temptation was to turn it down. It wasn't what I saw myself doing as my first opera with the Met. I didn't know if I could put my best foot forward with that piece, or if the situation was harmonious for me at that moment. But Ronald Wilford [Levine's manager] asked me a very interesting question: "Can you do *Tosca* better than it's going these days in these circumstances?" I said I thought I probably could, and he strongly advised me to do it because then I would have the chance to change something and develop it. His perception was absolutely right.

1970
NOVEMBER 12

General Manager Rudolf Bing signs James
Levine to conduct seven performances of
Puccini's *Tosca* during the 1971–72 season.

CONDUCTOR (Per Performance)

METROPOLITAN OPERA ASSOCIATION, INC.
STANDARD CONDUCTOR'S CONTRACT (Per Performance)

AGREEMENT dated _Nov. 12_____, 19 70, made in the City, County and State of New York by and between METROPOLITAN OPERA ASSOCIATION, INC. (hereinafter called "Association") having its principal place of business at the Metropolitan Opera, Lincoln Center Plaza, Broadway at 64th Street, New York, New York 10023

and_____James Levine_____

residing at_____c/o Ronald Wilford, Columbia Artists Management,_____
_____165 West 57th street, New York, New York 10019_____

WITNESSETH: In consideration of the mutual agreements herein contained, the parties agree as follows:

PERIOD OF ENGAGEMENT:

Association hereby engages your services as a conductor and you agree to render such services for a minimum of _____seven (7)_____ performances within the period(s):

From_____November 1, 1971_____ through_____December 17, 1971_____,

From_____through_____, and

From_____through_____,

inclusive.

COMPENSATION:

Association agrees to pay and you agree to accept the sum of _____seven hundred_____ ($_700._____) Dollars per performance. Any additional performances as elected by Association shall be compensated at the same fee.

REHEARSAL WEEKS:

In addition, you shall be available for _____two (2)_____ rehearsal weeks(s) from _October 18, 1971_____ to _____October 31, 1971*_____ without additional compensation.

*You will not be required to rehearse on October 18 and 19, 1971

REPERTOIRE:

It is agreed that the work(s) you will conduct will be _____TOSCA_____

provided, however, that if presently unforeseen scheduling or repertorial changes should occur which would make your conducting of the aforementioned work(s) impracticable, we shall have the right to substitute other works within your repertoire therefor, but only after prior consultation with you.

~~ROAD TOUR:~~

~~Association shall have the right to engage you following the close of the regular New York season for such number of performances as Association may elect within a period of not more than~~ _ ~~weeks on the same terms, by notifying you in writing not later than December 31st immediately preceding such tour. While on tour you will receive the per diem allowance set forth in the Basic Agreement between our Musical Staff and Local 802 for each day you are required by Association to be outside New York City in connection with its performances.~~

OTHER TERMS:

This agreement is subject to and includes all the terms and conditions contained in the Basic Agreement between Association and Local 802 and in Schedule A annexed hereto, which schedule is incorporated herein and made a part hereof in the same manner as if fully set forth herein.

IN WITNESS WHEREOF, this contract has been executed by the parties as of the date first above written.

METROPOLITAN OPERA ASSOCIATION, INC.

James L. Levine
(Signature)

By_____
(General Manager)

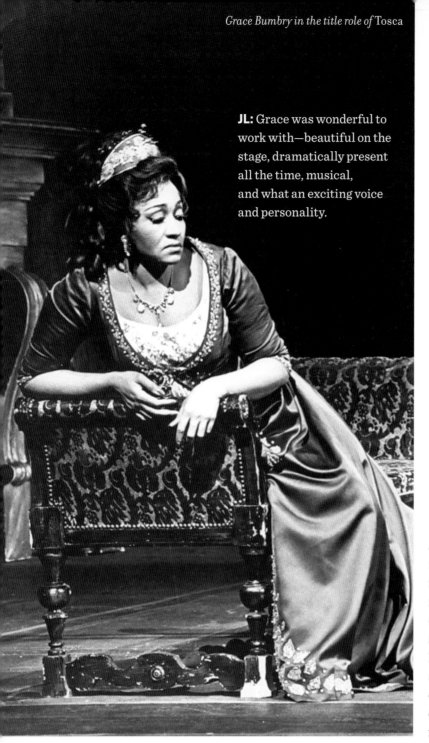

Grace Bumbry in the title role of Tosca

JL: Grace was wonderful to work with—beautiful on the stage, dramatically present all the time, musical, and what an exciting voice and personality.

JL: Richard Tucker was the last person to call me in my dressing room before I went to the pit for *Tosca*. He was a friend of mine from when I was a kid, a family friend. The phone rang at five minutes to, and when I picked it up: "Jim, it's Richard. Knock 'em dead." He gave me a little two-minute pep talk in the light speaking voice he used when he was resting, and it was so sweet. I was waiting for the stage manager's call to come, and I felt like a racehorse, raring to go. I wasn't nervous at all. It was a perfect case of somebody doing what they're put there to do. I was so excited and happy and so looking forward to it, that I couldn't find any nervousness.

1971
JANUARY 22

A new contract for two *Tosca*s in June 1971
moves his debut forward a season.

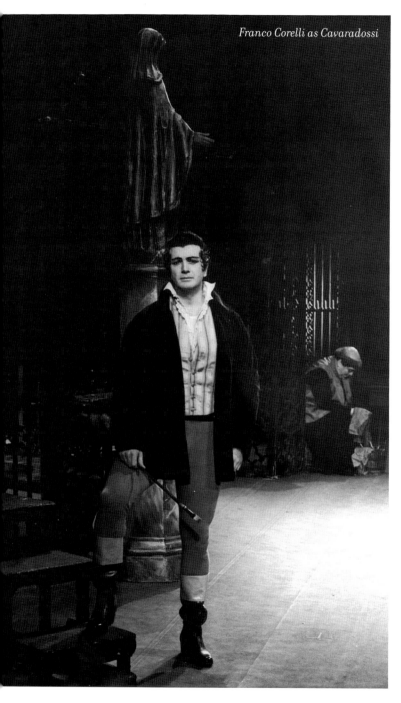

Franco Corelli as Cavaradossi

JL: Franco was an extraordinary singer in every respect, but sometimes very nervous, and I think it was important for him to know that I was there for him, that he wasn't going to have to fend for himself. We had an absolutely wonderful first session together. He was experimenting with something technical that wasn't really working well. But sometimes, working on interpretive content and communication can spill over into technique, and by the time we finished our session, he had modified things so that they worked. He was happy, and I was thrilled. That was the only time I conducted for Franco, and I wish I'd worked with him again. I used to just go and listen to him sing, and it burned on my brain. What a god of a tenor.

JUNE 5

Just short of his 28th birthday, he makes his Met debut conducting *Tosca,* starring Grace Bumbry in her role debut, Franco Corelli, and Peter Glossop in his House debut.

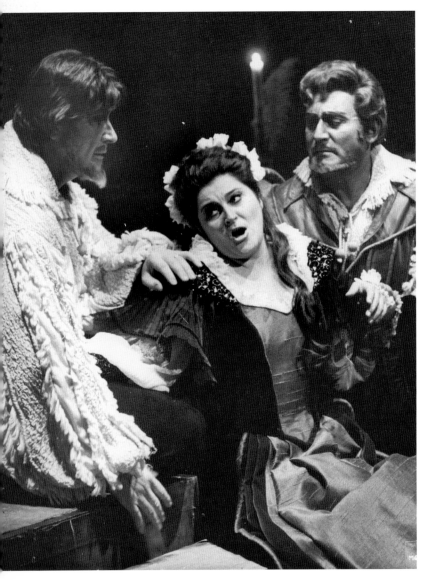

JL: I came at my repertoire at the Met from Italian pieces to German, but that was only a question of what they needed me to do. Fausto Cleva died that summer, so they needed a conductor for *Luisa Miller*. It was sort of my favorite of the then lesser-known and not-so-accessible Verdi operas. I loved Verdi as much as I love anything, and I had studied with Cleva and was close to him. I offered myself to Mr. Bing because I thought there wouldn't be any way he would know I had *Luisa Miller* in my head. And the minute he found out he said, "Please." It turned out to be a piece I did relatively frequently at the Met. That was an example of the kind of Verdi opera Mr. Bing added to the repertoire, thank God, because he had the most wonderful singers for it: Caballé, Tucker, and Milnes, and in this first revival, Adriana Maliponte sang the title role—beautiful singer she was. And also Tucker was there—my God, he was incredible! He was dressed in a doublet and black tights, and I tell you, he believed himself in it and sang marvelously with all his unique élan, style, and enthusiasm.

Sherrill Milnes as Miller and Richard Tucker as Rodolfo with Adriana Maliponte in the title role of Luisa Miller

OCTOBER 15

Luisa Miller is his first Verdi opera at the Met, starring Adriana Maliponte, Richard Tucker, Sherrill Milnes, Ruggero Raimondi, and Paul Plishka.

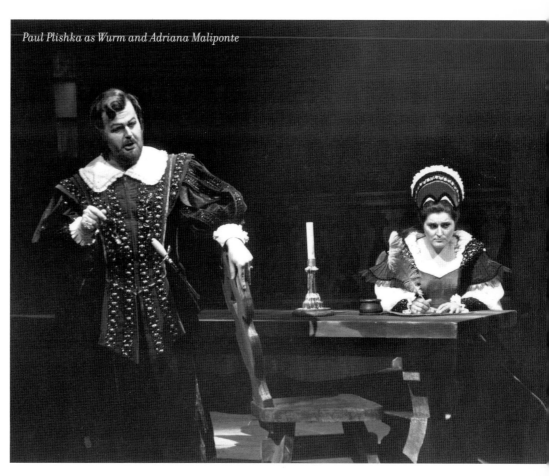

Paul Plishka: When Jimmy made his debut with *Tosca,* I sang the role of the Sacristan, and shortly after that I did Wurm in *Luisa Miller* with him. Fausto Cleva, a really tough old guy whom I was a little afraid of, was supposed to conduct, but unfortunately, he passed away a few months before, and Jimmy stepped in. I thought, "He's going to be cool, I don't have to worry."

Working with Jim over all these years—thousands of hours and more than 300 performances—is almost like working with a brother. It always feels like a collaboration. He has a wonderful way of convincing you without your even knowing that you're being convinced. Whatever it is, you're doing it together, and that's a nice feeling, that you have contributed.

Some nights you know that there's a flaw in the performance, that an element of the show is not right. Maybe a cast member is ill, and you think, "Oh God, we've got to get through this." Then Jim comes into your dressing room with this big smile, this attitude that it's going to be great. I look in his eyes and think to myself, "Are you pulling my leg? Do you really believe that?" And he does, he really believes that it's going to be a great night every single time, or at least that's what he projects to me. It feeds me—by the time Jim leaves the dressing room, I sort of feel, "Wait, maybe we have something good going here."

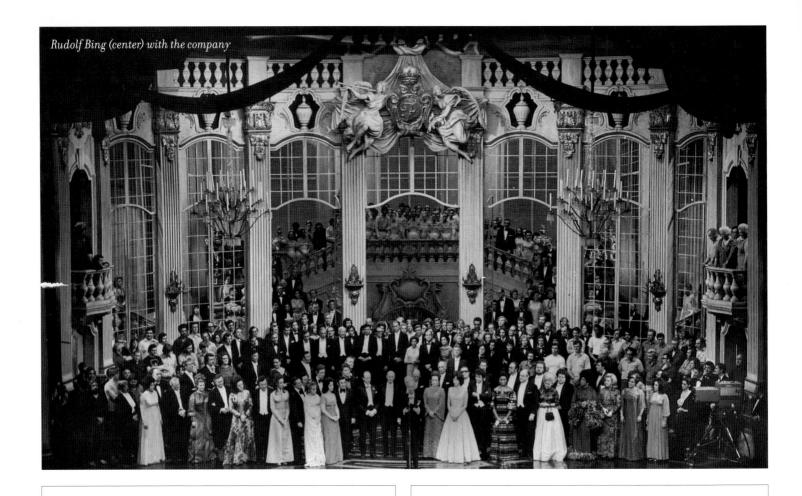

Rudolf Bing (center) with the company

Saturday Evening, April 22, 1972, at 8:00

Gala Performance

HONORING
SIR RUDOLF BING

Benefit
Metropolitan Opera Guild

FOR THE
METROPOLITAN OPERA BENEVOLENT
AND RETIREMENT FUND

PART I
In the set of DON CARLO, Act I, Scene 2
designed by Rolf Gérard

Luisa Miller: Overture	VERDI
Roberta Peters, Sherrill Milnes	
Il Barbiere di Siviglia: "Dunque io son?"	ROSSINI
Teresa Stratas	
La Bohème: "Donde lieta"	PUCCINI
Thomas Stewart	
Otello: "Credo in un dio crudele"	VERDI
Paul Plishka, Ruggero Raimondi	
Luisa Miller: "L'alto retaggio"	VERDI
Montserrat Caballé, Placido Domingo	
Manon Lescaut: "Tu, tu, amore? Tu?"	PUCCINI

Conductor: James Levine

Anna Moffo	
Manon: Gavotte	MASSENET
Martina Arroyo	
Il Trovatore: "Tacea la notte placida"	VERDI
Joan Sutherland, Luciano Pavarotti	
Lucia di Lammermoor: "Sulla tomba"	DONIZETTI

Conductor: Richard Bonynge

INTERMISSION

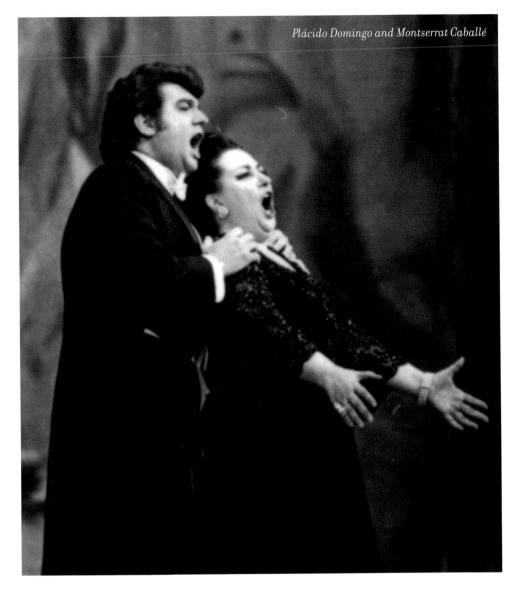

Plácido Domingo and Montserrat Caballé

JL: That was really a very emotional occasion because Mr. Bing had put a standard into his tenure at the Met that was absolutely extraordinary, giving New York a hell of an opera season year after year. Among other things, I did the real corker *Manon Lescaut* Act II duet with Montserrat and Plácido. And my, that was an extraordinary occasion. That gala was on Saturday night after the last broadcast of the season, and in the middle of the week, [artistic administrator] Bob Herman called me and asked if I would do that duet because one of my colleagues had discovered that there was no way to rehearse the singers together with the orchestra, so he threw it back at them. I had warmed to the occasion, so I said I would do it. That afternoon before the matinee, Montserrat came to the Met, and we met for the first time. We went through the duet with Plácido, and Jimmy Johnson played the piano. I remember very vividly that Montserrat was tickled— she smiled when I didn't rush her through high notes or high passages, which was sweet. The antecedent is that I had rehearsed the orchestra alone on Wednesday. At the gala, there was no way you would ever have known it was put together in separate pieces. It was one of those spontaneous combustion things— you can hear it on the recording.

1972

FEBRUARY 9

Named Principal Conductor, beginning in 1973–74, by newly-appointed General Manager Göran Gentele and Music Director Rafael Kubelik.

APRIL 22

Opens the Gala honoring departing General Manager Rudolf Bing with the overture to *Luisa Miller* and conducts eight other excerpts by Rossini, Verdi, Puccini, and Charpentier.

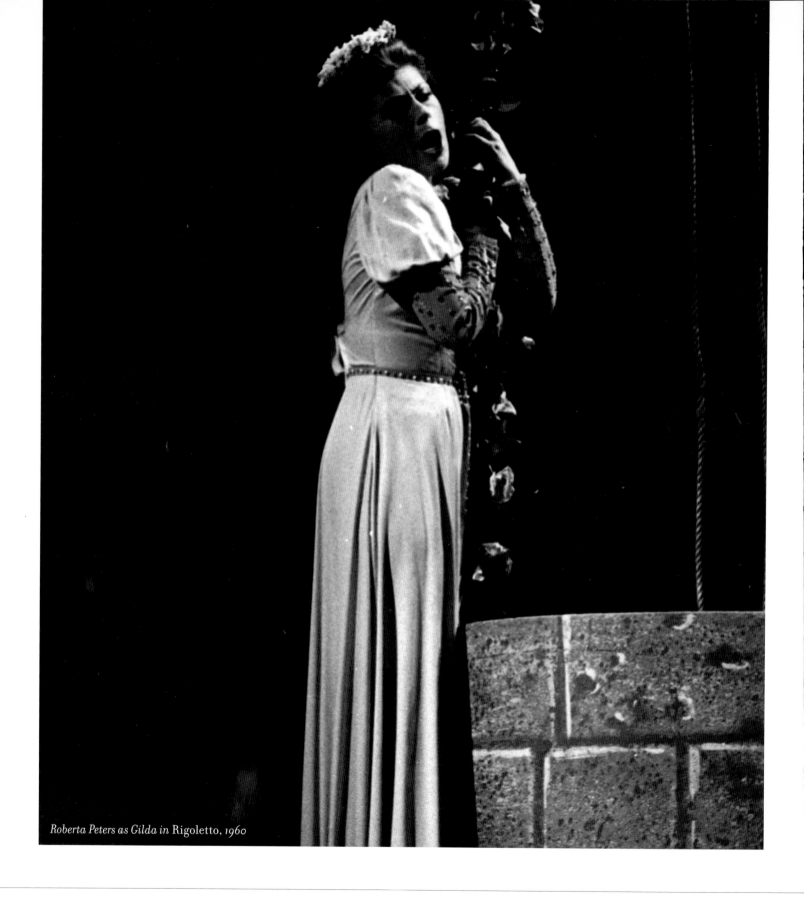

Roberta Peters as Gilda in Rigoletto, *1960*

Roberta Peters: The only time I worked with Jimmy in a complete opera at the Met was when I did Nannetta in *Falstaff,* and it was a wonderful experience. He has always had such a bond with music, and when he conducts, he makes it an intimate relationship between the singer and him.

I knew him from many years ago. When I was doing *Lucia di Lammermoor* at the Cincinnati Zoo opera, I got a knock on my door after the performance. There was a little boy with a score and markings. He had it open to the mad scene and knew absolutely everything about the opera. I was so amazed that I said, "Young man, how old are you?" And he said, "I'm 10. How old are you?" It was so funny. Of course, it was Jimmy Levine. A few years later, I was doing *Rigoletto* at the Met, and Jimmy came backstage. He was about 15 then, and he complimented me on the appoggiatura that I did at the end of "Caro nome."

He played a little upright piano that belonged to a friend of mine in Cincinnati. I wish I had used him as an accompanist, but I never thought of it at the time because he was so young. He was still a young man when I worked with him at Meadow Brook, the summer home of the Detroit Symphony, where he conducted *Rigoletto.* Even then, early on, he had such love for the music, and he was able to impart it to all his singers. What particularly impressed me was that I would walk away after a piece as familiar as the quartet from *Rigoletto* and discover something, that he mentioned to me, which I had never thought of before.

JL: During Mr. Bing's last June festival before leaving the Met, he had a cancellation of the title role, leading lady, and conductor for *Falstaff* (Gobbi, Tebaldi, and Dohnányi). He called me on vacation and asked if I could conduct it. I thought to myself, "My God, he wants me to jump in and do *Falstaff* on one day of theater rehearsal!" I said to Ronald [Wilford], "Well, I know how to do this, but should I?" I was curiously stubborn at that particular age, and I said I just didn't believe in *Falstaff* with one day of rehearsal, even though Mr. Bing had begged me to do it. But Ronald said, "I can think of a reason or two why you might consider it. Don't you think the company might be glad to know you can do something like that, and that you're willing to help them? Mr. Bing was good to you. Why don't you help him?" All of a sudden it made sense to me. I said yes, and we had an absolutely great time. My first three projects at the Met— *Tosca, Luisa Miller,* and then *Falstaff*— established a kind of energy flow between my work and the company's expectation, which was really extraordinary. I would have cheated myself out of it if I hadn't said yes. And who knows? Their future and mine might have been quite different.

JUNE 8

Conducts Verdi's *Falstaff* for the first time at the Met, starring Fernando Corena, Lucine Amara, Roberta Peters, Fedora Barbieri, Luigi Alva, and Matteo Manuguerra.

JL: I always regarded *Otello* as one of the greatest operas, one of my favorites, but I had no idea when I started to do it that I would have so many performances of it eventually— 82 performances with the Met. It's interesting that the lion's share were sung by three tenors. I did push our administration to keep doing it as long as we could have McCracken or Vickers, and then Plácido. That was the first thing Jon and I did together. Such a beautiful voice and such intensity in every respect! We went in the rehearsal room to go over the entire part and didn't emerge all afternoon. We established a strong rapport very quickly, and mostly we agreed like a house afire about everything. We did eventually come to just one place in the whole piece where we got stuck. It's where Iago first mentions the handkerchief. Otello says, yes, it was my first gift to Desdemona, my first love token. And Jon sang it so softly and slowly and dreamily—self-consciously, for me, in a way. I said, "Jon, you know Verdi writes five or six pianos sometimes, but this is almost a passing place." He said, "I know, but the thing that bothers me is Iago is going to make all that mischief with the handkerchief, and if I don't establish what that handkerchief meant to me, then it looks foolish." I said, "I hear you, but Verdi has written it in a matter-of-fact way, not projecting or imagining how much mischief Iago could make." But Jon was very conscious of Otello looking like a fool. It was great to discover that we were content to hear each other's opinions and discuss them. I didn't feel I had to press him to do what I wanted, and he didn't feel he had to press me. In the end, I would say he ended up taking a little exaggeration away, and he was still able to get what he wanted, while I felt this one line hadn't become distorted. With a great artist like that, the discussion itself is usually enough, because having registered the point, he's going to be careful not to make an impression of exaggeration. There was another thing about my relationship with Jon that was very satisfying. I always go to singers' dressing rooms before the performance, or call them on the phone, just to see how they feel and if they want anything. Jon was one of the few singers where we both had an instinct to pick out a couple of spots from the previous performance that we thought needed to be redirected and intensified or altered slightly. It gave us wonderful details to concentrate on and kept our performances very interactive and responsive.

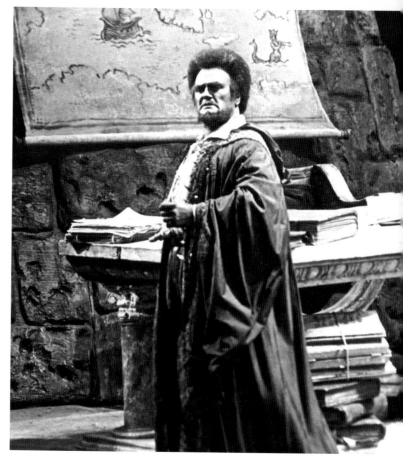

Jon Vickers in the title role of Otello

DECEMBER 5

His first Met performance of Verdi's *Otello*, heard this season with both Jon Vickers and James McCracken in the title role and Renata Tebaldi as Desdemona in her Met farewell performance.

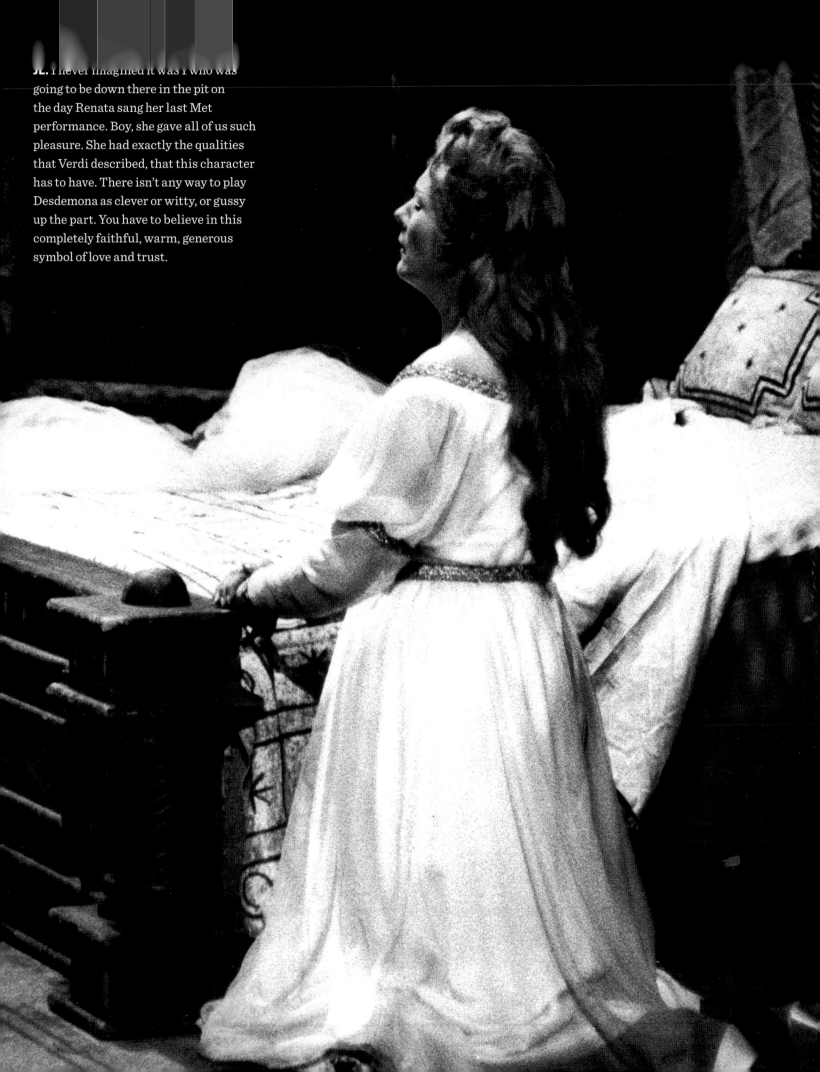

JL: I never imagined it was I who was going to be down there in the pit on the day Renata sang her last Met performance. Boy, she gave all of us such pleasure. She had exactly the qualities that Verdi described, that this character has to have. There isn't any way to play Desdemona as clever or witty, or gussy up the part. You have to believe in this completely faithful, warm, generous symbol of love and trust.

JL: This was something [General Manager] Göran Gentele put together. He had done something like it in Stockholm, and Danny Kaye was obviously the one for it because he had a lot of experience doing fundraisers with symphony orchestras, and these were operatic versions of those. Danny and I became good friends. What an amazing artist and amazing guy. This picture shows us each conducting our own side of the orchestra. Isn't that a riot? Look at the expressions on the musicians' faces! He was one of the most musical people ever to draw a breath. Didn't have to be able to read music, he just was music.

Danny Kaye and Levine conducting the orchestra

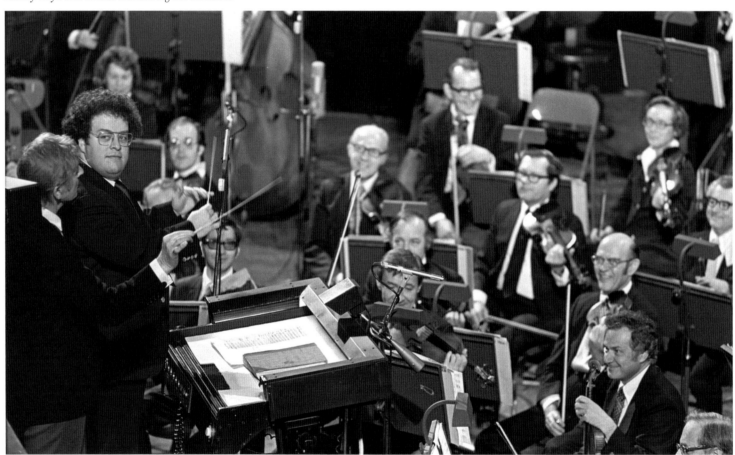

1973
JANUARY 4

Shares the podium with Danny Kaye for the Metropolitan Opera Guild's first Look-In for students.

JL: That production was new in 1954, so I'd grown up with it. Jackie [nickname for Marilyn Horne] is a unique artist, an unbeatable vocalist and musician and a one-of-a-kind personality. She had the kind of voice, technique, and personality for which composers write original music. If she had lived back in Rossini's time, she'd have been one of those people. She has insatiable curiosity about singers and music and style and everything. A joy on every level.

Cesare Siepi as Don Basilio, Fernando Corena as Dr. Bartolo, Enrico Di Giuseppe as Count Almaviva, Hermann Prey as Figaro (raised), Marilyn Horne as Rosina, and Jean Kraft as Berta in Il Barbiere di Siviglia

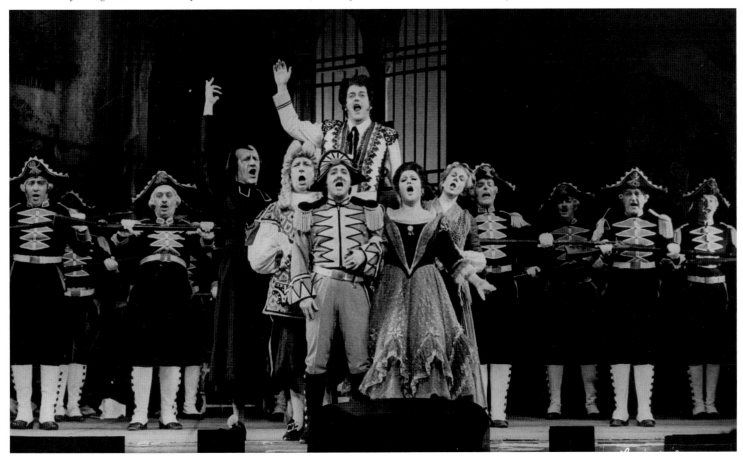

APRIL 2

Adds Rossini's *Il Barbiere di Siviglia* to his Met repertoire, with Hermann Prey, Marilyn Horne, Enrico Di Giuseppe, Fernando Corena, and Cesare Siepi in the leading roles.

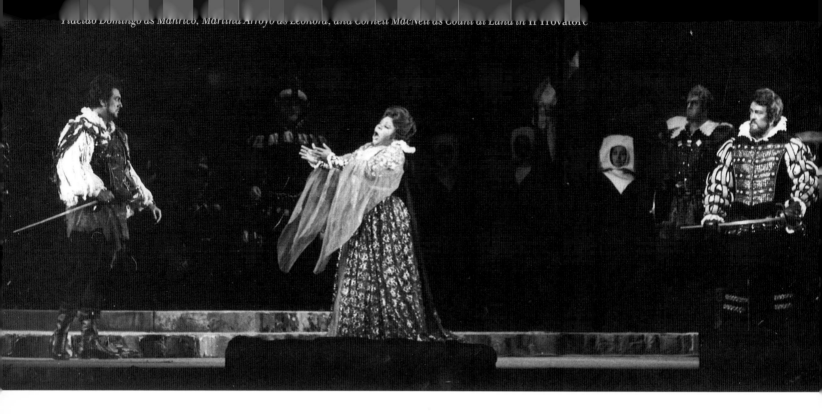

Plácido Domingo as Manrico, Martina Arroyo as Leonora, and Cornell MacNeil as Count di Luna in Il Trovatore

Martina Arroyo: From the very first time I sang with Jimmy, it felt as if we had been working together forever. He always put you at ease, which was especially valuable when you weren't in the best voice. When we did *Il Trovatore* on Opening Night of the 1973–74 season, I was a little under the weather. But my colleagues were all friends, and with Jimmy in the pit, I knew I could go on. Jimmy always knew if you needed to take a little time with a phrase—or if you needed to move ahead. He went with you, the orchestra went with him, and somehow it felt as if this were the way you had always done it.

Coaching with Jimmy was extra special. Even with a part I had done hundreds of times, there was always something to learn. He'd say, "Oh, look at this, doll. You know, this is nice."

I'm a little older than Jimmy, and by the time I started coaching with him I had worked on parts with many other seasoned conductors. Jimmy was kind enough to let me do certain things which wouldn't have been his first choice but which worked. He also accepted each singer's special abilities and that not all singers excel in the same areas. He wouldn't ask a person to sing especially *pianissimo* if that wasn't the singer's strength. But the moment he had someone who could do it, he played with it. He allowed the singer not only to sing at his or her best, but to be so musical that it seemed as if it were all organic. When I sang with Jimmy, I was not singing as Martina. I was singing as Leonora, or living those three hours in Aida's life.

JL: I always enjoyed working with Martina—such a beautiful voice and technique to match. She was indispensable in very important roles.

SEPTEMBER 1973

Becomes the Met's Principal Conductor, a position he holds through the 1975–76 season.

SEPTEMBER 17

His first Opening Night, with Martina Arroyo, Mignon Dunn, Plácido Domingo, and Cornell MacNeil starring in Verdi's *Il Trovatore*.

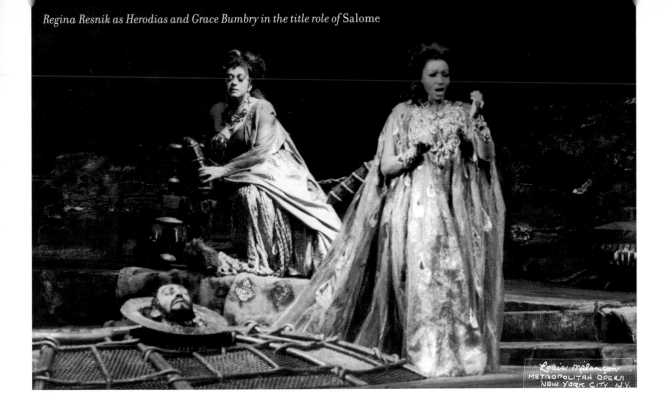
Regina Resnik as Herodias and Grace Bumbry in the title role of Salome

JL: Perhaps it is worth mentioning that Regina Resnik is one of the few great singers who literally had two successful international careers—first as a real soprano in roles as diverse as Alice in *Falstaff*, Leonora in *Trovatore,* and Sieglinde in *Walküre.* And then as a truly low-voiced mezzo/contralto in roles like Dame Quickly and Klytämnestra. This kind of full-scale artistic success in two totally different ranges is quite unusual. And of course she was a great musician and a great actress.

Regina Resnik: He has such a quality of openness. I worked with him only once at the Met, when I was Herodias in *Salome.* We hadn't seen each other for years, but when we greeted each other it was just as though we had seen each other the day before. The atmosphere was completely free and easy, and that made life easier for everybody performing.

There are very few conductors who've taken an opera house unto themselves and decided that there were things going on musically, dramatically, and in many other ways, that had to be corrected so that the various parts of the organization could come forward. That is what James Levine has done at the Met, little by little. He wanted the Met to be one unit, so that the chorus and the orchestra were as important as the soloists, and each got its due. I believe that in his truly musical heart and soul, he wanted the opera house to have all its parts in readiness to do anything that he—or any other conductor—wanted.

SEPTEMBER 19

Conducts Strauss's *Salome* **for the first time, with Grace Bumbry and Regina Resnik.**

JL: This was John Dexter's debut and my first new production at the Met, an extremely strong production. We were scheduled to do Göran Gentele's production of *Ballo,* but after he died, *Vespri* felt right to me for some simple reasons. The tenor engaged for *Ballo* was Gedda, and the nature of the tenor role in *Vespri* is very long and high, so I thought, "Aha!" And then I thought how the nature of the difficulties of the soprano role fit Montserrat perfectly. This was the first chance I had to bring forward one of the pieces that hadn't been part of the Bing regime, a great opera with a very strong cast and strong singers for revivals, too.

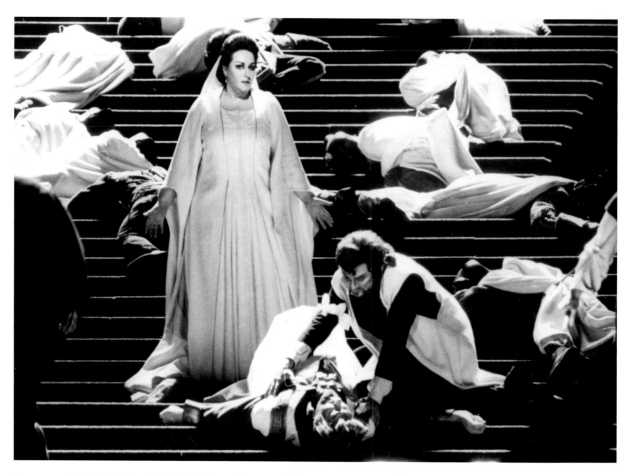

Montserrat Caballé as Elena, Nicolai Gedda as Arrigo, and Sherrill Milnes as Monforte in I Vespri Siciliani

1974
JANUARY 31

Introduces Verdi's *I Vespri Siciliani* to the Met, conducting Montserrat Caballé, Nicolai Gedda, Sherrill Milnes, and Justino Díaz in John Dexter's Met debut production.

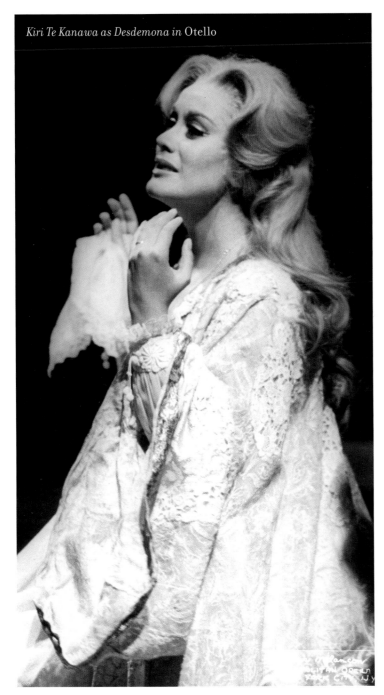

Kiri Te Kanawa as Desdemona in Otello

JL: That was my first experience with watching someone the audience had never seen before become a star right before their eyes. Kiri walked onstage, so beautiful, and then she opened her mouth, and it was just wonderful. Jon Vickers felt it, too; we could feel it while we were rehearsing that if she had to go on, that she had the quality ready.

Kiri Te Kanawa: My Met debut was on very short notice. I hadn't had a great deal of coaching with Jimmy. But throughout the performance he never took his eye off the ball. He was so kind to me—he didn't just plow on but helped me all the way through, even though I wasn't alone up there, and he had to be aware of everyone else, too.

Over the years, I was always amazed by Jimmy's impeccable timing. He always made us look good. It's a bit like playing tennis: he puts the ball in the right position so when you hit it, you look like a god.

FEBRUARY 9

Conducts the eleventh-hour Met debut of Kiri Te Kanawa in a Saturday matinee broadcast performance of *Otello.*

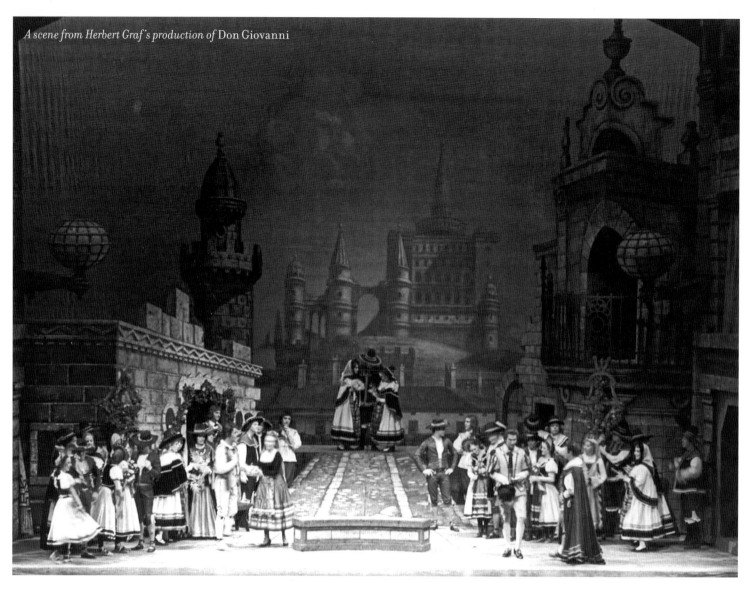

A scene from Herbert Graf's production of Don Giovanni

JL: It was supposed to be a new production, but they didn't have the money, so they decided just to refurbish the old production. Dr. Böhm [conductor Karl Böhm] said, "I'm withdrawing if you don't do a new production!" (even though, curiously, he himself had conducted the premiere of this production). So Schuyler [Chapin, General Manager] asked me, and I said if the cast would stay and rehearse it I'd do it in a minute. All eight of them said, "We'll do it with Jimmy, gladly." The refurbished production looked beautiful, and we had a wonderful time.

MARCH 28

His first Met Mozart performance is an all-star
Don Giovanni, with Sherrill Milnes, Leontyne Price,
Teresa Zylis-Gara, Teresa Stratas, Stuart Burrows,
Walter Berry, Raymond Michalski, and 27-year-old
James Morris as the Commendatore.

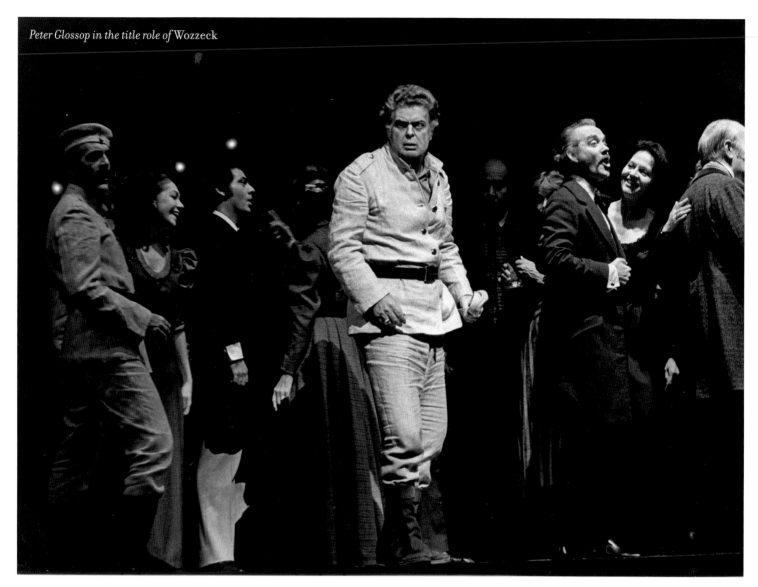

Peter Glossop in the title role of Wozzeck

JL: It may be one of the two or three greatest operas of the century, and it's written in a very specific idiom contemporary in its time. Our audiences were slow to catch on to operas like that, and we felt it was very important that they do, or we'd still be behind. Because I loved this piece a lot, and I knew it well, I was able to keep it in front of the public.

Same with *Lulu,* same eventually with *Moses und Aron.* I've always been very partial to operas that are driven by the music. That is to say, there are a lot of operas that are rather like film scores, and that's a perfectly valid approach, but to me it's not as interesting in the long run as an opera that uses great music for its vessel, its communication.

If somebody asked me about the greatest operas in a 20th-century idiom, I would say that *Wozzeck, Lulu,* and *Moses und Aron* are probably the most exciting for me. But of course I love many others: *Peter Grimes, Jenůfa, Rake's Progress,* etcetera, etcetera.

OCTOBER 7

Conducts Berg's *Wozzeck,* starring Peter Glossop, for the first time at the Met.

JL: *Forza* is a very difficult and fantastic piece—technically difficult, and with a conception that's hard to bring off. All the genre scenes are necessary so that there's context for the protagonists, but for years people cut those scenes and therefore threw the whole opera out of balance. If you do it right, this is nearly as big a conception as *Don Carlo*. We couldn't do a completely new production, financially, but John Dexter stripped the old one down and adjusted it so that it was much cleaner and clearer and had new costumes. We also restored the inn scene, which had been totally cut before, but for which the design existed. What thrilled me was the audience really loved it.

Cornell MacNeil: I sang often with Jim at the Met, beginning with his first season. He never surprised you with something you hadn't rehearsed. He never came to a rehearsal half-prepared, and he asked the same of everyone. His rehearsals were intense, but he never insisted on doing something that everybody didn't want to do. By the time you were done, the performance was ready to be immaculate.

In the 1960s, we had done a lot of concerts together, and as we traveled, he would ask me question after question. He'd say, "I notice that Bing is doing so-and-so at the Met. Do you have any idea why?" Even then, he was constantly searching out the ideas and the reasons at the Metropolitan Opera.

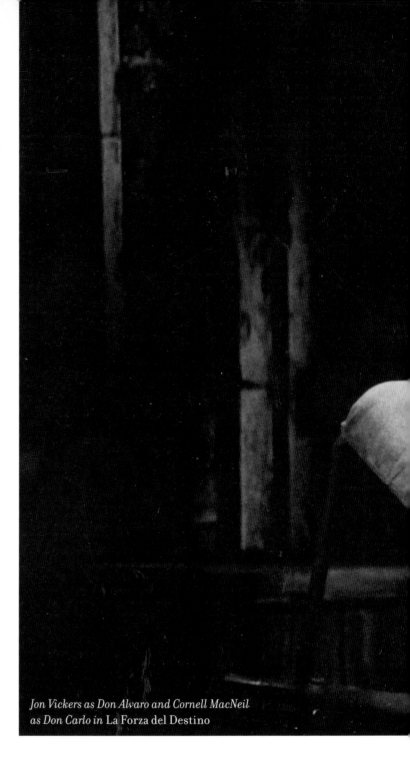

Jon Vickers as Don Alvaro and Cornell MacNeil as Don Carlo in La Forza del Destino

1975
JANUARY 17

His first performance of Verdi's *La Forza del Destino* stars Martina Arroyo, Jon Vickers, Cornell MacNeil, and Bonaldo Giaiotti.

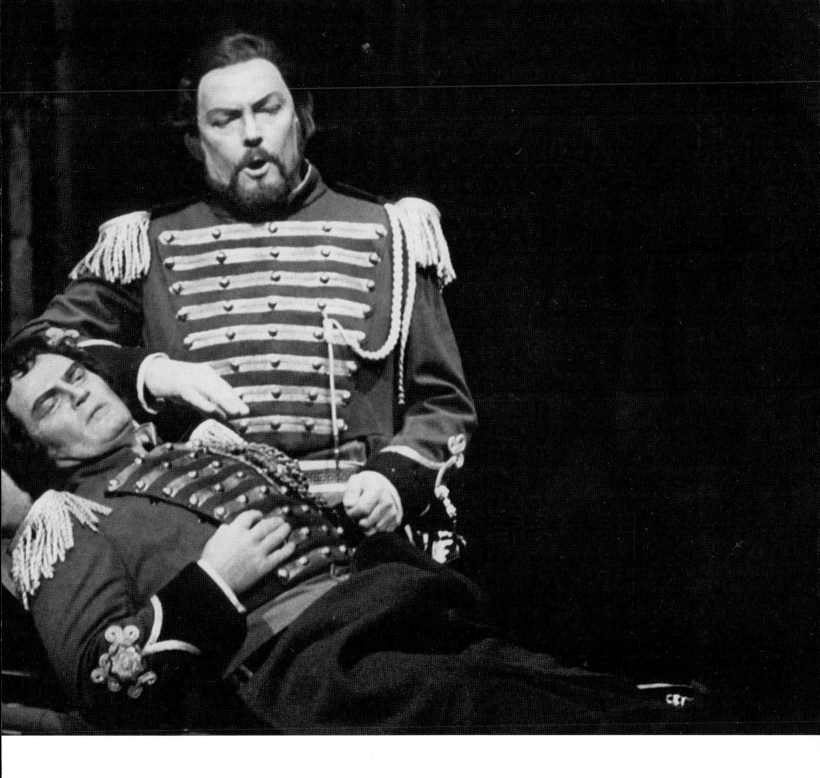

APRIL 10

Another Look-In with Danny Kaye, televised
by CBS, presents Adriana Maliponte and
José Carreras in Act I of Verdi's *La Traviata*.

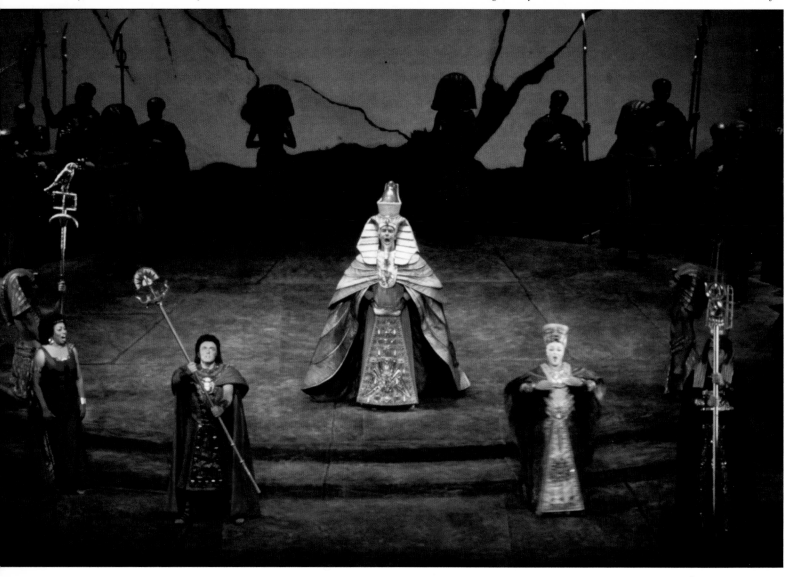

JL: Leontyne truly had the right psychological relationship to her own voice. She knew it was wonderful; she didn't have false modesty about it. She knew the voice was a vessel of expression to a very high degree, and she loved her own voice in the most healthy way.

1976
FEBRUARY 3

Leads a new production of Verdi's *Aida,*
with Leontyne Price, Marilyn Horne,
James McCracken, and Cornell MacNeil.

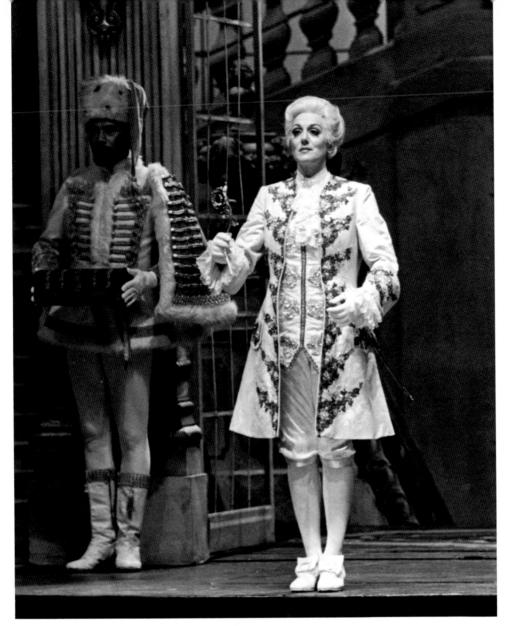

Tatiana Troyanos as Octavian in Der Rosenkavalier

JL: Tatiana made her Met debut that year in two Strauss parts, back to back: Octavian, and then the Composer in *Ariadne auf Naxos,* both of which we did together. God, what a wonderful artist. She had just about everything: brilliant onstage, a brilliant musician, a very striking vocal timbre, a tremendous stylistic range from Mozart to Berg to Bizet to Wagner to you-name-it... I mean, she sang everything and sang it really, really well. She got audiences excited because she was a heated performer, the opposite of cool and distant—she sang everything with a lot of passion and conviction. Boy, we lost her too soon!

MARCH 8

His first performance of Strauss's *Der Rosenkavalier* also marks the Met debut of Tatiana Troyanos in the title role.

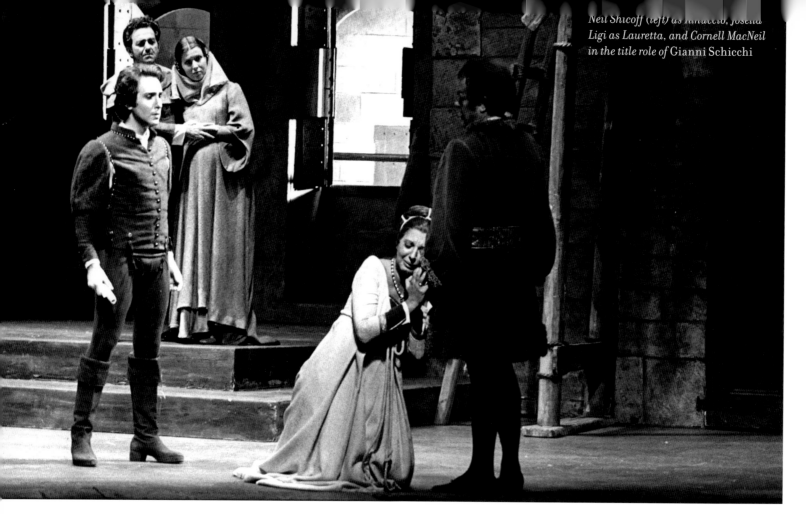

Neil Shicoff: Jimmy changed my life. It's that simple. He took a kid from Brooklyn who was going to be difficult—and I have a reputation for that—and he was able to galvanize me and focus me. I made my Met debut with him at 27, as Rinuccio in *Gianni Schicchi,* and I did a lot with him in the beginning of my career. Those were perilous times. I was in very good vocal shape, but the nerves were extreme, and he was able to help me utilize them. If he had stamped me as an uncontrollable, neurotic tenor, I don't know where my career would have gone. But he didn't,

and he was absolutely the key figure for me in those years. He gave me such a foundation.

It comes down to expression, and Jimmy was the first person to say that to me. Early on, he said, "There seems to be an imaginary curtain between you and the audience, and you have to learn how to break through that curtain and grab those people so they can experience things with you." For knowing and bringing out what is inside the mind and heart and soul of an individual singer, there is absolutely no conductor like him.

Jimmy is in a league of one when it comes to taking a risk; I never felt that if I made one wrong step, it was the end of the collaboration. He lets a singer find the visceral passion. He gave me something at the beginning that has lasted for my whole career, and indeed my life: the ability to express what is hidden, to go under the rock, to see what's there so you can share it, and other people can grow from the experiences that you're sharing with them.

SEPTEMBER

Becomes the Met's Music Director.

OCTOBER 15

Conducts Puccini's *Il Trittico,* in which Hildegard Behrens (as Giorgetta in *Il Tabarro*) and Neil Shicoff (as Rinuccio in *Gianni Schicchi*) make their debuts.

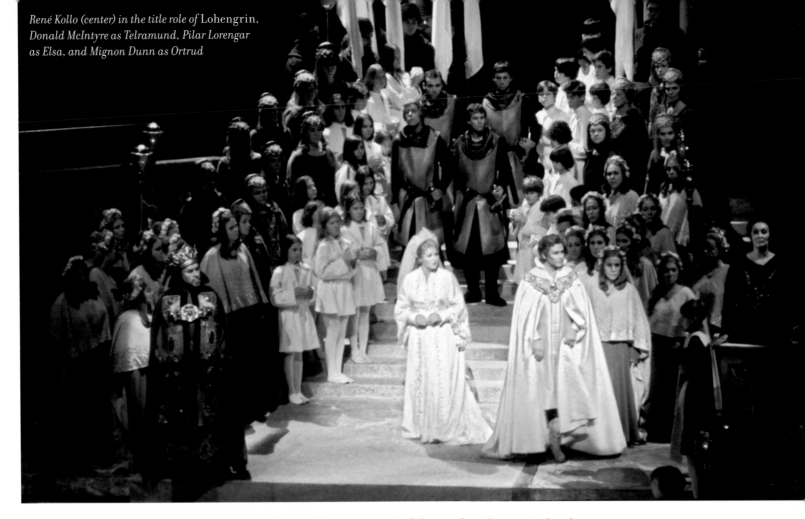

JL: Everding was wonderful to work with, practical and enthusiastic. The cast we had was thrilling, particularly Lorengar, who was a wonderfully affecting and moving soprano her whole career, and René Kollo, who had technical ups and downs but a beautiful voice and delivery of parts like this. He said to me after he'd been at the Met about a week, "It has the same kind of unpretentious warmth and energy as Bayreuth," even though it's in one of the biggest cities—New York. When you haven't been at the Met before, it seems kind of monolithic and forbidding, but it is really a warm company. Don McIntyre sang Telramund, marvelously, and Mignon Dunn sang Ortrud. She had really grown up in the house. She was a very valuable company member during her whole career.

NOVEMBER 4

His first Wagner at the Met, a new production of *Lohengrin* directed by August Everding, with René Kollo, Pilar Lorengar, Mignon Dunn, and Donald McIntyre.

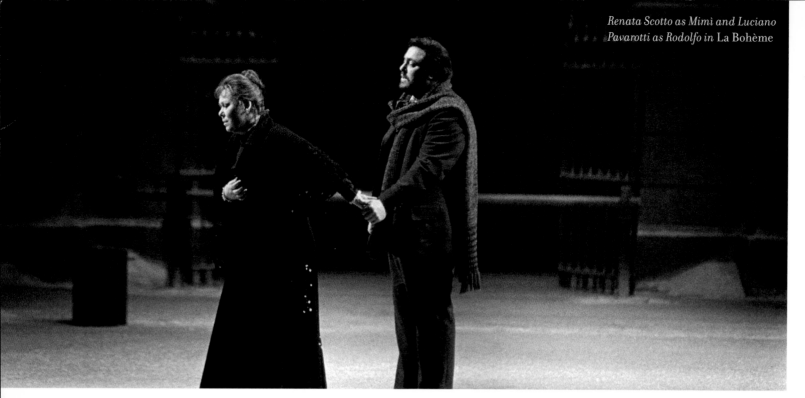

Renata Scotto as Mimì and Luciano Pavarotti as Rodolfo in La Bohème

JL: One statistic still rings in my ears: more people saw that telecast than had seen *Bohème* live in all of its performances worldwide since it was written. Can you believe that? The power of television. This telecast demonstrated that our company usually gets constructively excited at pressure moments. It really rises to every occasion with a tremendous concentration and energy, even now, when the exposure has only steadily increased.

Bruce Crawford, former General Manager: I first met James Levine in 1976. I had been recruited to join the Board of Directors and oversee the development of television, which was about to take a giant step forward with the origination of a series of live telecasts on PBS. The first production was *La Bohème* with Luciano Pavarotti and Renata Scotto. Jim was a fierce proponent of opera on TV and worked diligently and creatively to broaden the Met's media offerings.

He was also the single most important reason I became General Manager of the Met. In the early 1980s the company faced giant deficits and a plummeting box office. A search for a new General Manager was underway and I had been proposed as a candidate. It was Jim who convinced me and the search committee that I should be named to that position.

As General Manager, I witnessed firsthand Maestro Levine's total commitment to the art of opera and to the Met, as he labored tirelessly to raise the standards of the company. He coached artists, young and old, who needed help with difficult roles or vocal problems. Many singers, including Pavarotti and Domingo, insisted that he be in the pit for their performances. He was always attentive to the perfection of his own craft and alert to opportunities to gain insight and knowledge (never missing a Carlos Kleiber rehearsal, for example). The constant improvement of the Met's orchestra and chorus, his championship of contemporary composers, the 21 *Ring* cycles he conducted… These are the attributes of a great conductor and artistic director, and his efforts have attracted a devoted audience to the Met.

1977
MARCH 15

Conducts the first *Live from the Met* telecast, Puccini's *La Bohème* starring Renata Scotto and Luciano Pavarotti.

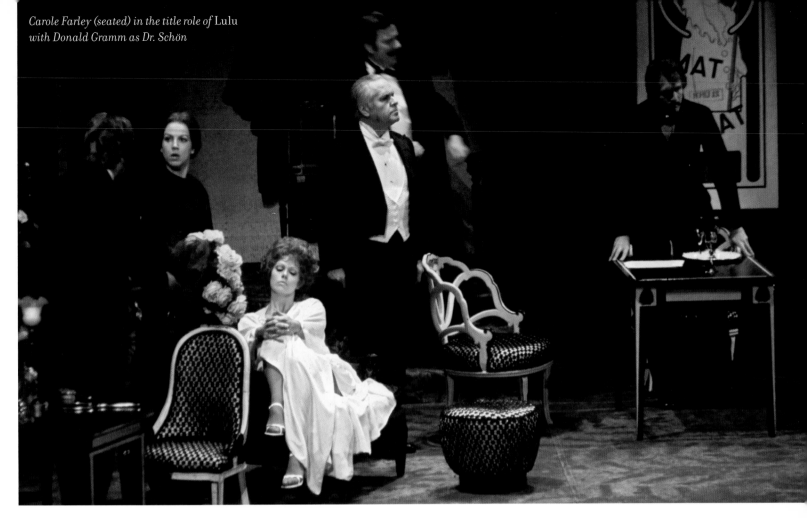

Carole Farley (seated) in the title role of Lulu *with Donald Gramm as Dr. Schön*

JL: We brought the two-act version, because there wasn't a finished, performable third act yet. *Lulu* is a very difficult piece, but so exquisitely written— it is easy to tell what Berg wants you to do; the indications are so clear. It does require a cast that can perform it in a way which is digested and natural, so that the public has a way in. Carole Farley was a damn good singer, as was Donald Gramm, who had done the American premiere at Santa Fe. I think it's important to understand that nothing about *Lulu* or *Wozzeck* is going to attract a tired-businessman audience. But for audiences that go to the theater or to opera and let themselves have enough exposure, these are incredible pieces. I don't think it's the music per se that makes them hard for an audience, but the dramatic side. They are unusually disturbing pieces if you get into them. And don't you think that pieces so dramatically truthful and about such difficult subjects can't be, after all, like *La Fille du Régiment* or *Don Pasquale*? They don't have such easy access. But they're masterpieces, and therefore part of the Met's function is to do them well so that they're there for people. And that's what we've tried to do. For me it's a real labor of love.

MARCH 18

Demonstrates his commitment to modern masterpieces by adding Berg's *Lulu* to the Met repertory.

JL: *Pelléas* is a one-of-a-kind piece, not something in a row of similar masterpieces by a Rossini or a Donizetti. Debussy worked so hard on it to try to get it right. He kept revising and watching the way they did it and sharpening details all the time. I never get enough of this piece. The most important thing about doing it, from the performer's point of view, is that "impressionism" is in the eye and ear of the beholder. It has nothing to do with what we are doing; it's an effect created by what we're doing. The audience's experience is impressionistic, but if we played it without clarity, it wouldn't arrive at that. That's a kind of illusion. I had an experience as a kid, when I went to a traveling art show at our museum in Cincinnati. There was a fantastic El Greco of Christ bearing the cross, and he had the most unbelievable expression on his face and in his eyes. I looked and looked and looked, and finally I couldn't stand it. I walked up to it, because I wanted to see how he got that look. And right in each eye was—psht, psht—of white. I gradually walked away from it and got about 10 or 12 steps away, and it looked again as it did before. I thought, "This is what one has to be able to learn. If you're an artist, it doesn't do any good to be excited by a work of art and not understand it." If you fear that knowing about it will spoil it for you, you've got the whole thing backwards.

José van Dam: I have sung such difficult operas with him, like *Wozzeck* and *Pelléas et Mélisande,* but working with him is so easy. He goes with the music—he doesn't try to force the music to go with him. The music is like a big river, powerful yet simple, and he swims with the current. We have almost no need to speak because we're on the same wavelength. Because of that I'd even say it's not work any more; it's a pleasure. We let the music carry us away.

He's a very kind person, very calm. I've never seen him angry. To have the humility to serve music and be guided by it, one has to be calm, because music is an art of peace. Also, James is sure of himself, with good reason. It's the ones who have doubts about their abilities that get worked up.

He works very hard and analyzes everything he conducts, but in the end, what is important is not intellect but instinct. And James has such a great instinct for music that he never makes a mistake. You feel that there is someone confident supporting you in the music. When he's in the pit, he always smiles when he makes eye contact, and he shows with this smile that he is with you.

OCTOBER 6

Performs Scott Joplin's *Maple Leaf Rag* on the piano as part of a Met Marathon fundraising concert.

OCTOBER 11

Conducts Debussy's *Pelléas et Mélisande* for the first time at the Met, with Teresa Stratas, Raymond Gibbs, José van Dam, and Jerome Hines.

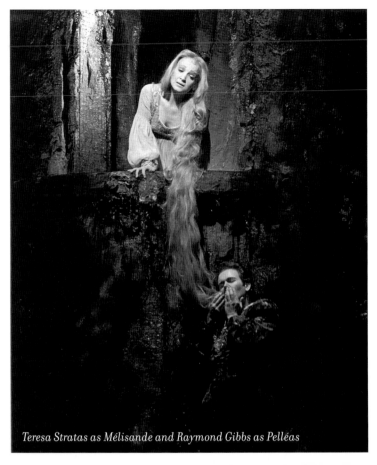

Teresa Stratas as Mélisande and Raymond Gibbs as Pelléas

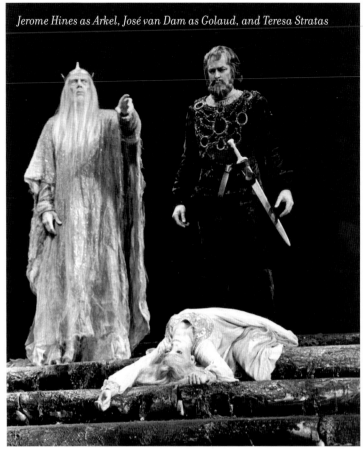

Jerome Hines as Arkel, José van Dam as Golaud, and Teresa Stratas

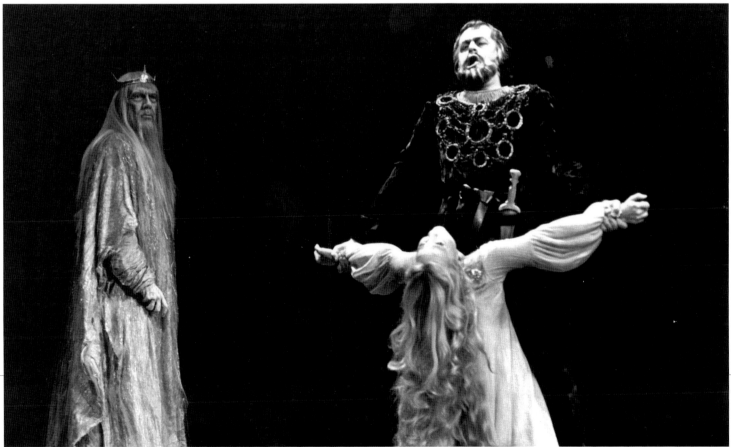

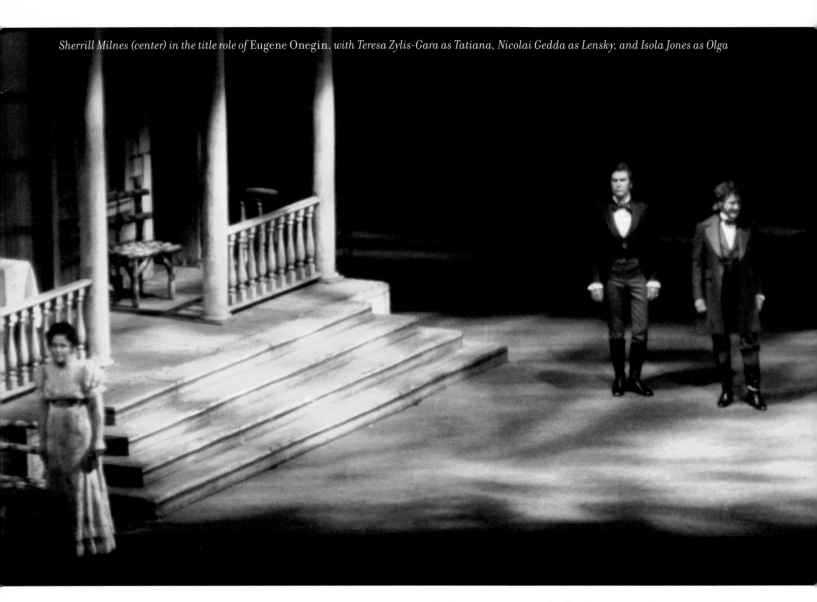

Sherrill Milnes (center) in the title role of Eugene Onegin, *with Teresa Zylis-Gara as Tatiana, Nicolai Gedda as Lensky, and Isola Jones as Olga*

JL: The cast was wonderful. Some were Russian-speaking, but not Sherrill, and he worked very hard. The role was excellent for him. It didn't use his spectacular high voice the way the big Verdi parts did, but he was very, very good. Zylis-Gara had a beautiful voice, and she was so sympathetic. And Nicolai Gedda was one of my favorite singers of all time and indispensable in this opera—passionate, elegant, phenomenal.

OCTOBER 15

Conducts Tchaikovsky's *Eugene Onegin,*
sung in Russian for the first time at the Met,
with Sherrill Milnes in the title role.

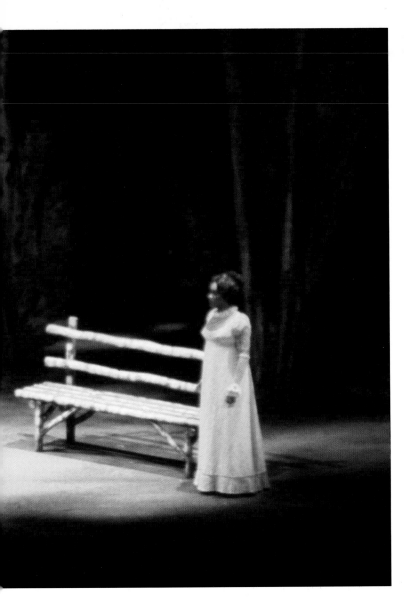

Sherrill Milnes: For me, Jim was the first "love conductor," versus the old-time "fear conductors." I'm old enough to have worked with Karajan, Böhm, Bernstein, Solti, Leinsdorf, Reiner... They were great conductors, but when you looked down at the pit, you would not think that's your friend. Whereas when Jim came into the pit, you had the feeling, "Here's a friend; we're going to do this together." I saw some of those older conductors annihilate certain singers. You had huge respect for them, but you were a little afraid. With Jim you have huge respect—and love.

Jim has a wonderful sense of humor. One week, back in 1978, I was juggling three operas at the Met: *Eugene Onegin, La Favorita,* and *Thaïs.* On a night I was off, I got a call at home that the baritone who was singing Iago in *Otello* couldn't go on for the second act, which was about to start, and there was no one else around who knew the part. I had a little bit of a cold, and I had a performance the next night, but I raced down there. It had been a while since I had done *Otello,* so the stage director was in the wings, and he would point at this and that to help me out. There's an orchestral passage at the opening that comes to a conclusion and then is repeated. At the end of the repeat, Iago sings "Non ti crucciar." All during that first part, I was kind of watching the director and moving the books and lifting the case and futzing with the map, thinking, "Oh, yeah, right! I remember that!" Except when the orchestra got to the end of the first passage, where I wasn't supposed to sing, I did. I wasn't keeping track because I was too busy doing the stage business. I sang, "Non ti crucciar," and Jimmy put his hand up to stop me and just started to laugh. I looked at him, shrugged my shoulders, and went on moving the books. When I got to the point where I was supposed to sing, he kind of put his baton down and said, "Okay, your turn now!" It was all I could do to keep a straight face. That's what I mean by fear and love. All the fear guys would have *glared,* but Jim laughed.

JL: This production was a real consensus success. It succeeded in showing very old imagery with contemporary technique. In fact, this production was the reason we asked Günther Schneider-Siemssen to design the *Ring.* People argue about versions of *Tannhäuser,* Dresden or Paris. I never understand this, because I'm so vehemently of the opinion that great composers make their works better. That's why they revise them. I know not a single case of a great large piece being better in its original form than it is in the form the composer developed. So for me, it's the Paris version all the way. It's a very hard opera to do well—the roles are difficult to sing, and the dramatic intensity is unrelenting. You need a pretty large, great cast. This was the first time I worked with Leonie. Heaven. Wonderful, passionate, funny, very hard-working. We had a very easy rapport. And she brought it all—the character, the voice, the commitment—to every performance, a real phenomenon. For me, Leonie was a reason to buy a ticket to any opera.

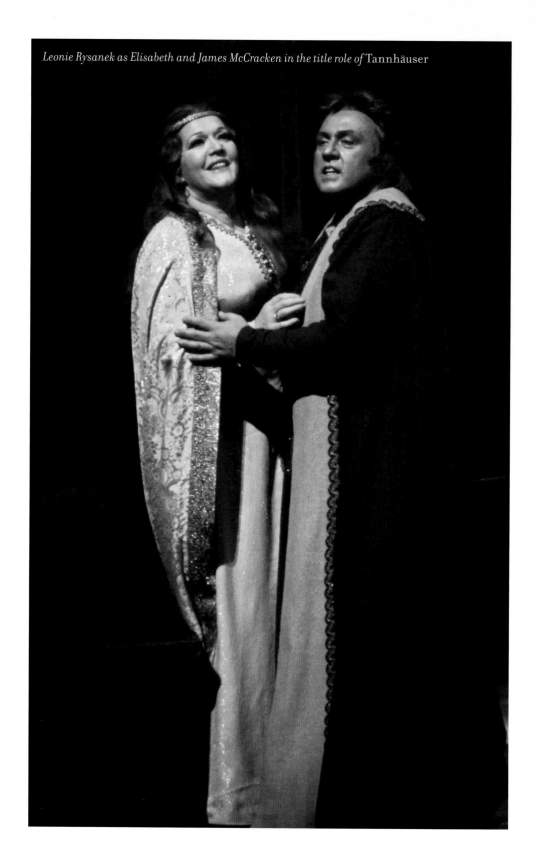

Leonie Rysanek as Elisabeth and James McCracken in the title role of Tannhäuser

DECEMBER 22

Conducts Wagner's *Tannhäuser,* directed by Otto Schenk, with a cast led by James McCracken, Leonie Rysanek, Grace Bumbry, and John Macurdy—with Bernd Weikl and Kathleen Battle in their Met debuts.

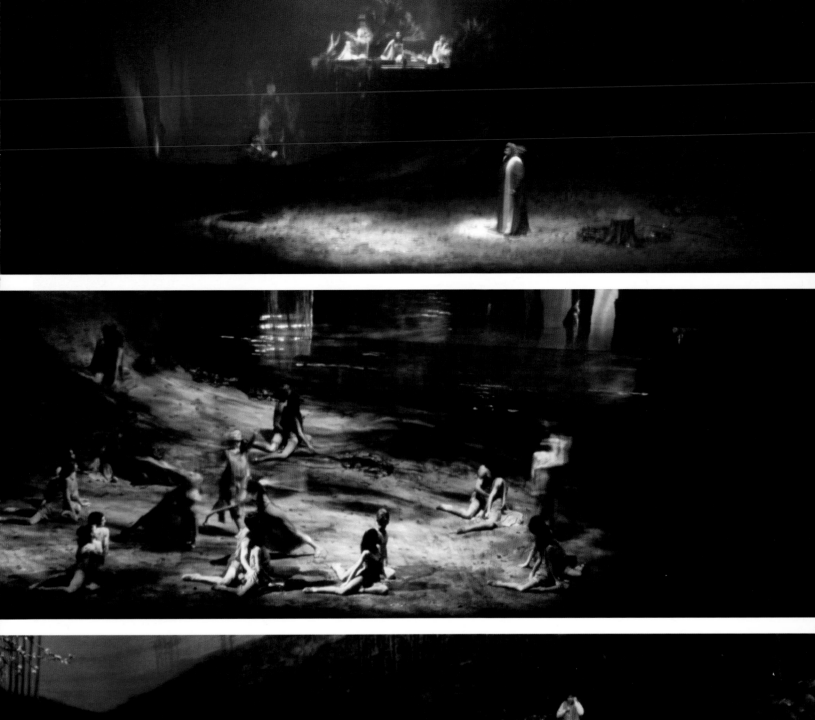

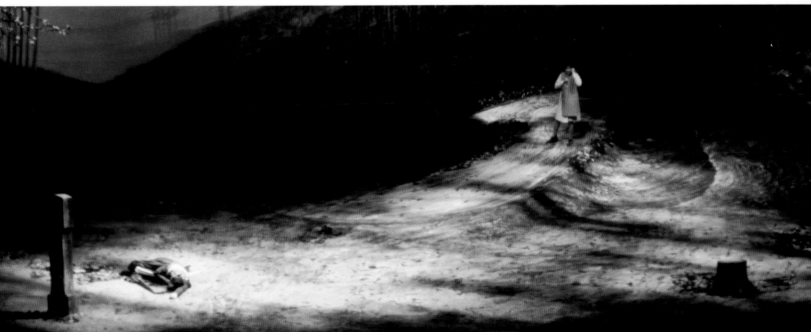

Scenes from Otto Schenk's production of Tannhäuser *with sets by Günther Schneider-Siemssen*

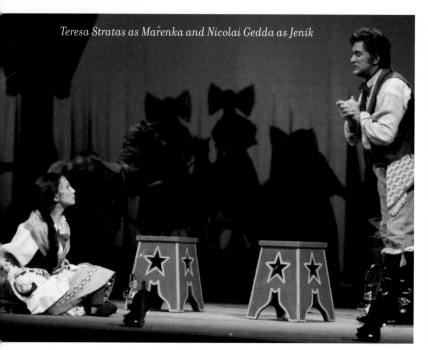

Teresa Stratas as Mařenka and Nicolai Gedda as Jeník

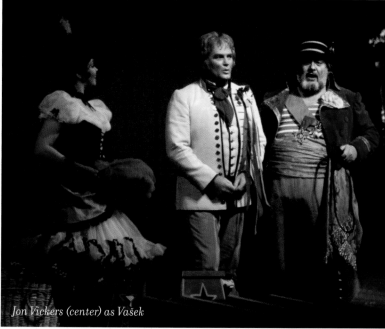

Jon Vickers (center) as Vašek

JL: This was one of the most wonderful productions the Met's ever had. *The Bartered Bride* is one of the great opera scores, and also one of the human comedies, those large pieces like *Rosenkavalier* or *Meistersinger* or *Figaro* or *Don Pasquale* that teach us a lot of things about human beings through comedy. At one time, it was a fairly standard piece of the repertoire, but then it went out of fashion in America, probably precipitated by the problem of either using an old translation or performing in Czech, which the company had not yet done back then. When I said to John Dexter, "Here are some operas I wish we had in the repertoire," he lit up about *The Bartered Bride.* He had a couple of ideas right off the bat. One was to get Tony Harrison, an English poet who was fluent in Czech, to write a new translation. Josef Svoboda and Jan Skalicky, who are Czech artists, gave us a design for a clean-lined, full-scale production that was atmospheric but not ornamental. Dexter and I both knew, sort of spontaneously, that we wanted Stratas and Gedda, and we thought of Martti Talvela because of how big and imposing he was in tragedies. He was not a natural comedian, but of course his part would be funny because it would be played seriously. The piece of casting which was particularly exciting was that Dexter wanted to cast Vašek against type: Jon Vickers, whom the Met associated with intensely dramatic roles like Florestan and Canio and Grimes. And, by God, we offered it to Jon, and he grabbed it—he was tickled. It made Nicky Gedda into a kind of folky hero and Jon into this adorable, heartbreaking character. It was a wonderful, very successful performance, a completely joyous, creative thing. We performed this piece quite often, televised it, took it on tour, and the audiences ate it up.

1978
OCTOBER 25

Conducts a new production by John Dexter of Smetana's *The Bartered Bride,* starring Teresa Stratas, Nicolai Gedda, Jon Vickers, and Martti Talvela.

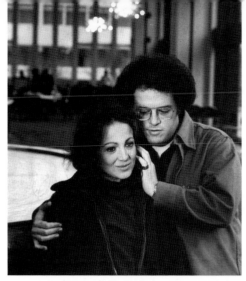

Levine and Teresa Stratas

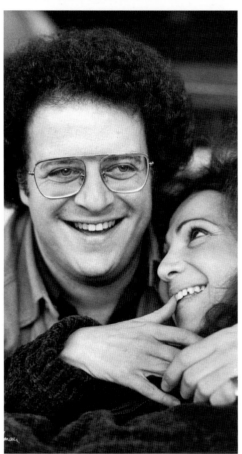

Teresa Stratas: Jimmy? It's very hard to talk or write about him. I love and admire him beyond words. In our work together we needed few words. Our communication was through the music. Jimmy's music always reveals his enormous depth of spirit. This allowed me to do what I did best on stage: express the utter joy and grief of life. We served the work. No egos in the way. Some of my fondest memories are from after performances, when we just sat in the dressing room not talking. There were periods of my life when I was profoundly discouraged. Jimmy always managed to pull me back so I could soar on the strength of his musical wings. For two complicated people it was never complicated. It was clear and pure. A communion.

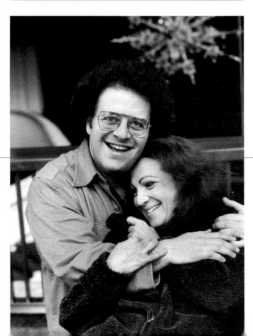

A scene from John Dexter's production of Don Carlo

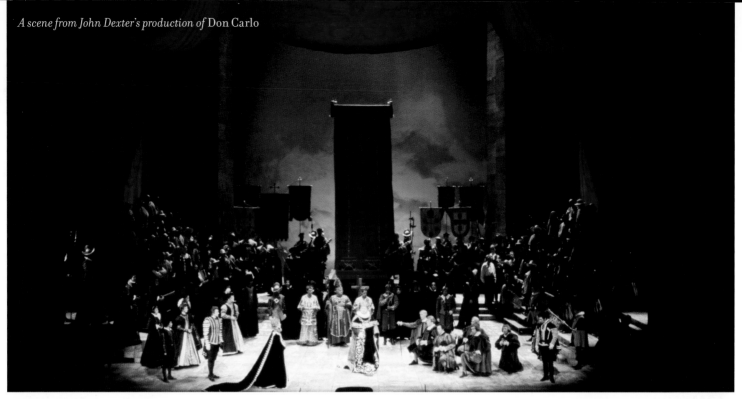

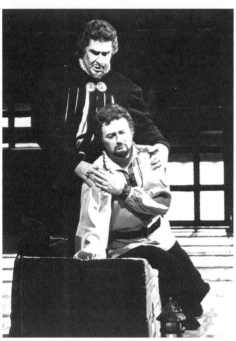

Sherrill Milnes as Rodrigo and Giuseppe Giacomini in the title role of Don Carlo

JL: We were finally able to do what I'd always wanted to do: five acts, without cuts—some people who did the five-act version cut so much out, they might as well have done a four-act version to start with. A complete five-act version is the ideal one for a big opera house.

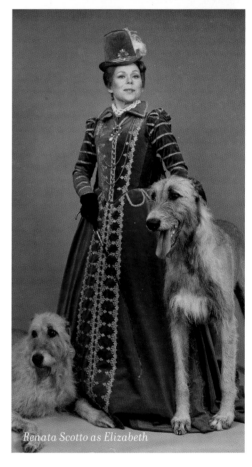

Renata Scotto as Elizabeth

1979
FEBRUARY 5

Conducts another Dexter production, Verdi's *Don Carlo,* presented in five acts for the first time at the Met since 1921, starring Giuseppe Giacomini, Renata Scotto, Marilyn Horne, Sherrill Milnes, Nicolai Ghiaurov, and James Morris.

A scene from Jean-Pierre Ponnelle's production of Der Fliegende Holländer

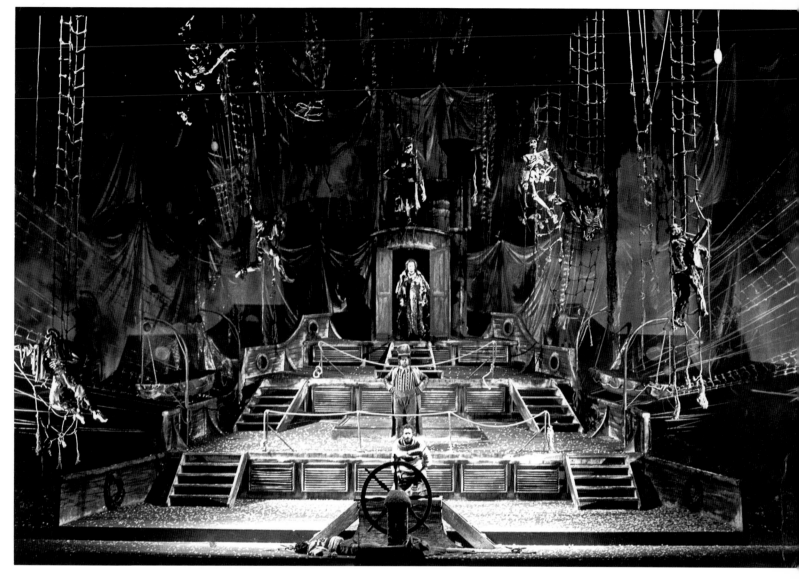

JL: This was a controversial production. I remember hearing a sound when the curtain came down at the end that I had never heard before: half the audience, "Yay!" and half the audience, "Boo!" It was unbelievable. The company performed it hotter and hotter from one performance to the next, because they believed in it very much. Why was it so controversial? A lot of good reasons. It had real imagination. It had a point of view. Ponnelle dared to put it up on stage the way he saw it, as a kind of a dream, so that he could use fantasy imagery, which is part of the legend. I mean, a realistic *Fliegende Holländer* isn't exactly much of anything.

MARCH 8

Conducts Jean-Pierre Ponnelle's production of Wagner's *Der Fliegende Holländer,* borrowed from the San Francisco Opera, with José van Dam, Carol Neblett, William Lewis, and Paul Plishka.

Christa Ludwig: Jimmy has an instinct for how the voice moves. Whether it's heavy or tiny, he makes the orchestra sound like the voice. When we worked together, it was always as if there were an electric wave between us, where the music went—sometimes floated—from one to the other. We fit together like an old married couple—or two horses! I once said to him, "You know, Jimmy, you are round, and I am round, and we are making round music." This is music-making which is 10 percent intellect and 90 percent body—it is the heart, the soul, the belly. Music is erotic, and we shouldn't forget it.

Jimmy is a very warm person, and although I worked with many great conductors in opera, he was the only one who called me in the dressing room during intermission and said, "Of course, you were great." He did it every time.

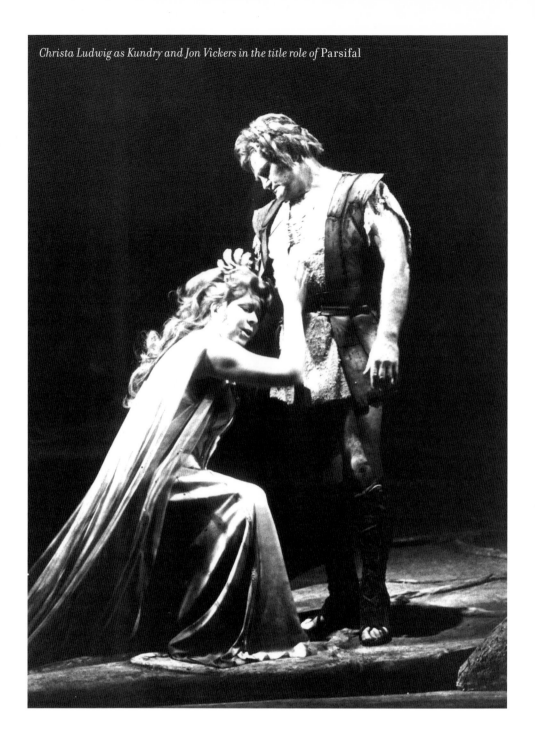

Christa Ludwig as Kundry and Jon Vickers in the title role of Parsifal

APRIL 2

His first Met performance of Wagner's *Parsifal*, with Jon Vickers, Christa Ludwig, Bernd Weikl, and Martti Talvela.

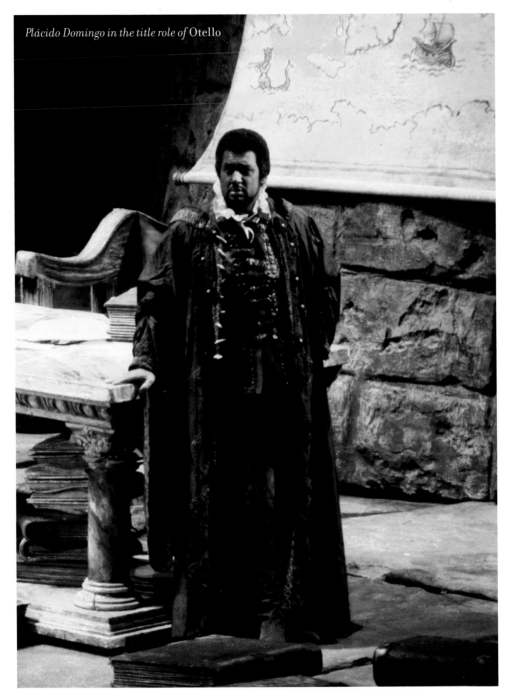

Plácido Domingo in the title role of Otello

JL: Plácido brought to this role such bel canto and such comprehension and Italianate intensity. Everything Plácido does is the work of a great artist, of a person who is sensitive to the whole spectrum of artistic criteria. He's aware of the vocalism, the technique, the language, the style, the physique, what's strong and weak about the performance, what contributions his colleagues are making... It's a great artistic consciousness. We have an extraordinary relationship, and we've grown in an almost perfectly parallel way. At each moment, whether we did something new or repeated something, we were ready for each other in every way, to every detail, with almost no words.

SEPTEMBER 24

On Opening Night, Plácido Domingo brings his Otello, first performed in Hamburg under Levine, to the Met.

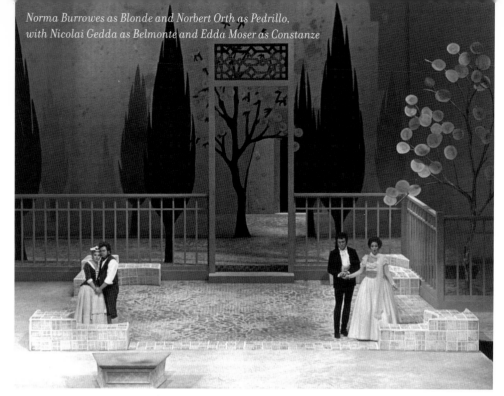

*Norma Burrowes as Blonde and Norbert Orth as Pedrillo,
with Nicolai Gedda as Belmonte and Edda Moser as Constanze*

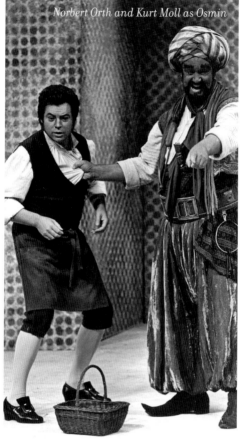

Norbert Orth and Kurt Moll as Osmin

JL: A new *Abduction* [*from the Seraglio*] was important because it had only been played, in the history of the Met, five times in 1946–47, in English. Jocelyn Herbert was the most sensational theater designer there ever was, her sense of style and proportion... And Dexter had the sense to leave this production mostly to Kurt Moll, who was sensational!

Kurt Moll: We have been friends for 40 years. We did so many things together—Wagner, Verdi, Mozart, Strauss—and I had a lot of fun every time. It is a duty to have fun on stage— not laughing, but fun in the music and the interpretation. Jimmy's specialty is kindness, and his complete friendliness on the podium always makes it easier to collaborate. As performers, we must take what is inside us and show it on the outside. With Jimmy it always works.

OCTOBER 12

Begins building the Mozart repertoire with a new production of *Die Entführung aus dem Serail,* not heard at the Met since 1947, starring Edda Moser, Norma Burrowes in her Met debut, Nicolai Gedda, and Kurt Moll.

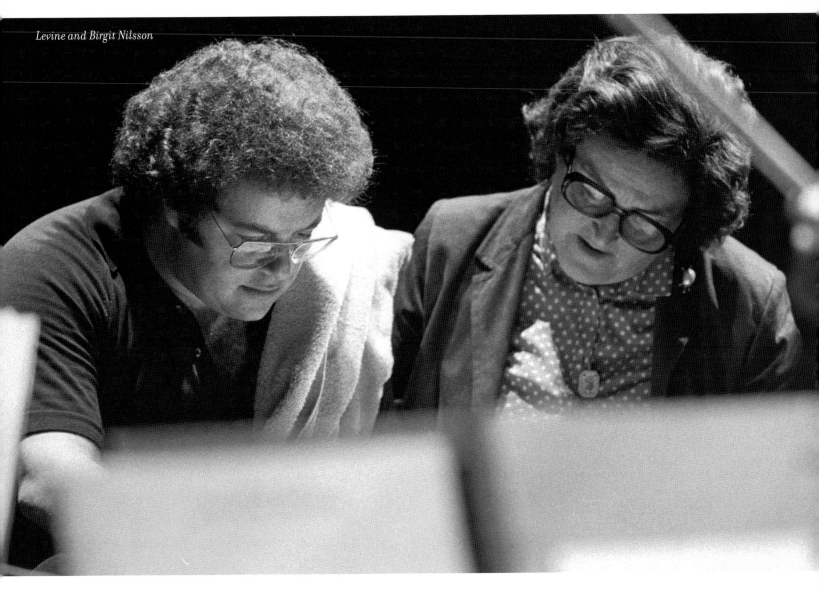

Levine and Birgit Nilsson

JL: Do you believe that, with the horn-rimmed glasses and
the whole routine? We finished a rehearsal for this concert,
and the orchestra left, and we were talking, and she said,
"I made too many mistakes in that. We should look at it."
So she sat down with me on the floor of the podium and opened
the score and reached in her bag and got those glasses. I said,
"If I ever write a book, can I use this photo?" And she laughed
and said, "Of course! Why not?"

NOVEMBER 4

Leads a solo concert by Birgit Nilsson,
returning after a four-season absence with
a program including music from *Tannhäuser,
Götterdämmerung,* and *Salome,* with
Brünnhilde's battle cry as an encore.

JL: John Dexter was an amazing director, a real theater guy. He only did a piece when he knew exactly how he wanted to put it on the stage. And the great hallmark of all his productions was that he was always burning about the essence of it—he was centered on the center. But he could also drive me nuts as a collaborator. Whenever you needed to ask him a question or suggest something, you were inopportune—too early or too late. He would sometimes try to spread his central idea across a whole piece without being sure that the details were going to work. But boy, when the details did work, he wound up with a production that you could put on today, and it would still be a classic. I noticed that almost every great actor I met who had worked with him said the same thing: the most difficult man to work with and the most brilliant. I found that difficulty, but I also found a lot of humor, and a lot of edge. I loved working with him, and we did a lot of very good productions together. I think his most successful ones were some combination of contemporary or native-language: *Mahagonny, Dialogues of the Carmelites, Billy Budd,* the French and Stravinsky triple bills, *Lulu...* It was fun to talk to him about everything. We had fun planning lots of things that we knew we couldn't do! But we succeeded in actually doing this *Mahagonny* with this extraordinary cast.

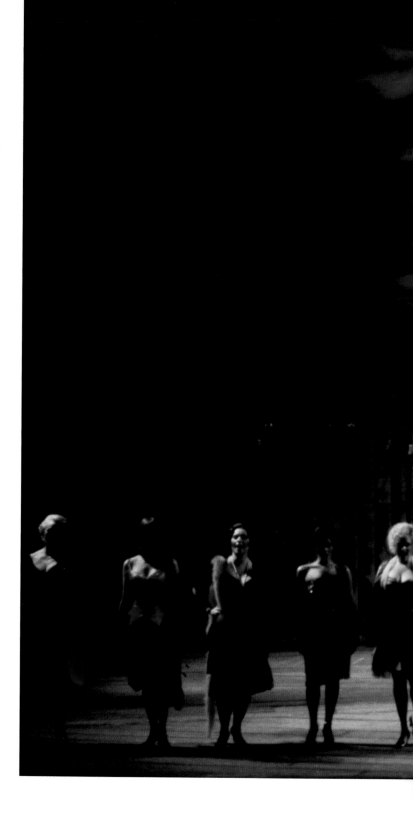

NOVEMBER 16

Conducts the company premiere of Kurt Weill's *Rise and Fall of the City of Mahagonny,* starring Teresa Stratas, Astrid Varnay, Richard Cassilly, and Cornell MacNeil.

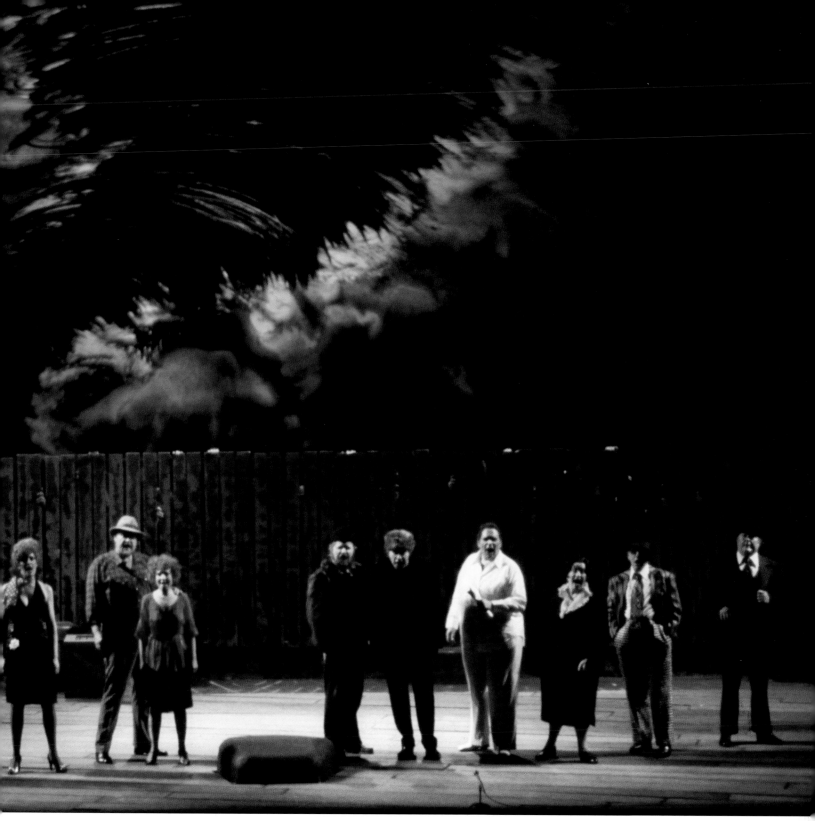

Klara Barlow, Gwynn Cornell, Joann Grillo, Isola Jones, Louise Wohlafka, Nedda Casei, Richard Cassilly, Teresa Stratas, Paul Plishka, Vern Shinall, Arturo Sergi, Astrid Varnay, Ragnar Ulfung, and Cornell MacNeil in Rise and Fall of the City of Mahagonny

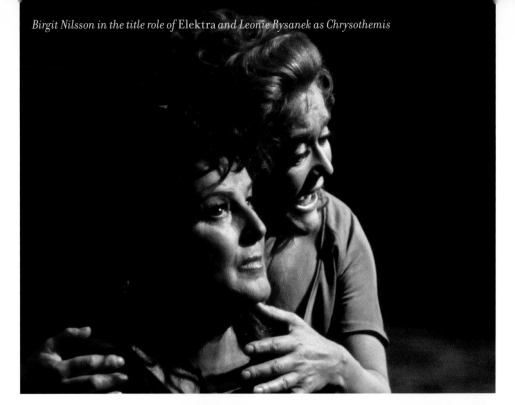

JL: Nilsson came back after five years away. The Met was scheduled to do a run of *Lohengrin*s, but we persuaded the people who were singing some of them—Rysanek, Dunn, McIntyre—to switch to *Elektra*s. That way, we were able to get Nilsson quickly. Leonie would have sung Elsa, but she was perfectly happy to sing Chrysothemis.

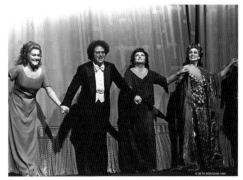 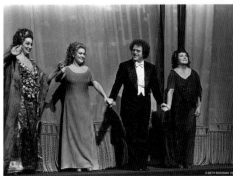

Levine with Birgit Nilsson, Leonie Rysanek, and Mignon Dunn

1980

FEBRUARY 1

His first Met performance of Strauss's *Elektra* features the classic pairing of Birgit Nilsson and Leonie Rysanek.

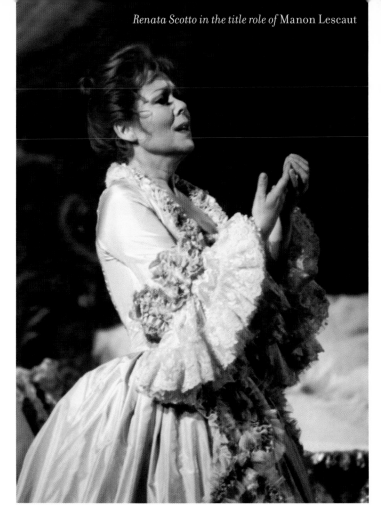

Renata Scotto in the title role of Manon Lescaut

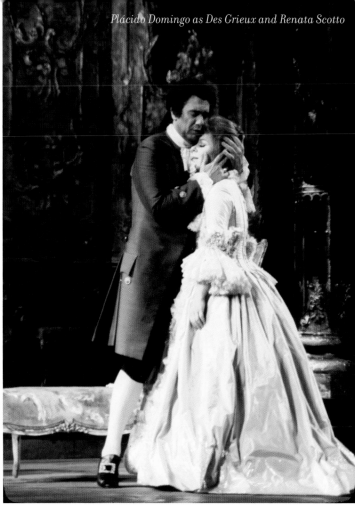

Plácido Domingo as Des Grieux and Renata Scotto

Renata Scotto: With *Manon Lescaut,* I was lucky to have not only Maestro, but Gian Carlo Menotti as the director. Gian Carlo let me do a lot of what I wanted, like being in my underwear in the second act, and jumping around on the bed. Musically it was different, because Maestro was in charge of *not* letting me do everything I wanted. *Manon Lescaut* is not easy vocally because it's very dramatic, sometimes melodramatic, and you must never forget to control your voice. I was involved more as an actress than as a singer, but Maestro didn't tell me immediately that I was sort of sloppy musically. We just rehearsed and rehearsed and rehearsed, until it was

fine. To be able to work on this with Maestro, to go through every line, even a little line, was such a joy.

I will never forget the moment I met Maestro. I was doing Elena in *I Vespri Siciliani,* and at the first rehearsal I saw him smile. It was like *un filo magico,* a magic thread between us, and it still is. I was very well known in Italy then, but I was considered a soprano leggiero [a light soprano], and I was very unhappy about that path. I wanted to sing what I liked and what I thought I was good at. Maestro understood what I could do. And so I found freedom, but with guidance, with a friend I could really trust. When he conducts a singer, he's

the guide, not the accompanist. He has thought of everything before he begins. He doesn't stay with a note because the singer likes it—he stays on it for a reason. The beauty of working with Maestro is that you can really talk and explore—get inside the music. For me rehearsing with Maestro was even better than performing. You could try everything! The performance was for the audience, but the rehearsing was for us, to try to discover every possibility that the composer gives us through the music. I would go back only for those rehearsals that we had.

MARCH 17

Leads a new production of Puccini's *Manon Lescaut,* directed by Gian Carlo Menotti, starring Renata Scotto and Plácido Domingo. The March 29 performance marks the first live telecast transmitted to Europe.

The Next Generation:
Lindemann Young Artist Development Program
Founded in 1980

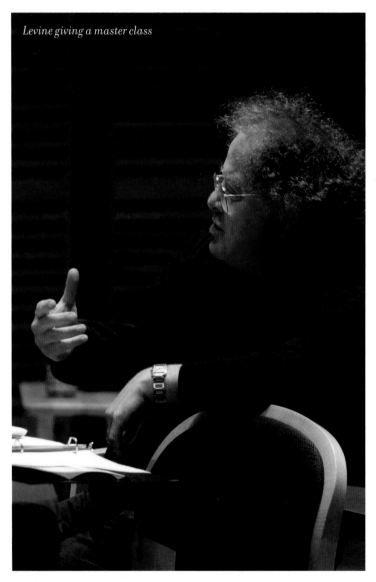

Levine giving a master class

JL: We could feel the operatic traditions weakening, and it was clear to me that if we didn't train some singers of our own we were one day going to be in trouble. I was very aware of the fact that each young singer I heard who was talented always had something to learn: language or technique or acting skills or musical comprehension... I wanted a situation in which we could use the resources of the Met to help very promising singers get through that gap between school and "career." The program was designed to help each singer with what he or she lacks. I didn't want to take singers whose careers were already in the bag. What's the point of that? We wanted to take the singer with the big talent who might not arrive if we didn't help them.

Our program still has a couple of hallmarks from the way I started it. One is a rule that singers cannot accept engagements without our approval during their time in the program. That way, we can at least keep them from running around singing things they shouldn't. Second, we sometimes offer them small roles on stage, which they do not have to accept. Some singers learn a lot by being on stage with a role that doesn't have to hold up the whole evening, and that is a hands-on experience that they need.

When you examine artists the first time, you cannot be certain at all which one has a talent that won't grow and which one has not yet manifested anything like the talent that they've got. But if you work very diligently at it, you get some amazingly gratifying results. The roster of singers who are working in the world who came through our program is a very diverse group who do very good work.

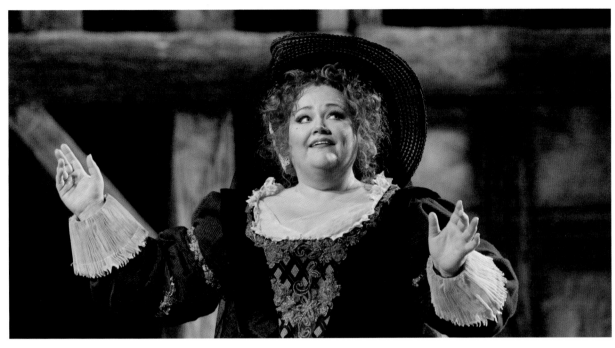

Stephanie Blythe as Dame Quickly in Falstaff

Stephanie Blythe: During the Metropolitan Opera's 1995–96 season, I was given a major role assignment: the cover for Marilyn Horne as Quickly in Verdi's *Falstaff*. It was a daunting task for a young singer in only her second year in the Met's young artist program, but I was excited at the prospect and ready for the challenge. The cast was truly brilliant, and the conductor was James Levine.

I had taken part in many of the principal rehearsals, and when I wasn't rehearsing, I was watching. Levine has a particular love of *Falstaff*, and I can hardly blame him. Marilyn Horne told me during this time that she considered this the leanest and most economical of Verdi's operas, and I quite agree. It was Maestro Levine's reading of this score that convinced me, and watching him conduct this music is witnessing pure joy.

One late afternoon, as I sat on my voice teacher's sofa, I received a phone call from the Met that I was going on. When I recovered my senses, we headed down to the theater. About an hour or so before the curtain, there was a knock at the door. There was Jim, smiling at me. He came in, sat at the piano, told me he knew I was ready and gave me advice about

how to look at him without looking as if I were looking at him. He asked if there were any spots where he could be of any extra help, and I said that basically, I felt fine. We agreed to keep close contact, and he wished me a great show. His ease and generosity made me strangely calm, and as I prepared to go onstage, I told myself: "Don't let a moment of this go; remember every bit of this night and keep it in your heart."

It was an amazing experience, and I recollect every second of it. I barely looked at the Maestro at all. You could just feel the energy coming from the pit, and every time I did look at him, I got that wonderful smile and a thumbs-up. What a feeling!

After the curtain call, he walked me back to my dressing room. My voice teacher was waiting there for me. The door closed and I just screamed with glee. I couldn't do anything but smile and laugh. 15 minutes later, I was just sitting there taking off my make-up, in contented shock, when there was a knock at the door. "I can't leave you yet," Jim said. "That was just too much fun!"

And so I say now, "Thank you, Jim—thanks for all the fun!"

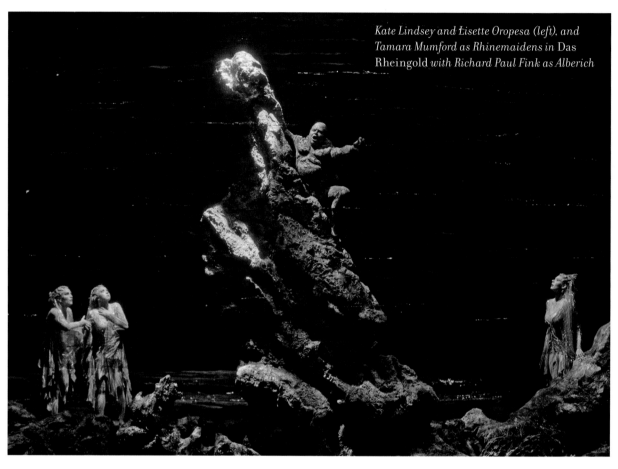

Kate Lindsey and Lisette Oropesa (left), and Tamara Mumford as Rhinemaidens in Das Rheingold *with Richard Paul Fink as Alberich*

John Fisher, former Met Director of Music Administration: "Isn't that something?" or "What an incredible thing!"—two of countless phrases I have heard uttered by James Levine on so many occasions, enthusing about practically every piece of music he happens to be rehearsing or performing at the time. I think it is this extraordinary, unbridled passion and true love of all music, theater and drama, which makes him unique— along with his ability, through his huge talent, to pass on that love to others. Part of my job at the Met was to work with Jimmy on running the LYADP. I witnessed what a consummate "singers' conductor" he is: he understands the voice and— a rarer and more important ability—the psychology of singers. In rehearsals, one becomes aware of how much his dramatic and theatrical instincts inform his creative process. Whether he is coaching a singer or rehearsing the orchestra, every note, phrase, word, or rest has a motivation and energy, and he always conveys that principle in such a logical and clear way, but again with his unique brand of joy and enthusiasm.

Kate Lindsey: It was 2004, my first year in the LYADP, and I was preparing the "Dunque io son" duet from *The Barber of Seville*. At the master class, Maestro Levine really got on me, and I was having trouble figuring out what was going on. I thought I was doing what everybody had told me to do. Finally he said, "Kate, you're mugging. It's not real." I was really upset, and I thought, "I've let him down, I'm cruddy, I don't know what's happening any more." And then it came to me, that everything you do has to come from a really honest core inside you. I needed to prepare for the day when I would take full ownership. Your coach and your teacher don't get up on stage with you. Maestro Levine made me see that you have to find the place from which you can get up on stage and own what you sing.

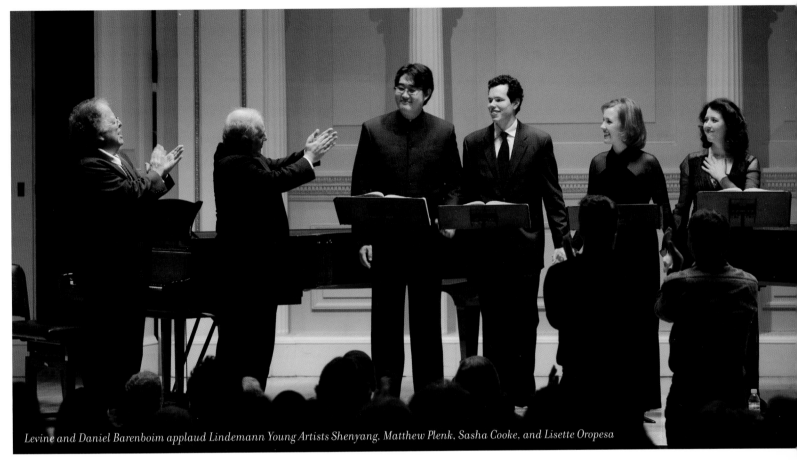

Levine and Daniel Barenboim applaud Lindemann Young Artists Shenyang, Matthew Plenk, Sasha Cooke, and Lisette Oropesa

Lisette Oropesa: Being in the LYADP is kind of like being in the womb: all the nutrients come to you, and you just grow and try to stay healthy. Maestro Levine handpicks everybody and handpicks pretty much everything we do and tries to keep as closely involved as he can. Towards the end of my time with the program, we found out that three of us were going to be cast as the Rhinemaidens in the *Ring* in the spring of 2009, and it was really exciting. It's not a long part but the music is really challenging, and the text is of course extremely important. Maestro Levine was at every rehearsal, very involved, so we were able to get a lot of input about how this should be done. It was also fun. One time we got to the part where we all sing, "Rheingold, Rheingold." In between, he joined us, singing, "Rheingold, I said Rheingold, oh yeah!" He just cracked everybody up. It seemed as if he didn't have a care in the world; he just wanted to make music. By the time opening night came around, it already had such energy behind it. When the orchestra began, it was so amazing I thought I was going to have a heart attack.

I would never hesitate to bring him anything, in any repertoire, because his specialty is *everything*. He always has something fresh to say. He'll ask what you think, and you can share ideas and have a conversation about a piece. He doesn't get bored, and he doesn't get stale. He's never going to encourage you to do anything that's going to hurt your voice. I remember someone asking him, "What's the right tempo for this piece?" And he said, "The right tempo is the tempo that works for you." Even if he hasn't heard you in months, he remembers the last thing you sang and how you sounded, and he comments on that. He says, "Oh, your voice is changing. I'm hearing some new colors for this," or, "Let's work on that. How about…?" He's like a doctor: he can diagnose perfectly, and he's always right on. The time that we get with him is gold. I write down what he's saying, and I try to remember everything. He's a voice teacher, and a therapist, and a coach—all rolled into one.

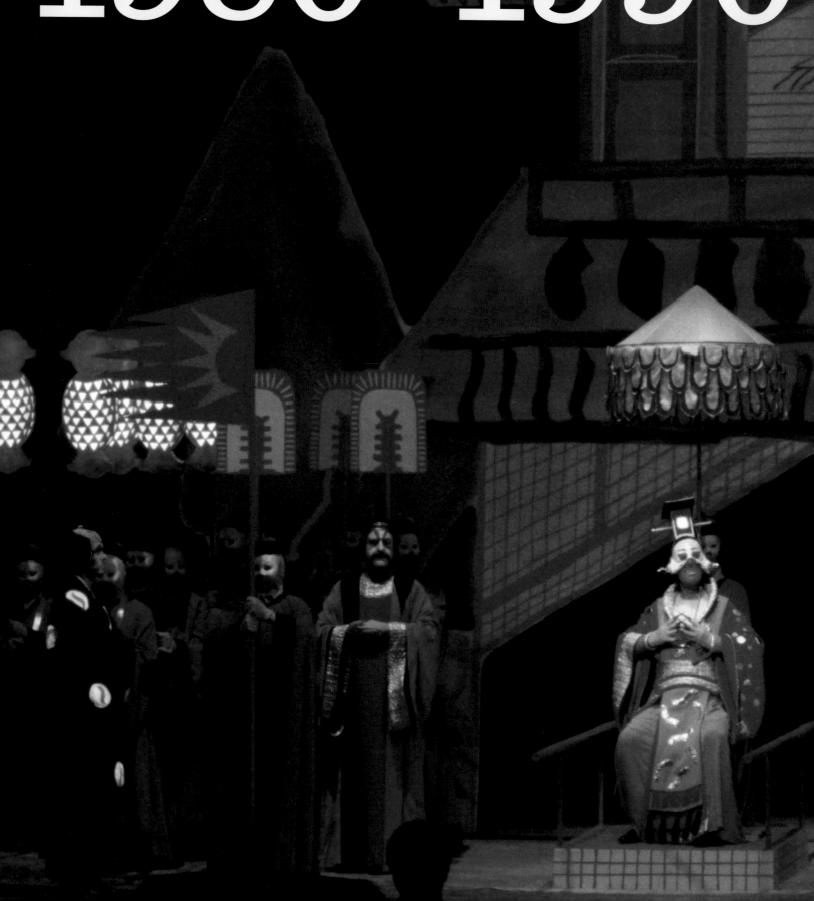

1980–1990

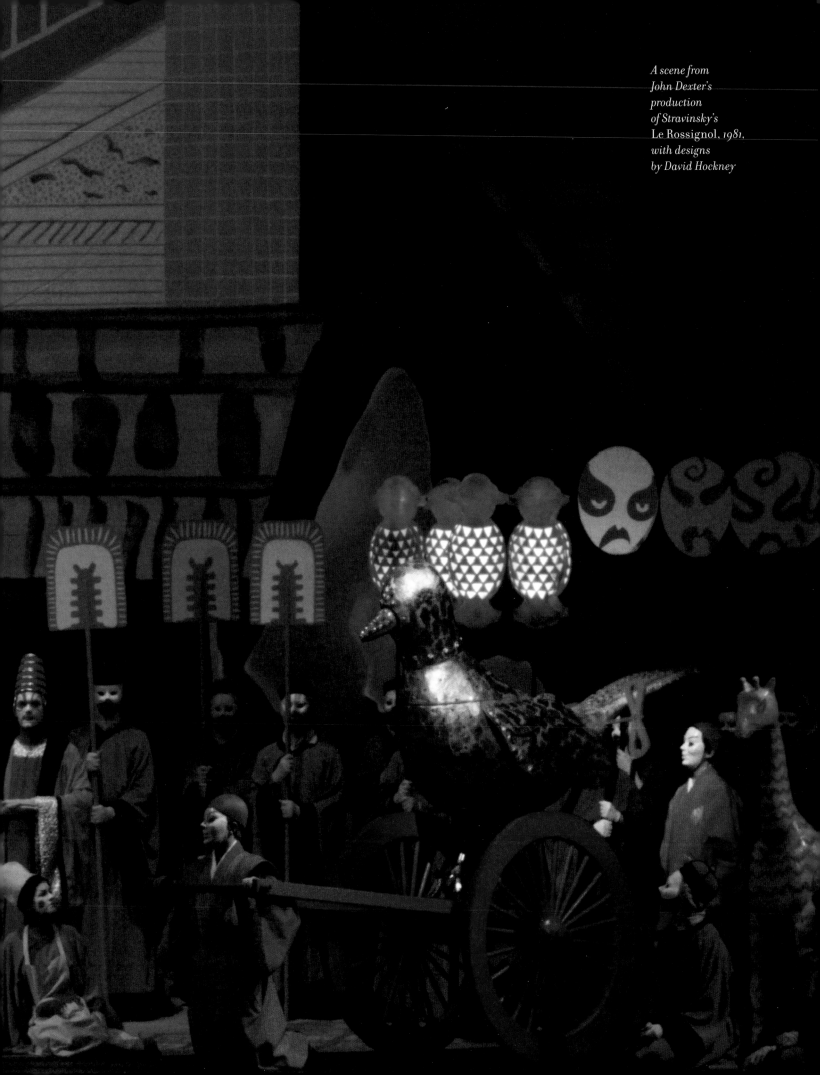

His Own Best Pupil

RICHARD DYER

Two little stories tell you a lot about the kind of conductor James Levine is because they tell you the kind of musician he is, and the kind of man.

The first dates back to the mid-1960s, when he was the assistant conductor of The Cleveland Orchestra under George Szell. One of Levine's first assignments was to rehearse Chopin's Second Piano Concerto, and he vividly remembers a little oboe solo near the beginning: "The oboist played it more beautifully than I could ever have imagined on my own. There was nothing I could have done that would have made it any more beautiful. I realized immediately that it was not my job to control every element of the performance, but to allow the musicians to bring the best of themselves to an overall conception of the piece."

The second revealing incident took place 40 years later at Tanglewood, when Levine was supervising reading rehearsals of Mozart's *Don Giovanni* with fellows of the Music Center—singers, conductors, and orchestra. No performance was scheduled; this was a learning experience. The conducting fellow was propelling an ensemble at an exciting tempo that was flustering the Donna Elvira. Levine stopped him. "What are you doing that for?" he asked. "Can't you imagine how well she could sing it at a slightly slower tempo? What do you have to gain by making her uncomfortable? What does *Mozart* have to gain?" Once again, Levine was talking about enabling performers to give their best, about how a conductor's job is not just to lead but also to listen. ("Jimmy hears *everything*," a player once said to me, with mingled admiration and panic.)

The statistics of Levine's tenure at the Metropolitan Opera are staggering: 40 years, nearly 2,500 performances of 85 different operas, and counting. But the significance of his service lies behind and beyond the statistical record. Statistics define quantity, not quality, and they don't tell anything about the process through which quality is achieved.

Everyone comments on how the orchestra, under his direction, has become one of the great ensembles of the world.

One of his strategies has been to encourage the members to play chamber music, and to turn them loose on the symphonic repertory—just as in posts he has held with symphonic ensembles, Levine has programmed operas. He doesn't believe in specialization, for himself or for the institutions he works with; all music unfolds on a continuum, and different parts of the continuum inform and instruct one another. An orchestra must emulate the phrasing, breathing, colorations, vibrancy, and emotional impact of a great singer in full flight; a singer should emulate the precision, ensemble skills, and coloristic range of an instrumentalist.

Another great legacy is Levine's widening and freshening of the Met repertory, from less-performed works by established composers to 20th-century masterworks to brand-new compositions. And he adds to his own repertory all the time—in the last few years he led his first *Madama Butterfly* and first *Don Pasquale*. There are works one wishes he would conduct—*Der Freischütz, Boris Godunov, Capriccio, La Gioconda,* or *La Fanciulla del West,* for example—but their absence is as much a question of timing or availability of suitable singers as it is of personal taste. One of his strengths is utilizing the changing interests and abilities of each generation of singers as it comes along. Of course, he also knows better than to conduct works for which he feels no real affinity, or that he feels others can do better.

Like a clerk in a Dickens novel, Levine maintains elaborate ledgers of his performances; the ledgers reinforce his instincts about when to return to central works for his own artistic development, when they have grown in his subconscious and it is time for new insights to assert themselves. And he strategizes repertory for the orchestra the way he strategizes for himself—how often it needs to ground itself in Mozart, for example. He didn't program Berg's *Lulu* before he brought back *Wozzeck,* and he didn't attempt Schoenberg's *Moses und Aron* before the orchestra had played both *Wozzeck* and *Lulu*.

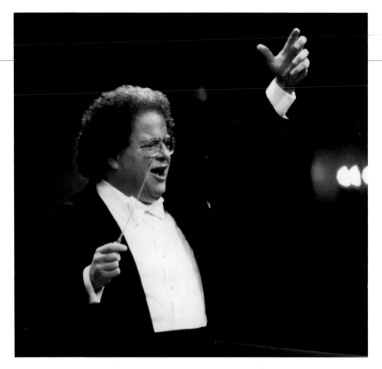

Levine's formal musical education was as comprehensive as he could make it—general studies under Walter Levin of the LaSalle String Quartet, famous for its mastery of the Second Viennese School and contemporary music; solo piano instruction with Rosina Lhevinne; chamber music with Rudolf Serkin and others; French repertory with Jean Morel at Juilliard; German repertory with Szell. At the Aspen Music Festival and School he sought out composers like Darius Milhaud and established singers like Jennie Tourel and Phyllis Curtin. One of his early idols was Toscanini, and he made it a project to work with as many singers as possible who had performed under Toscanini. Levine has coached countless singers, but it is equally important to point out how many singers he has made it a point to learn from. He is his own best pupil.

From the beginning Levine knew what his core repertory would be. Back in Ohio, he created an orchestra at the Cleveland Institute of Music and gave concert performances of *Don Giovanni, Don Carlo,* and *Simon Boccanegra.* Mozart and Verdi—Wagner came later, first at the Met, and then at the Bayreuth Festival. To these composers one should add Berlioz and Berg, as well as *The Bartered Bride, Pelléas et Mélisande,* and Strauss's *Elektra, Der Rosenkavalier,* and *Ariadne auf Naxos.* Anyone who has heard Levine conduct these works must have indelible memories of his way with them.

Of course, Levine wants each performance to be as good as it can be, but he is at least as interested in process, in the whole movement from developing a conception prior to rehearsal, building on what happens in rehearsal, and watching interpretation develop through a series of performances—even foreseeing what might happen in future seasons that will build upon the present. He is not afraid to say "Sorry, my mistake" in rehearsal, and he knows when he has not operated on his own best level. I once heard him muse ruefully about a Sirius re-broadcast of a Mozart opera, "What a great cast, and I let them down."

Singers love Levine. "It is never easy to sing," the late Lorraine Hunt Lieberson told me, "but James Levine makes you believe you can do things you never thought you could." There are very few singers of the front rank over the last 40 years who have not worked with him, and his collaborations continue today with a younger generation.

For all of Levine's presence in a starry firmament, he lives in the real world and works within the complex conditions of a major modern opera house. The curtain does not invariably rise on an ideal cast in an ideal production, and vocal cords are subject to the various physical and emotional ills the flesh is heir to. But he has the imagination, ability and true grit to make the best of every situation so no one goes home after a Levine performance with an empty heart.

Often as conductors grow older, their tempos become slower, as if they are reluctant to let go of the music, or accelerate, as if they are trying to outpace time itself. Levine is a collector and student of time-pieces, and he has avoided both extremes, just as he charts a course that avoids complacency and routine at one extreme, and egocentric eccentricity for its own sake at the other. The public has learned to depend on a high level of quality when he is on the podium. But even after 40 years, the public also knows to expect surprise.

Richard Dyer wrote about music and the arts for The Boston Globe *for 33 years. His involvement with James Levine continues through his writing of weekly podcast scripts for the Boston Symphony Orchestra and his teaching at the Tanglewood Music Center.*

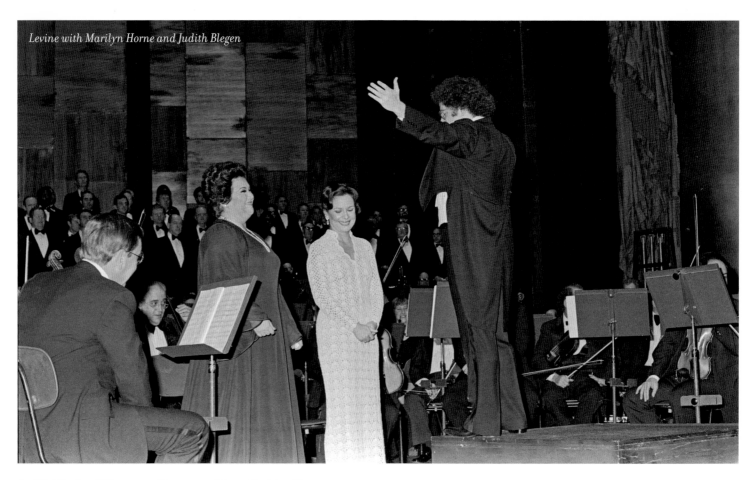

Judith Blegen: Whenever Jimmy and I met in his office, no matter what, I always came back feeling that everything was fabulous. He suggested a lot of repertoire to me, and I wish I could subtract about 30 years from my life and say yes to a lot more things! Especially because Jimmy knew me and knew my voice. It has been such a privilege to watch him work. He is the biggest sponge I've ever seen. He grasps everything and understands its significance right away, but he never stops thinking about it. That's the way to make a mountain: take a little tiny thing and work on every detail.

1980
DECEMBER 10

After a completely dark autumn due to labor disputes, Levine opens the Met season with Mahler's Symphony No. 2, "Resurrection," featuring soloists Judith Blegen and Marilyn Horne.

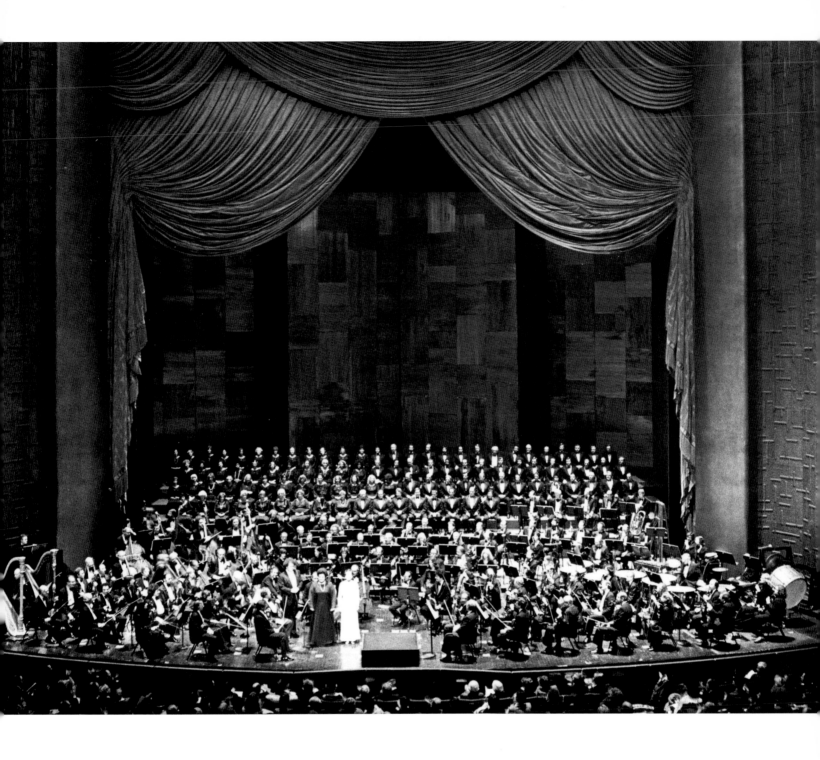

JL: John Dexter and Jocelyn Herbert's production from 1977 was brilliant, and it easily accommodated the third act, that Friedrich Cerha had just completed. When you've got all three acts, the form of *Lulu* is represented properly: the ascent and descent of Lulu are each three scenes—the middle of that shape is the interlude between the two scenes of the second act. It was one of the great experiences of my operatic life to work with Teresa on this part. She had the voice, the musicianship, the stagecraft, the experience, and the human being for this part—and for any of the parts that suited her, which covered a huge stylistic range. She has a temperament that doesn't quit, but she always talks with extraordinary lucidity. She was so powerful onstage, by instinct, that you might think she had an intellectual weakness. But no one is more lucid than Teresa when she needs to explain or articulate something—she's aware of everything.

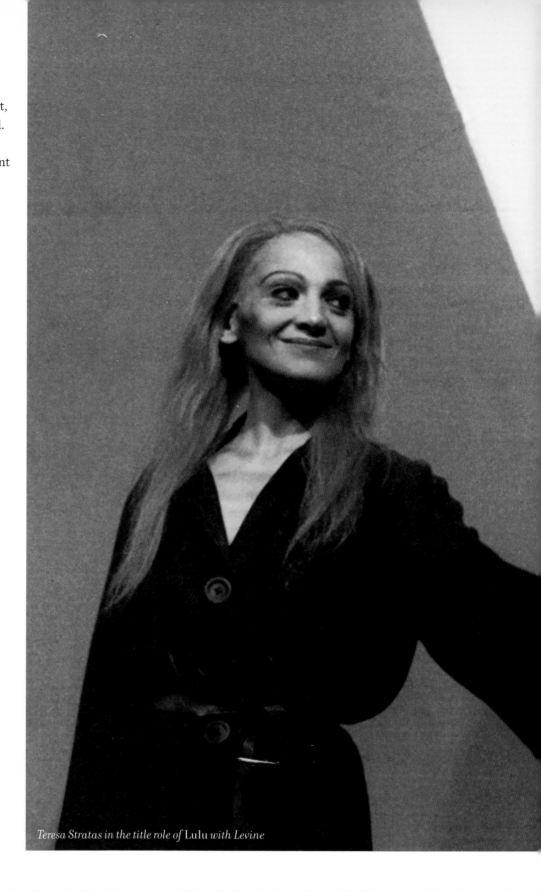

Teresa Stratas in the title role of Lulu *with Levine*

DECEMBER 12

Leads the first Met performance of the complete three-act *Lulu,* with Teresa Stratas in the title role.

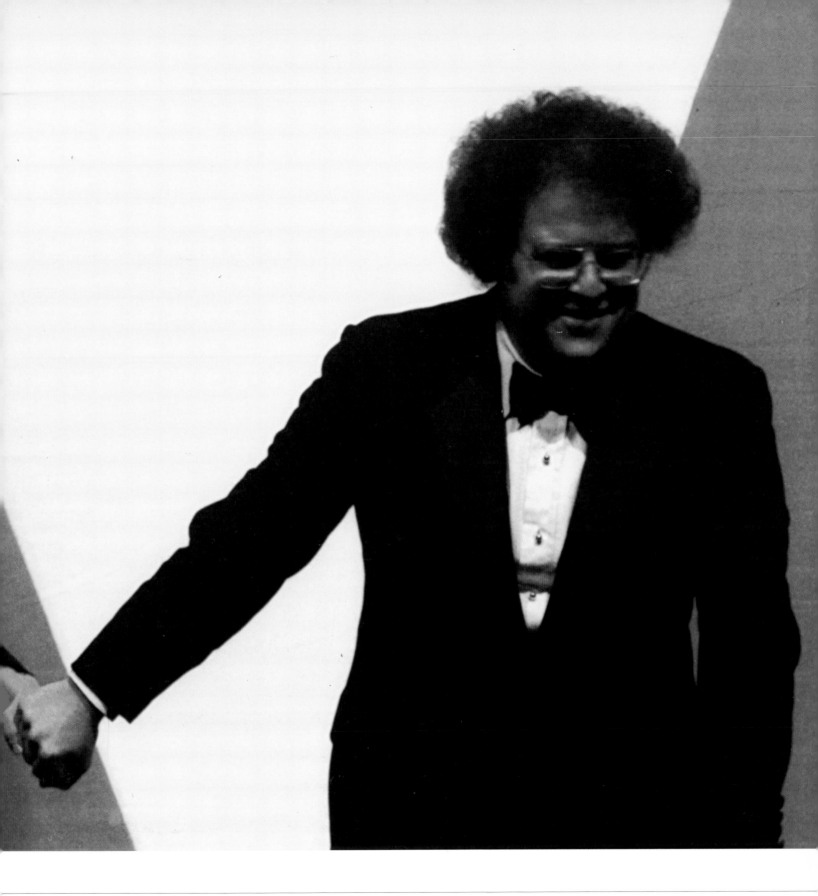

JL: We were just coming out of a terribly depressing labor dispute—the house was dark the entire autumn, and we reopened in December. The entire schedule had been shot, we had to give up the singers because we couldn't guarantee the contracts. It was the singular low point of my entire artistic life. As Music Director, I don't have a function if we are not performing. I could do nothing because the issues were financial and structural, not artistic. When we finally opened, Joan Ingpen, the artistic administrator, and her staff had to cobble together what was left of the season.

The first opera we actually did was *Lulu,* with Stratas. But trying to get a sophisticated, detailed performance of *Tristan* had me in a situation I had never been in before—there was no way to rehearse properly. All the work I would have done with the company in advance, all the pre-season time, was gone. And of course it is normal for us, when putting on a large opera like this in a repertory system, to have a much bigger and more complex rehearsal schedule than, say, for *The Barber of Seville.* And by that time I had conducted *Tannhäuser, Lohengrin, Dutchman,* and *Parsifal,* but had not yet done *Tristan, Meistersinger,* or the *Ring* operas at the Met. I had been building a way of working with the company in this repertoire with continuously better results, but this situation was a nightmare.

As it turned out, there was eventually a happy ending, as it forced us, coming out of that dark autumn, to pull out every drop of company esprit to keep the Met in the best form, and to keep going. And the Met ended up doing lots of *Parsifals* during those years but very few *Tristans.* The balance began to be redressed with our new production of *Tristan* in 1999, when the long-term ripples from the labor dispute were far behind us and we had had lots of Wagner time since then for *Meistersinger* and the *Ring,* as well as revivals of *Tristan, Parsifal, Lohengrin,* and *Dutchman.*

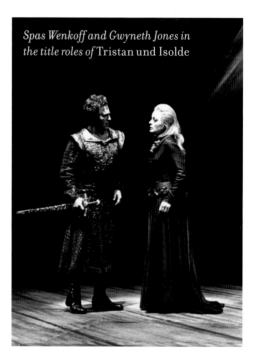

Spas Wenkoff and Gwyneth Jones in the title roles of Tristan und Isolde

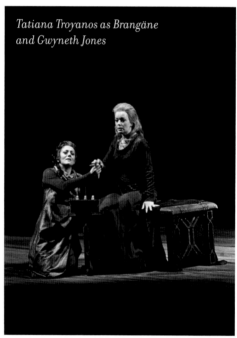

Tatiana Troyanos as Brangäne and Gwyneth Jones

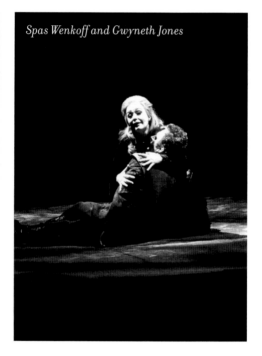

Spas Wenkoff and Gwyneth Jones

1981
JANUARY 9

Adds *Tristan und Isolde* to his Met repertoire in the company's first uncut performances of the work, starring Gwyneth Jones, Spas Wenkoff, Tatiana Troyanos, and Matti Salminen.

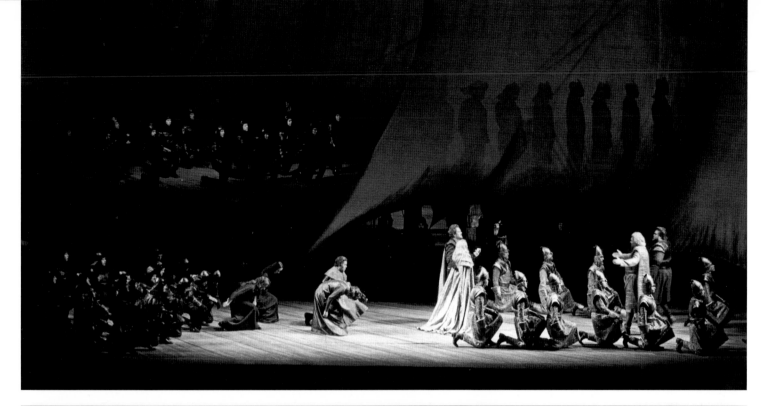

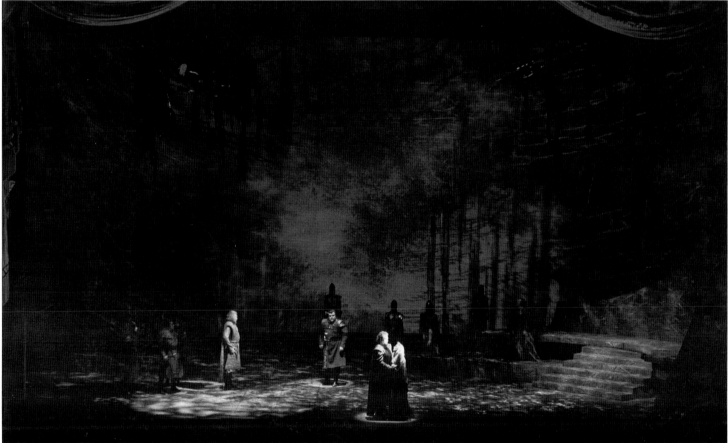

Scenes from August Everding's production of Tristan und Isolde

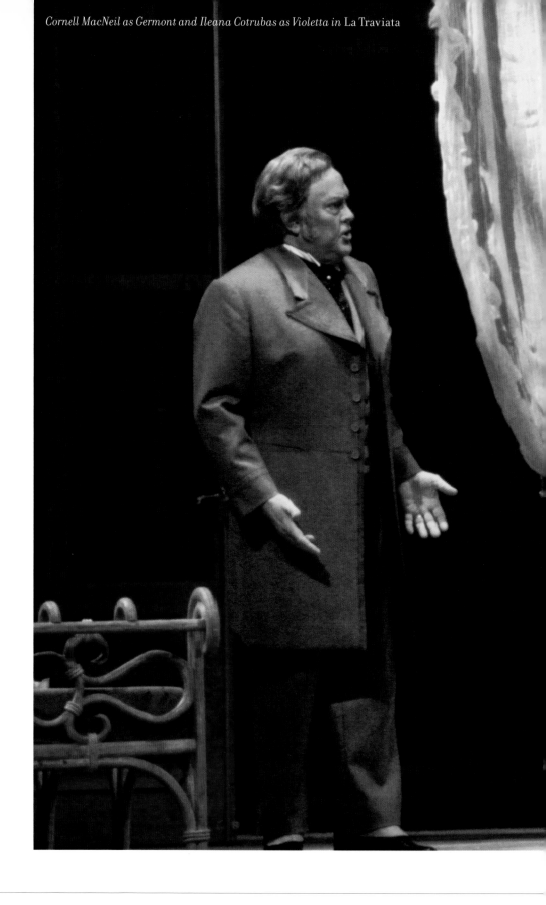

Cornell MacNeil as Germont and Ileana Cotrubas as Violetta in La Traviata

Adds Verdi's *La Traviata* to his Met
repertoire, in a new production starring
Ileana Cotrubas, Plácido Domingo,
and Cornell MacNeil.

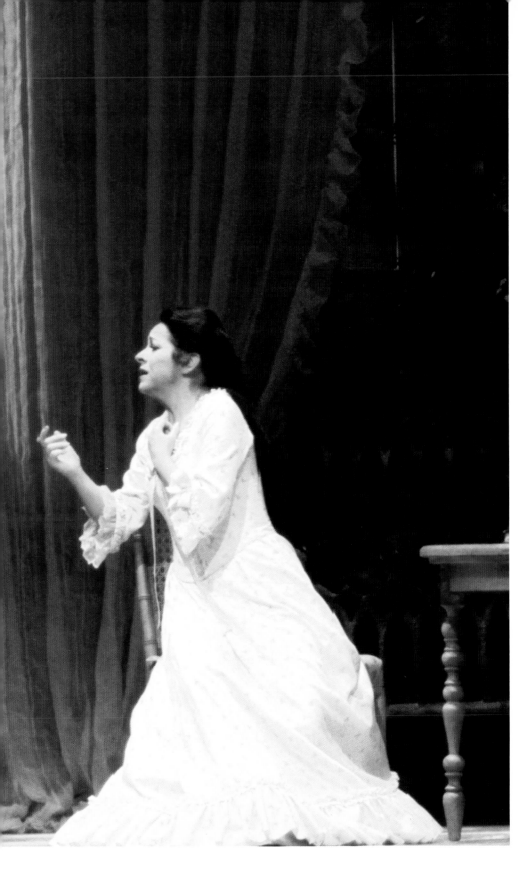

JL: I first got wind of Ileana because MacNeil was in an Otto Schenk *Traviata* with her in Vienna, and he wrote me a letter saying, "Here's the genuine article. You should hear her." I ended up doing a lot of work with her. Wonderful girl, wonderful artist, with a special gift for being expressive and communicative in an ideally detailed way.

JL: *Trittico* is unique in that all three operas are masterpieces of their type. It's one thing to do a comedy and a tragedy, but here we have a Grand Guignol-type melodrama, followed by an intense religious drama, then a comic masterpiece. I think the whole is most successful when the performers concentrate on doing justice to each opera with its own discrete qualities. Renata was an artist with a deep understanding of the communication of various kinds of roles. She was particularly dynamic as Giorgetta and Angelica, and then it was wonderful to have the lady who went through all that do Lauretta, a sweet part with a sweet aria. Renata and I did a huge range of operas together, and she was a joy to work with, both tremendously imaginative and tremendously hard-working. Her presence at the Met made it possible for us to keep the Italian style wonderfully alive and well in a period when it was gradually declining worldwide.

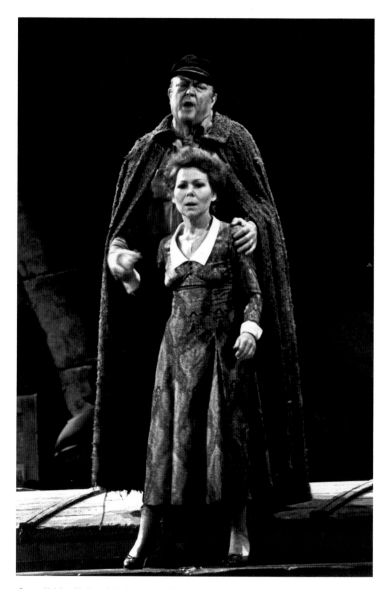

Cornell MacNeil as Michele and Renata Scotto as Giorgetta in Il Tabarro

OCTOBER 30

Conducts Renata Scotto in all three leading roles of Puccini's *Il Trittico*.

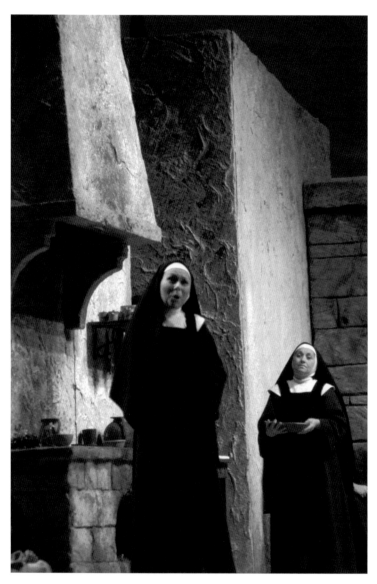

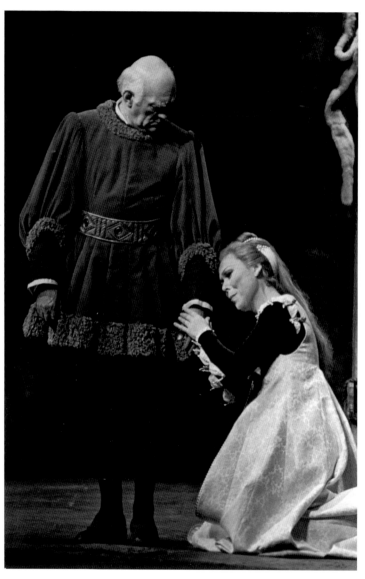

Renata Scotto in the title role of Suor Angelica
and Loretta di Franco as an Alms Collector

Renata Scotto as Lauretta and Gabriel Bacquier
in the title role of Gianni Schicchi

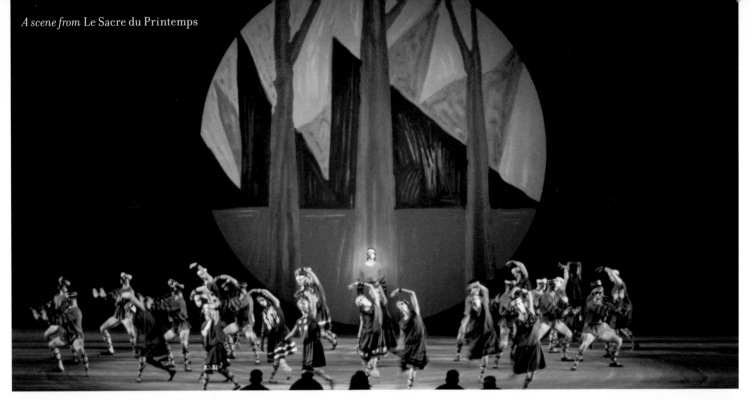

A scene from Le Sacre du Printemps

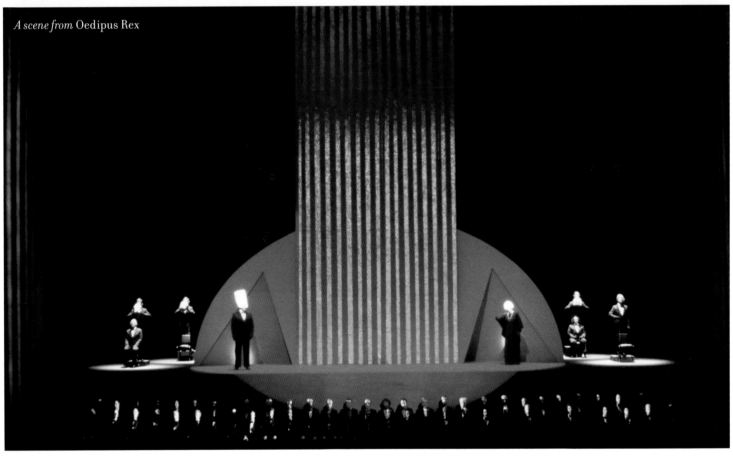

A scene from Oedipus Rex

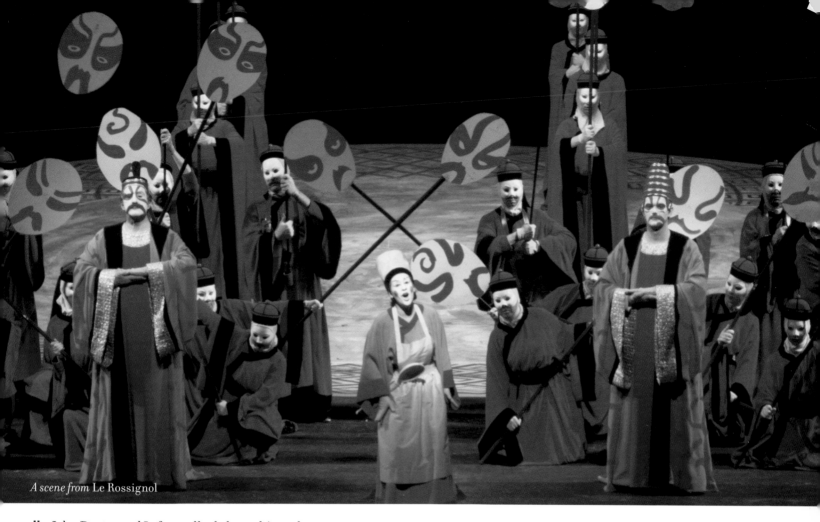

A scene from Le Rossignol

JL: John Dexter and I often talked about things that were difficult to produce at the Met, like operettas and one-act operas. There are many great and powerful one-act operas, but the problem is finding a combination that works well together and can draw an audience. In the previous season, John had dreamed up a French triple bill, a ballet followed by two operas. Having succeeded with that, he wanted to do a triple bill in honor of the Stravinsky anniversary. I was always kind of fascinated by the idea of *Sacre du Printemps* as an opener—the first sound you hear. John proposed *Oedipus Rex,* I proposed *Rossignol,* and Hockney designed the three pieces as different kinds of ritualistic-symbolic mask dramas. It was an intense and exciting evening, and the response from the audience was excellent.

DECEMBER 3

Leads a Stravinsky triple bill, staged by John Dexter and designed by David Hockney, that combines the Met premieres of *Oedipus Rex* and *Le Sacre du Printemps* with *Le Rossignol.*

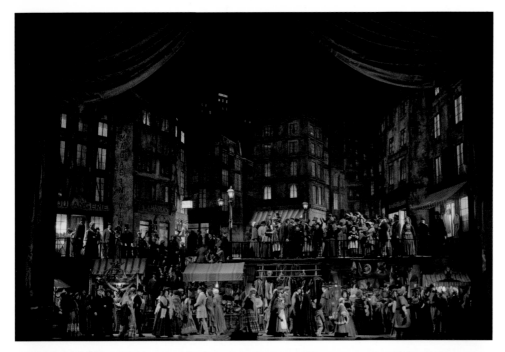

Franco Zeffirelli: Jimmy always commits himself to finding something new, something different, something that he has not spotted before in an opera. When we worked together, he communicated these things not by telling me, "This is what I have done here," but just by looking at me, right in my eyes, at the end of a rehearsal. Even if it was something I had heard many times, he would reveal new emotions to me. Every performance, every rehearsal is a moment to rediscover secret vibrations. We need geniuses like Levine to grab hold at every performance, to revisit scores with new eyes and ears. I have worked with a lot of great conductors, but I really would jump out of bed at midnight to go work with Jimmy.

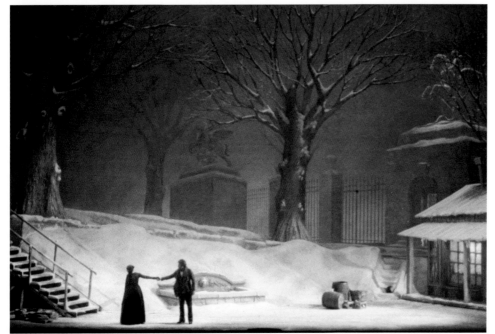

Acts II and III of Franco Zeffirelli's production of La Bohème

JL: In Franco's work, the milieu, the atmosphere, and the acoustics are always brilliant, and every one of his productions has certain scenes that are ideal operatic art—things like *Bohème* Acts II and III, *Falstaff* Act III, *Otello* Act III, *Turandot* Act I, etcetera.

DECEMBER 14

Conducts Franco Zeffirelli's new production of *La Bohème,* starring Teresa Stratas and José Carreras.

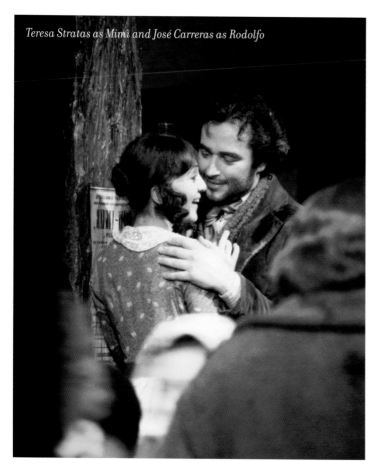

Teresa Stratas as Mimì and José Carreras as Rodolfo

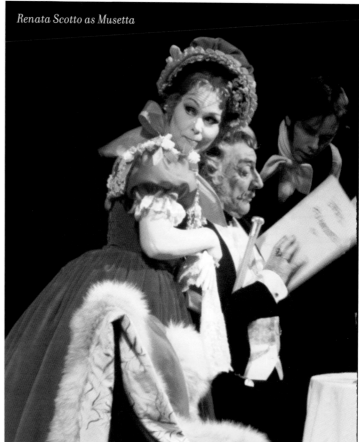

Renata Scotto as Musetta

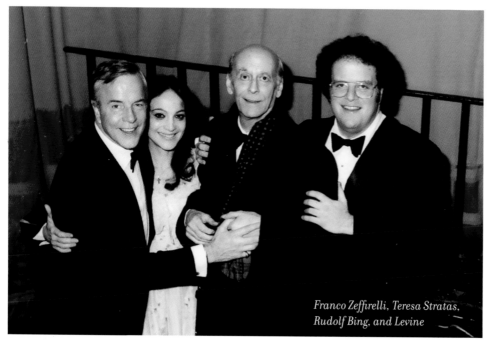

Franco Zeffirelli, Teresa Stratas, Rudolf Bing, and Levine

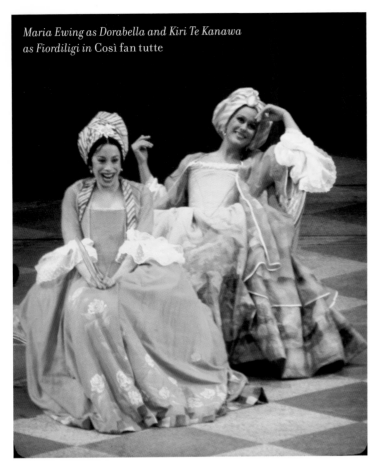

Maria Ewing as Dorabella and Kiri Te Kanawa as Fiordiligi in Così fan tutte

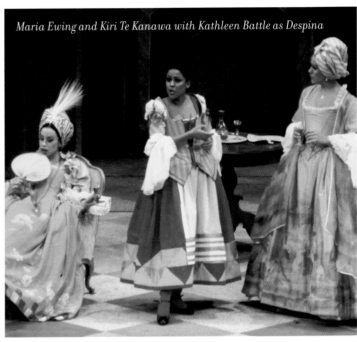

Maria Ewing and Kiri Te Kanawa with Kathleen Battle as Despina

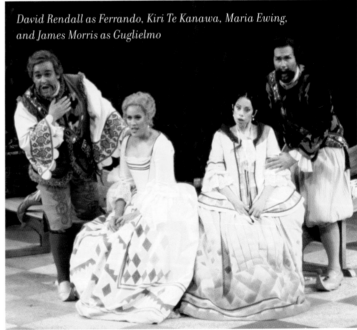

David Rendall as Ferrando, Kiri Te Kanawa, Maria Ewing, and James Morris as Guglielmo

JL: Maria Ewing was the funniest, most stylish Dorabella you could imagine, absolutely sensational. She had the whole gift: brilliant on the stage, brilliant musician, brilliant linguist, very striking timbre. Maria started off with maybe the most full-scale and versatile gifts of any artist I ever worked with, able to sing every language, every style, recital, oratorio, opera, the whole business. And she was such a persuasive Dorabella, perfect with Kiri because they sparked each other. They made each other more beautiful and funny than they would've been separately.

1982
JANUARY 29

His Mozart cycle continues with Colin
Graham's new production of *Così fan tutte,*
starring Kiri Te Kanawa, Maria Ewing,
Kathleen Battle, David Rendall, James Morris,
and Donald Gramm.

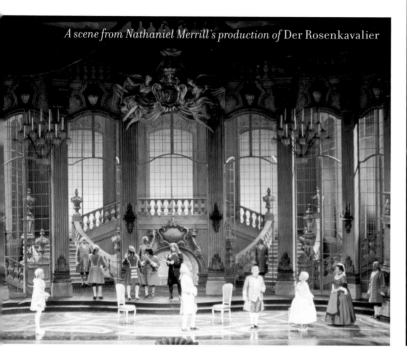

A scene from Nathaniel Merrill's production of Der Rosenkavalier

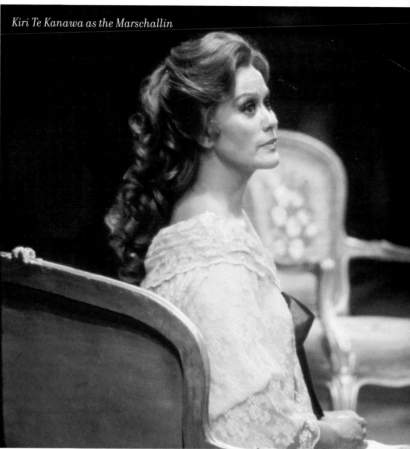

Kiri Te Kanawa as the Marschallin

JL: Kiri was not an egghead, over-intellectualized Marschallin—she was a beautiful, young one who brought just what was needed at every moment. She coached with people who made her work on details, and she ate it up and performed brilliantly. She always took her artistic work very seriously. What a wonderful personality altogether—warm and radiant, a fantastic sense of humor. And her voice was just perfect for... well... beautiful voice repertoire!

SEPTEMBER 20

Opens the Met season with *Der Rosenkavalier,* starring Tatiana Troyanos, Kiri Te Kanawa, Judith Blegen, and Kurt Moll, with Luciano Pavarotti performing the Italian Singer in subsequent performances.

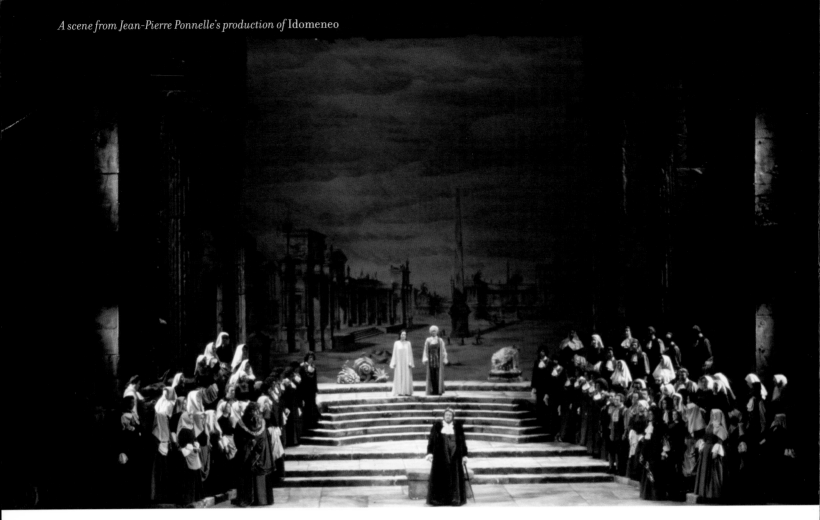

JL: When I was a kid, the only Mozart operas played regularly in international repertoire were *The Magic Flute, Don Giovanni,* and *Figaro.* When the others were played, they were cut or made into weird versions. But Mozart wrote seven masterpieces, besides quite a lot of other good operas. Two of these masterpieces were opera seria: the first was *Idomeneo,* and the last—written in the last year of his life—was *La Clemenza di Tito.* Jean-Pierre appreciated these pieces and approached them with great perception, flair, and brilliance. He also managed to use the same fundamental chorus costumes and physical frame to do both, so that it was economically sound. *Idomeneo* is a piece of extraordinary dimension, and expressive range. There are only three ensembles in this huge, gigantic opera. The rest is arias, recitatives, choruses—unbelievable in a piece of that scale. It's a very difficult opera, but Jean-Pierre put in on stage in such a persuasive, apt, and detailed way. And these singers were more than ready to get into it and do it. It was a wonderful cast, and then we had a series of wonderful casts in revivals, too.

OCTOBER 14

Introduces Mozart's *Idomeneo* to the Met, in a production by Jean-Pierre Ponnelle, with Luciano Pavarotti in the title role, alongside Ileana Cotrubas, Hildegard Behrens, Frederica von Stade, and John Alexander.

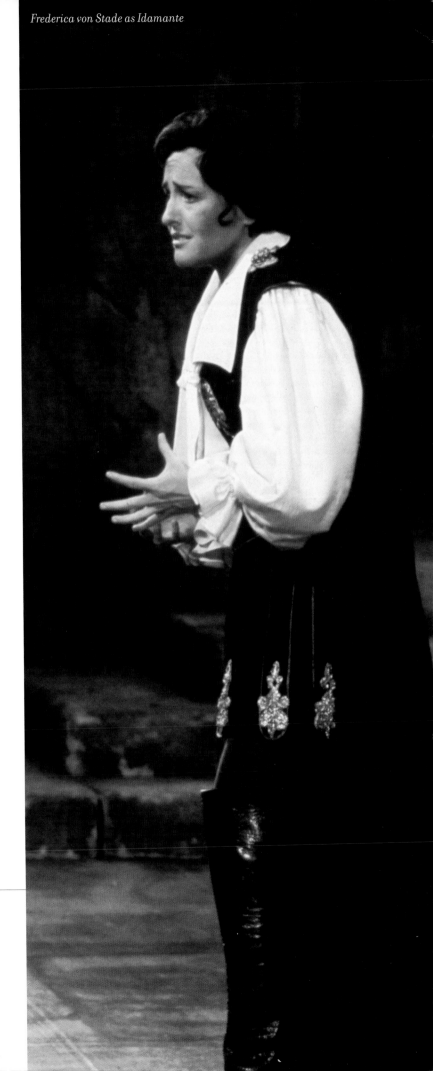

Frederica von Stade: Long before I met him, I had heard of Jimmy Levine, this wunderkind, this amazing guy, but I first worked with him for the Met premiere of *Idomeneo.* I had never done Idamante before. It's a difficult role, and it came at a difficult time in my life. Jimmy led me through it with such care, and I will forever adore him for that. The discovery of that piece for all of us was amazing. I was too ignorant to feel the tremendous responsibility of presenting a Mozart work for the first time. I think Jimmy cushions his singers a great deal, so that you don't feel any of the weight; you just feel the pure joy of singing. I always had the feeling with Jimmy that the music is safe, I'm safe, my colleagues are safe, the director is safe—we are all in an unbelievably safe place. Jimmy would take away my worries and replace them with something I had never conceived of. It's like when you're teaching a kid to ride a bike: your heart is in your mouth because she's about to fall over, and then you see the look on her face when she knows that she can do it. Jimmy does that with artists, saying, "You can do it this way, you know. Watch yourself—you're going to love this!" He makes the miracles happen. But I think that kind of goodwill has to cost him an enormous amount of energy. He really loves his singers, and we're imperfect, so that love has to include a lot of forgiveness. He makes space for all levels of musicality and musicianship. Working with Jimmy is like playing tennis with someone who is better than you; it elevates your playing. You sing better because he has that magic devotion to what he is doing. It's like a laser beam, and you get in the light and the energy of that and do better than you even thought you could.

I can see in Jimmy the confidence and strength that comes from learning music as a child and getting good at it, as if it's no big deal. But of course it is a big deal. Jimmy is American-trained and he has a kind of openness about him. It's as if there's nothing he can't do, because he has done it. He's fearless, and unbelievably generous with his gift. He creates a space filled with love of what he's doing, as if he would rather be doing that than anything in the world, and he makes you part of it.

JL: Michael Walsh, the music critic for *Time* magazine, proposed a piece on Herbert von Karajan. But Martha Duffy, the arts editor, said, "There might be a better story right here in your backyard. I think you should do a piece on James Levine." So he listened to a bunch of my recordings for a couple of weeks and got all turned around and wanted to do it. When I found out, first of all I was very surprised because I didn't understand what possible point of view they would have. But it turned out to be one of the most wonderful nonmusical experiences I ever had. It renewed my faith in what could be done in that field. I look at the cover photo, and by God, not only do I think they got an image that was actually organic, but they also got these people who were also organic: Pavarotti, Stratas, Scotto, Blegen, Carreras, Milnes, Troyanos, Domingo, Hofmann... it wasn't a random sample. There are two facts about the article that are interesting in retrospect. One, it may have been the first time that any treatment like that had come to a conductor who wasn't spending time primarily with a symphony orchestra—so for opera it was a first. The other thing is, it was also a last. If you look at the annals of the *Time* cover you will see that up until 1983 or so, you could find classical artists on the cover with fair regularity. If you look at the annals since 1983, they have barely been represented on the cover at all, and there were numerous times when there existed a phenomenon that could easily have been documented that way. I think it's a telling symptom of the culture going in the wrong direction, where nowadays you turn on the television and it's as though the more trivial it is, the more it's up there. I feel bad for the kids because I think they could just as easily have something that excites them about all kinds of very constructive things, and I don't see it. The whole thing worries me a lot because it's as though gradually the source material is disappearing for the next generation. Everybody wants to convince everybody that the watered-down version will do, but of course that's the very thing that won't do. The amount of didactic information people need in order to enjoy opera and classical music is almost none—so many things come just from getting the right exposure.

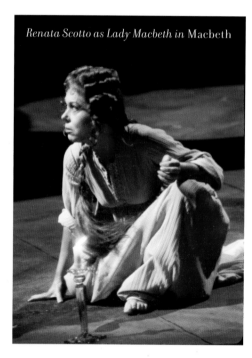

Renata Scotto as Lady Macbeth in Macbeth

Renata Scotto: Of all the Verdi I did with Maestro, my favorite was *Macbeth*. In Lady Macbeth's sleepwalking scene, there has to be no movement at all with your body; your voice has to express everything, and this is something that I learned from Maestro.

1983

NOVEMBER 18

JANUARY

Conducts a new production of Verdi's *Macbeth*, directed by Peter Hall, starring Sherrill Milnes, Renata Scotto, Giuseppe Giacomini, and Ruggero Raimondi.

Appears on the cover of *Time* magazine in a profile that declares him the premier American conductor on the international scene.

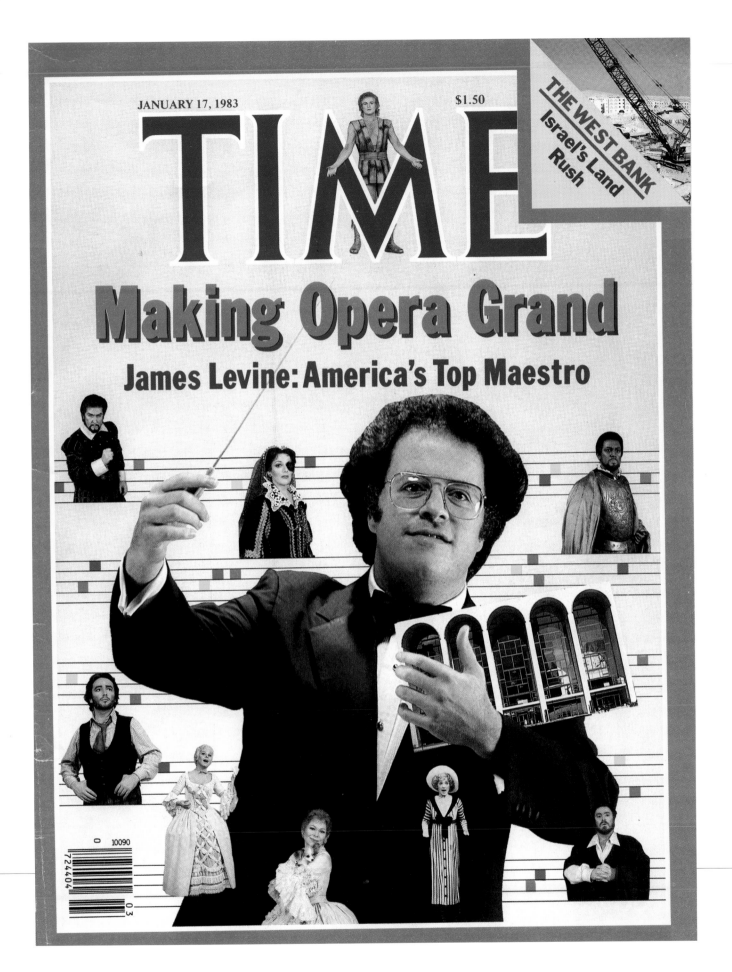

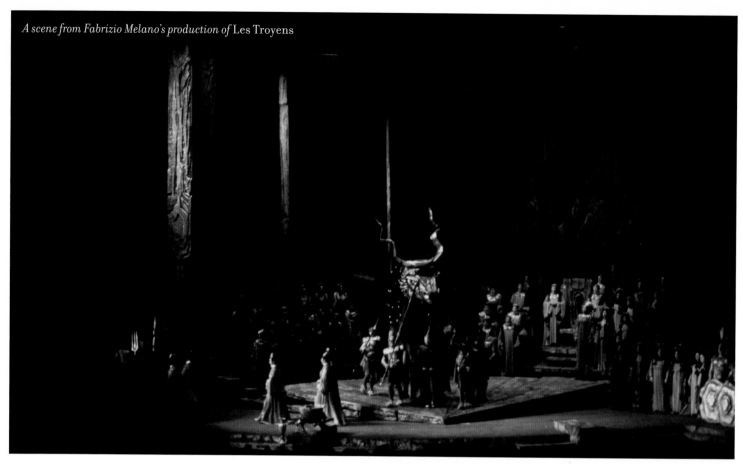
A scene from Fabrizio Melano's production of Les Troyens

JL: *Troyens* was the perfect piece to open the centennial season because we were looking for something that said large scale, epic drama, big Met... We had opened with *Faust* in 1883, and here it was 1983. I said to everybody, "What do we want to open with? *Faust* again? No. We want an opera that best presents what the Met can do that smaller companies with fewer resources can't do." We'd played Wagner operas, and *Don Carlo*... Clearly, *Troyens* was the piece to elevate to that status, an epic masterpiece that plays in one evening. The management and the board decided that the old production hadn't had enough performances to justify throwing it out and doing a new one. But we changed it—lightened it and took some pieces away to make it look airier and more open.

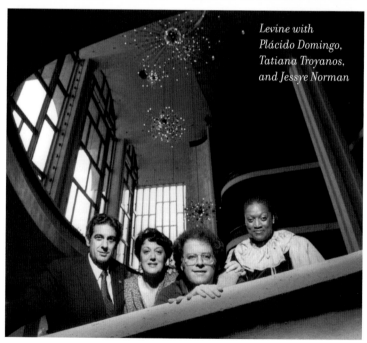
Levine with Plácido Domingo, Tatiana Troyanos, and Jessye Norman

SEPTEMBER 18

Appears with Leontyne Price on "In Performance at the White House," a televised concert with President Reagan in the audience and a number of young Met artists also performing.

SEPTEMBER 26

Opens the Met's centennial season with Berlioz's *Les Troyens,* with Jessye Norman making her Met debut as Cassandra, and Tatiana Troyanos and Plácido Domingo as Dido and Aeneas.

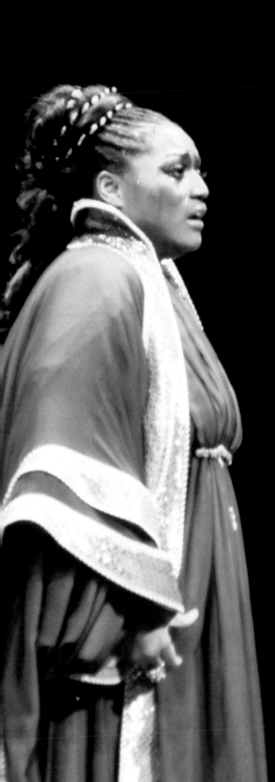

Jessye Norman as Cassandra

JL: I worked with Jessye from the very beginning, conducting her first American opera performance, as Aida at the Hollywood Bowl. And we were close right away—we just hit it off. We must have gone to dinner two or three times just to try to determine an approach to a Met repertoire for her, because she was an extraordinary combination of elements. For her opening role at the Met, she could have sung anything from Erda to Ariadne— that's just the nature of her voice. Eventually, we hit on her doing the Cassandra, and then later also Dido. She wound up doing both parts on a couple of occasions. She was wonderful, going straight for the jugular of the expression the way she would in a song or a recital or an oratorio. It was always a profound joy to work with Jess, a searcher and an extraordinary musician. Ultimately her Met repertoire reflected her special artistic qualities and voice range. It wasn't a pigeonhole of standard vocal or dramatic type: Cassandra, Dido, Jocasta, Ariadne, Elisabeth, Madame Lidoine, *Bluebeard's Castle, Erwartung,* Sieglinde, Kundry, Emilia Marty.

Jessye Norman: The rehearsals with Jim were a wonderful and exciting revelation in how such a vast work should and could be prepared in a relatively short period. It is a pleasure working with someone so sure and prepared and focused. All of our work together, whether in opera productions or with him at the piano, has been inspirational and infused with the joy of music-making. The rehearsal time just rushes away because one is having such a grand time exploring and discovering the magic of these tremendously demanding scores. And then came the performances, where we often did things in ways we had never rehearsed, because we were so at one with the music and with each other.

OCTOBER 22

Performs in the Met's two-part Centennial Gala, leading excerpts from operas including *Der Rosenkavalier, Otello, La Fanciulla del West,* and *Tristan und Isolde.*

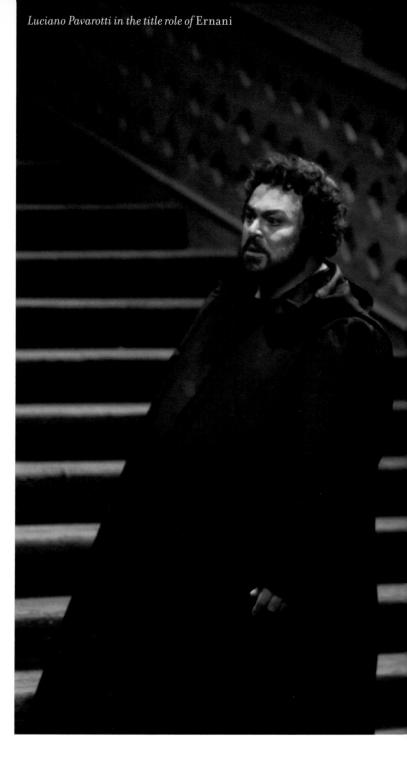

JL: One day in 1979, Luciano asked if I would come to his apartment and have lunch with him. There was one little point of back history. The first time I did a broadcast with Luciano was *Rigoletto* in 1973. We had established that there was one arguable interpolated top note that he was not going to do. And all the other tenors singing in that series had done what we asked. Cut to: he came on the stage and sang the note he wasn't supposed to. Results? It took a long time before he was convinced that he hadn't blown my respect for good. [Acting General Manager] Schuyler Chapin wrote him a letter and said, "We don't run the Met that way—if there is a second incident, it'll be the last one." In the next several years, we did do other things, but he was singing more bel canto pieces and other operas that were not what the management deemed necessary for me to do—they wanted me to spend time on larger pieces that developed the company as a group. But on this day that Luciano made lunch for me, he said, "You don't work with me, and I'm losing artistically because of that. I need to work with you." And I said, "I'd be happy to work with you, but look at the repertoire you choose and the repertoire I choose." He said, "You choose it because Plácido sings it so musically with all the imaginative details..." "No!" I interrupted. "As a matter of fact, it's the other way around. I need for us to do that repertoire, and because of Plácido we can." Everything from *Otello* to *Troyens*—all kinds of things that would have been unthinkable for Luciano. And Luciano said, "You're still angry at me about that *Rigoletto* thing, aren't you?" I said, "No, I'm not. I think that was silly, but I don't keep grudges, and you know I love the way you sing. What would we work on?" He said, "Whatever you want. My favorite opera is *Idomeneo*. I sang Idamante in Glyndebourne years ago. What about Idomeneo?" I said, "Tomorrow, if you want." He said, "What about some Verdi that is right for my voice, like *Ernani*?" I said, "Now you're talking my language." We came up with three or four things, and we started to work together more, including a wonderful and carefully prepared recital onstage at the Met, which gave us a chance to develop an even closer communication. Our closeness, our artistic success, our rapport with one another never flagged from then on. He made continuous stunning artistic development, and he turned out to be a miraculous guy as a friend, one of the closest friends I had in my life.

NOVEMBER 18

Leads a new production of Verdi's *Ernani,*
with Luciano Pavarotti, Leona Mitchell,
Sherrill Milnes, and Ruggero Raimondi.

JL: It occurred to me that just as there had been a very strong bel canto revival, the veristi were also due to have their operas heard again. Beyond Puccini, the verismo repertoire internationally is rather limited to a couple of Giordano pieces, a couple of Cilèa, *La Gioconda,* and *Cavalleria Rusticana/Pagliacci.* But the great array of pieces that came after Verdi, including works by composers like Boito, Mascagni, Ponchielli, Montemezzi, and all these Puccini successors—some of these pieces were really good on the stage. We started with *Francesca da Rimini* because Zandonai was a voice that had not been recently paid much attention to. We also made it a point that we would only do these pieces if we had appropriate singers or could approach them in some valid way. And in the case of *Francesca,* it was possible because Scotto, Domingo, and MacNeil were virtually ideal. And the production [directed by Piero Faggioni with sets by Ezio Frigerio] turned out to be one of the most beautiful we ever had on our stage.

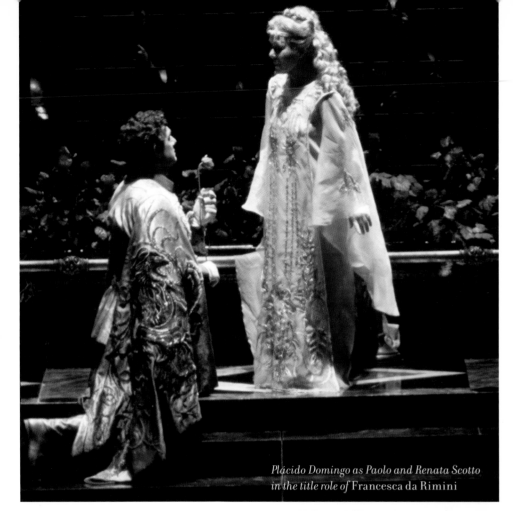

Plácido Domingo as Paolo and Renata Scotto in the title role of Francesca da Rimini

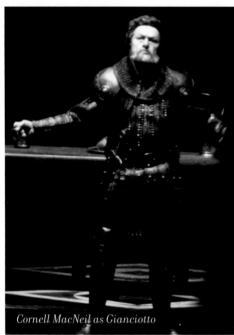

Cornell MacNeil as Gianciotto

1984

FEBRUARY 26

Celebrates the 25th anniversary of Leonie Rysanek's Met debut with a gala concert of Wagner: Act I of *Die Walküre* and Act II of *Parsifal.*

MARCH 9

Brings back Zandonai's *Francesca da Rimini,* unheard at the Met since 1918, in a run that marks Cornell MacNeil's 25th Met anniversary, opposite Renata Scotto, Plácido Domingo, and William Lewis.

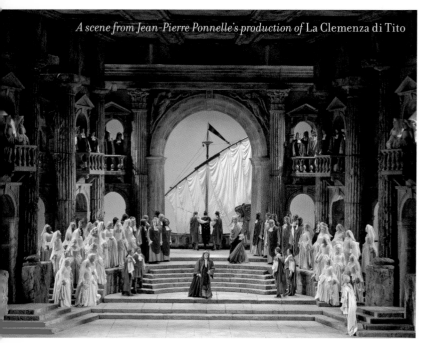

A scene from Jean-Pierre Ponnelle's production of La Clemenza di Tito

JL: I had this limitless rapport with Jean-Pierre Ponnelle—musically, dramatically, stylistically, and in every way. I wish he'd lived to be an old man, and we could have kept going, because this was work on some unbelievable level. And had he wanted to stop producing and start conducting, he could have done it tomorrow—he was that musical. I would not have added *Idomeneo* and *Clemenza* to the Met at that time if he hadn't been available. In the end, Jean-Pierre did parts of the whole operatic repertoire, regardless of the language and style. Watching him rehearse was a virtuoso thing. It was in all languages at once—he had the expression he wanted in whatever language the person understood. And he worked always from the orchestra score, which he had in his head. He had studied the whole panorama of the art form with brilliant people and absorbed everything. I appreciated that he said he could always count on my eyes. In fact, I remember a funny thing that happened one time when he was staging a recitative in *Figaro*. After they'd run it a couple of times, I said to him, "You know, this isn't your best version." He said, "It isn't? What did I do before?" I said, "If you go away for 20 minutes, I'll show you." So he went away, and I picked it up with the people and redid it, based on something I'd seen him try in an earlier series with different singers. And he came back and sat in the first row and watched it, and he was in hysterics. He laughed so hard and said, "It's better. We should leave it!" It was not part of his aesthetic that there was one version that was the best. But having stood there and watched him improvise different versions with different people through countless rehearsals and performances, I had become aware of which things were working better than others. It's the same thing when you make musical choices with tempi and rubati and that sort of thing.

APRIL–JUNE

Conducts *Francesca da Rimini, Die Walküre, Die Entführung aus dem Serail,* and *Tosca* on a North American tour at the conclusion of the Met's centennial season.

OCTOBER 18

Adds Mozart's *La Clemenza di Tito* to the Met repertoire, with Kenneth Riegel, Renata Scotto, Gail Robinson, and Ann Murray stepping in for Tatiana Troyanos.

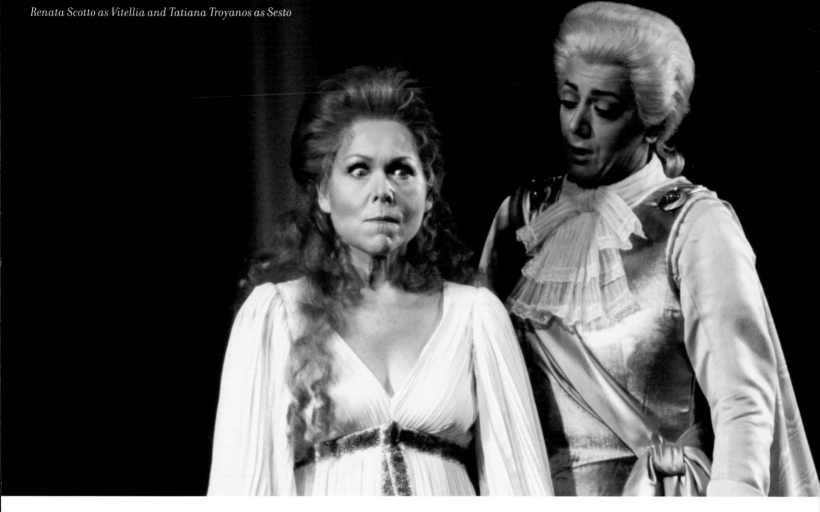

JL: One interesting thing about Mozart's operatic output was that at his first chance to write a singspiel, he turned out *Abduction,* and at the end of his life he turned out *The Magic Flute,* which was a kind of super-special singspiel. Contrarily, after having composed the big opera seria *Idomeneo* relatively early in his career, at the end he wrote *Clemenza di Tito.* What almost always is the case with great composers is they start off making a banquet of it, then learn how to distill it. So, *Clemenza* is a more concise and subtle version of the kind of piece he composed with *Idomeneo.* And with Scotto as Vitellia in *Clemenza* and Luciano as Idomeneo, audiences had a chance to hear those wonderful recitatives, secco and accompagnato, from the mouths of great Italian artists.

NOVEMBER 23

Adds Verdi's *Simon Boccanegra* to his Met repertoire, in a new production starring Sherrill Milnes, Anna Tomowa-Sintow, Vasile Moldoveanu, and Paul Plishka.

Dear Maestro Levine,

It was a pleasure to have made such beautiful music with you in so many different venues. The most lasting and personal experience for me was my final performance of *Aida* at the Metropolitan Opera, in 1985. It is as fresh in my mind today as if we had just finished the performance. Your sensitivity to the human voice as an instrument has never been more apparent. From the opening through the final curtain we were performing as one. Your ability to create an atmosphere in which we could excel is praiseworthy. For me this was a singular moment and one of the most poignant in my career. Our artistic merging was palpable and total. I thank you for that once-in-a-lifetime experience. You are truly an International as well as a National Treasure. May your next 40 years be filled with the total gratification that comes from your art. God bless you and keep you.

Sincerely,
Leontyne Price

JL: Leontyne did one of the most amazing things that I ever witnessed that night. This is going to sound academic, but it's the exact opposite: she put every note where it belongs—with full breath, full tone, full expression, full communication. Nothing slipped away, nothing was wishful thinking. You could have knocked me over with a feather—I was absolutely riveted. She sang the whole role that way, but particularly the Nile aria, which is an iconic piece that sort of embodies the difficulty and beauty of the part. I'd heard her sing Aida a lot and we'd done it together often, but for her to be able to stand up there in front of God and everybody and do it that way on the time she had decided was going to be her last... It was unbelievable, like a reaffirmation of where she had come to since she first sang it, and first sang at the Met [*Il Trovatore*, 1961].

1985
JANUARY 3

Conducts Leontyne Price in her farewell performance as Aida, telecast live across North America, with Fiorenza Cossotto, James McCracken, and Simon Estes.

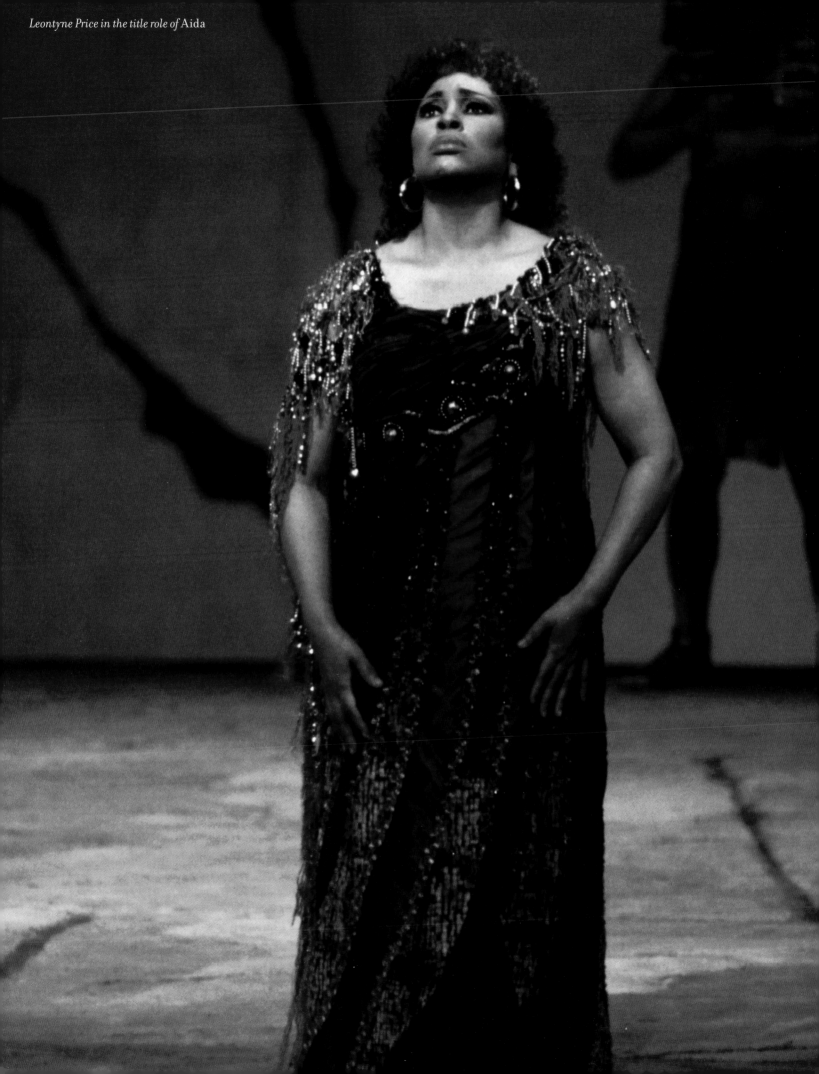

Leontyne Price in the title role of Aida

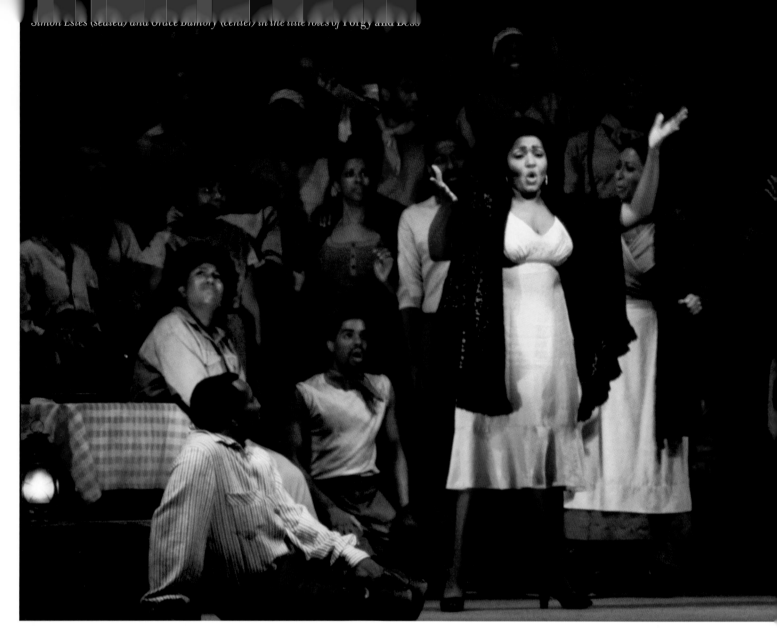

JL: There is no other work like *Porgy and Bess*. It's a huge three-act conception which Gershwin was fond of saying had come from three role models: *Boris Godunov* because of the chorus, *Meistersinger* because of the community, and *Carmen* because of the hit tunes. Like a Wagner opera, it was written with accompagnato, no dialogue. And it was written in three acts, not the customary two for Broadway musicals. It is a gigantic piece, with a title role that has the dimensions of Hans Sachs or the Flying Dutchman. But at the time Gershwin finished it, no one had much of a response to the conception of it as an opera. Instead, the Theatre Guild took it and produced it as a Broadway musical. They got rid of recitatives and made

dialogue, and he aided and abetted that. If the Met had done it, what would the version have become? What cuts would he have had to make? I took a position which was, admittedly, very one-sided, but I had to do it once: if the Met was going to do *Porgy and Bess* 50 years after Gershwin wrote it, then we were going to play every bloody note. The piece had never been played in an opera house without a microphone and without a cut. We played it 32 times over the first two seasons, and it sold out. If I did it again, I would probably use my experience and try to estimate the few cuts Gershwin would have made. If he'd been preparing it for a Met premiere, he'd have known what to do, because this would have been duck soup for him.

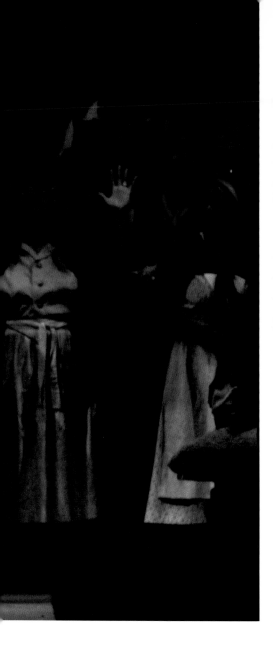

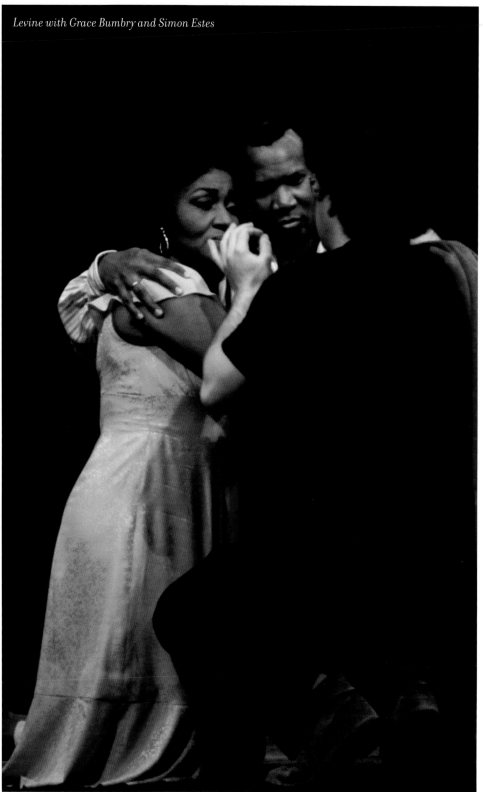

Levine with Grace Bumbry and Simon Estes

Brings Gershwin's *Porgy and Bess* to the Met,
50 years after its world premiere, with Simon
Estes and Grace Bumbry in the title roles.

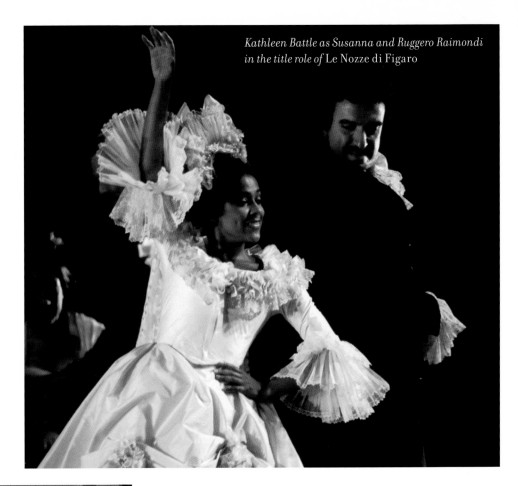

Kathleen Battle as Susanna and Ruggero Raimondi in the title role of Le Nozze di Figaro

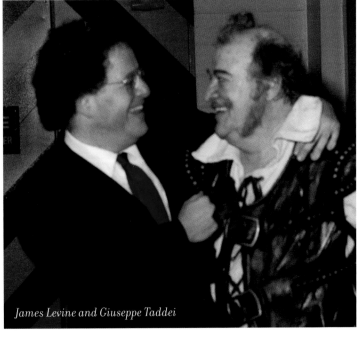

James Levine and Giuseppe Taddei

JL: What a special thrill Peppino [nickname for Giuseppe Taddei] gave to all of us at the Met, debuting at nearly 70 years of age. What a great case of "better late than never." Whew!

SEPTEMBER 25

Conducts *Falstaff* **with 69-year-old Giuseppe Taddei making his Met debut in the title role.**

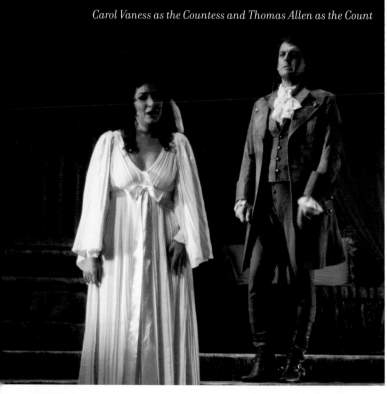

Carol Vaness as the Countess and Thomas Allen as the Count

JL: I think this production was a high-water mark for this sort of piece, with its difficulties and its brilliance. The style was so committed and defined, the storyline set forth so unequivocally, without general nonsense. And the cast was extraordinary. I choose the operas that I do in any season partly based on whether I can get a cast with which I can achieve the right rapport. This, I think, represents a standard of ensemble that is quite amazing for a repertory theater in the middle of a season.

Thomas Allen: Apart from Jimmy's obvious skills and talent as a conductor and communicator, it's clear that he just loves what the human voice can do and knows what the requirement is at any particular time in any particular opera. *The Marriage of Figaro* was the first time I worked with him at the Met. When you're on stage at the Met, you realize you're dealing with castle-sized proportions, and it makes you play big. In the way that Jimmy makes Mozart work in that house, it's very, very dynamic and very powerful.

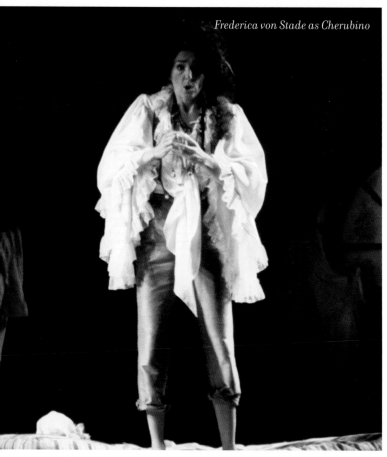

Frederica von Stade as Cherubino

Frederica von Stade: I always felt that the character of Cherubino was very close to Mozart—dear, enthusiastic, young—and I felt that Jimmy understood that so clearly, that underpinning of the dazzling energy of youth. When kids ask me about Cherubino I say, "Well, boys that age never stop moving. If you stop them moving, they'll perish." Jimmy gave that to me in his approach to the music. Whenever Cherubino was singing—even something a little slow—there was that underlying, "Any minute I am going to burst wide open, and I don't know why." Just listening to the overture, the way Jimmy did it, my heart would start beating faster. I felt like a soccer player who just couldn't wait to get out there and kick the ball.

NOVEMBER 22

Continues the Mozart cycle with his first Met performances of *Le Nozze di Figaro,* starring Ruggero Raimondi, Carol Vaness, Kathleen Battle, Frederica von Stade, and Thomas Allen, in a production by Jean-Pierre Ponnelle.

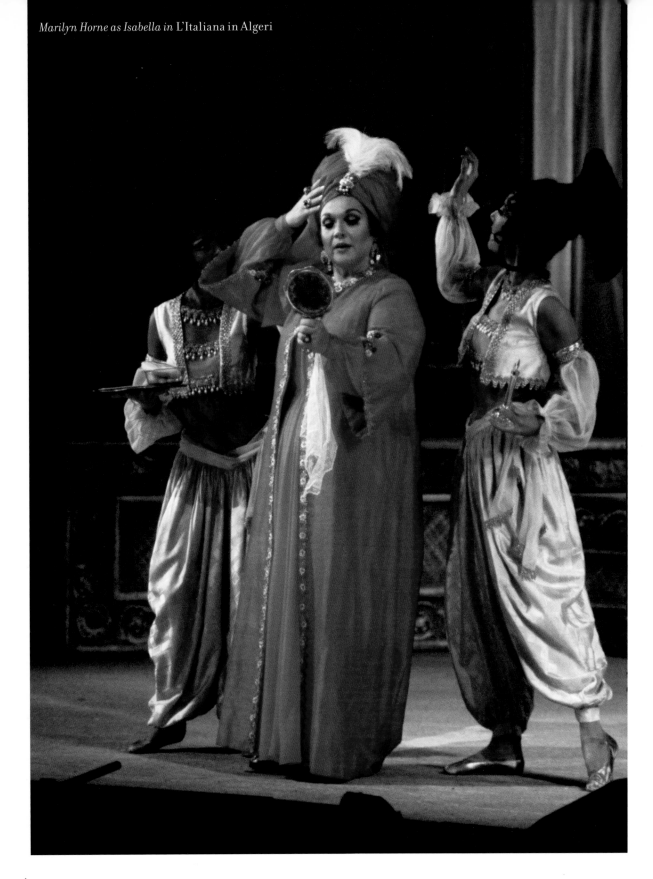

Marilyn Horne as Isabella in L'Italiana in Algeri

Rossini's *L'Italiana in Algeri,* starring
Marilyn Horne, becomes the 48th work in his
Met repertoire, making it larger than any
other conductor's in Met history.

Maria Ewing: When I was 18, I went to the Meadow Brook Music Festival in Michigan to audition for Maddalena in *Rigoletto.* I was nervous because I had prepared the role on my own. Jimmy looked up with those flashing beautiful blue eyes and the trademark towel at his shoulder and said, "Maddalena?" When I sang, he got sort of animated and said, "Your Italian is terrible—well, we can work on that—but your expression is just..." I knew I got the job. A month or two after the concerts, I got a postcard from Paris. It said, "If you work hard, you will be one of the best singers one of these days." And then I realized it was from Jim. He became my mentor, and his influence on me was huge. I went to his conducting classes at the Cleveland Institute and was in a group of musicians who went to Aspen for the summer, which Jimmy had arranged. One day, he walked in with about 10 or 15 brand-new opera scores—*Carmen, La Cenerentola, The Barber of Seville*—and said, "Here, these are things I think you will do." When I did *Carmen* with him at the Met, it was just like going home.

Jimmy really looked after me when I was young, suggesting repertoire, recommending that I coach with Jennie Tourel. He never pigeonholed me, and I made some of my most important debuts with him. His sense of rhythm, of the right tempi, of the dynamics, of the dramatic shape, all made sense. If he said, "Do this, don't do this, breathe here," you'd listen. It didn't mean that you were being blindly led along; you knew that you were being nurtured.

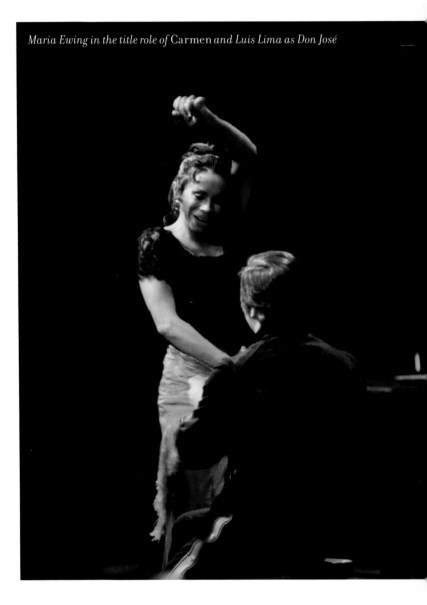

Maria Ewing in the title role of Carmen *and Luis Lima as Don José*

1986
MARCH 10

Adds Bizet's *Carmen* to his Met repertoire, in a new production starring Maria Ewing and Luis Lima.

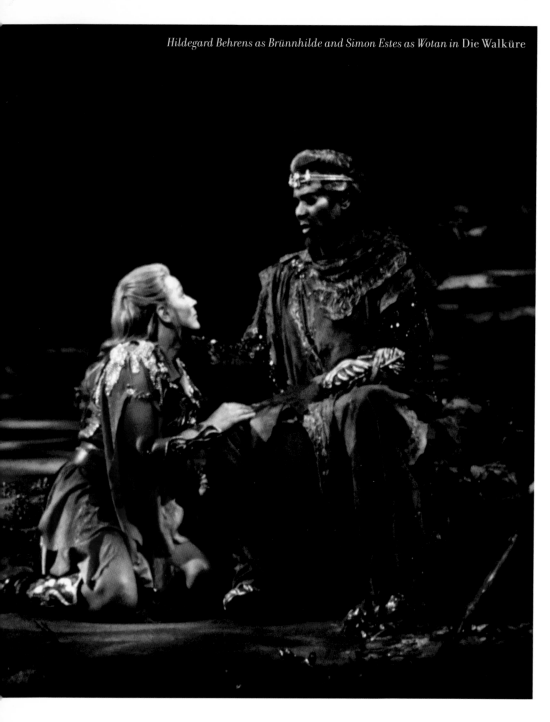

Hildegard Behrens as Brünnhilde and Simon Estes as Wotan in Die Walküre

JL: We decided that it was time for a new *Ring* cycle for a very simple reason: the old one was falling apart. Schenk had done our very successful *Tannhäuser* production, with Günther Schneider-Siemssen. It was representational, but it used a new set of techniques, with very magical effects. Traditional Wagnerites liked it, but new people could also get into it. One day, as my colleagues and I were sitting around talking about the *Ring,* I heard myself say, "We ought to do a *Ring* that's like that *Tannhäuser.*" I meant just the basics, the techniques. Schenk had never done the cycle before, so his ideas would be fresh, while Schneider-Siemssen, having done half a dozen of them, would know what we needed. Little by little I saw in [Technical Director] Joe Clark's face that he agreed with what I was saying, and then the others did, too.

SEPTEMBER 22

In his first season as the Met's Artistic Director, conducts the Opening Night performance of *Die Walküre,* the first part of a new *Ring* cycle, directed by Otto Schenk and designed by Günther Schneider-Siemssen, with Hildegard Behrens, Jeannine Altmeyer, Peter Hofmann, and Simon Estes in the principal roles.

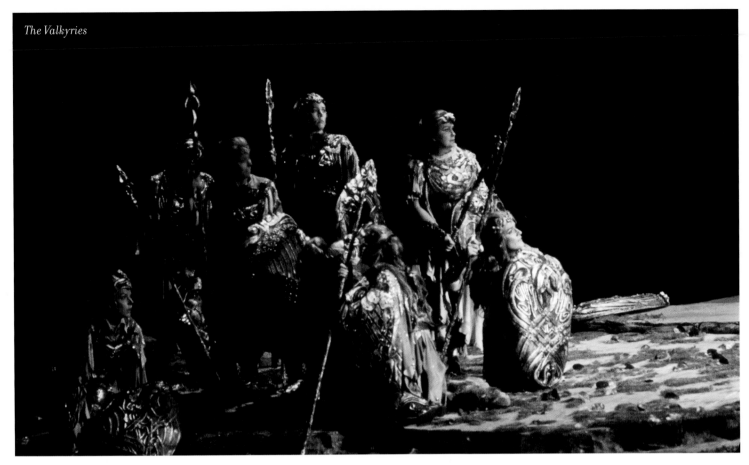

Otto Schenk: James Levine was clever in seducing me to do the *Ring*. He's a great seducer! I didn't dare to do the *Ring;* I wasn't sure that I could do it as well as I wanted to. He said, "You can do it," and we sat together and had funny talks, and he seduced me with humor. We always laughed a lot when we talked together, and he has his boyish laughter. When you look in his face you've already gone his way. He is like a *kobold,* a naughty little sprite, but a good sprite.

I did mostly Wagner with him, and he has such a feeling for Wagnerian breathing and Wagnerian words. I think we were from the same Wagnerian mafia. As a director, I never had the slightest feeling that I wanted something different. We worked together, and we made some jokes, but we didn't have to talk about anything in our productions. It was all natural and as it should be.

He has a magic baton. I don't know how it works, but you have the feeling that his heart comes directly through the baton, to the strings, to the brasses, to everybody in his orchestra. Everyone understands even his littlest movements. Jimmy is always interested in what is on stage, too. He has such a dramatic sense for music. When we got to the rehearsals with orchestra, I always got a carpet of music that was ready for acting, and it was heaven.

One thing we had together was "the gesture." When we saw each other in the morning at the Met, we made a funny, helpless gesture, one to the other, lifting our arms in a shrug as if we were saying that we don't know anything, how to do anything, how to start. This was instead of saying "Good morning" and starting the work with optimism—but we knew it wasn't true. The luckiest time I had in opera was with James Levine.

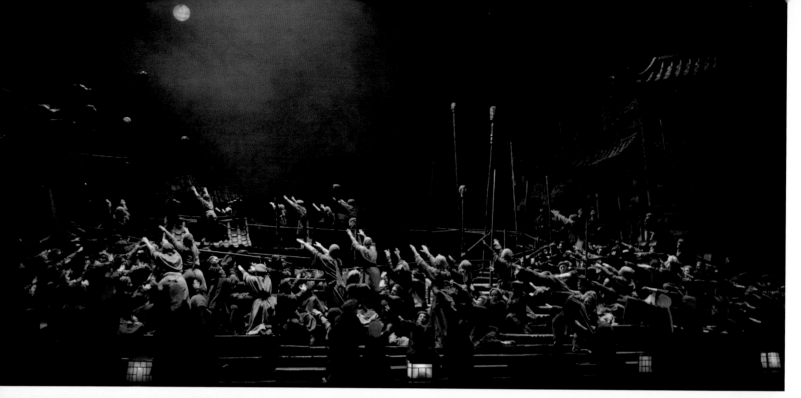

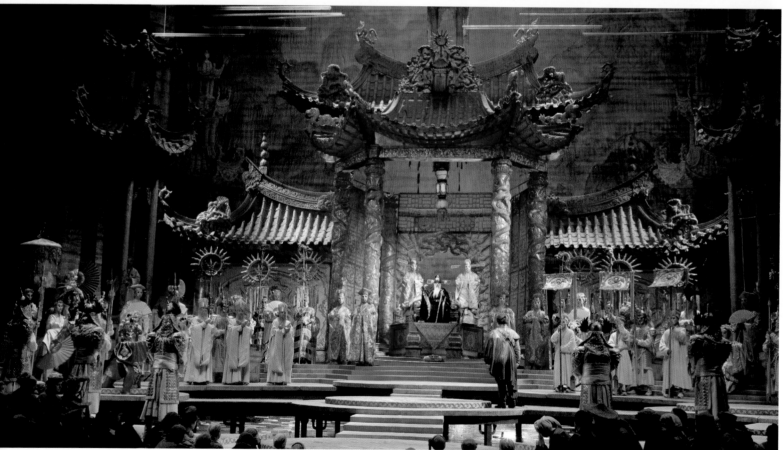

Acts I and II of Franco Zeffirelli's production of Turandot

Eva Marton in the title role of Turandot

Franco Zeffirelli in rehearsal, with Plácido Domingo as Calàf

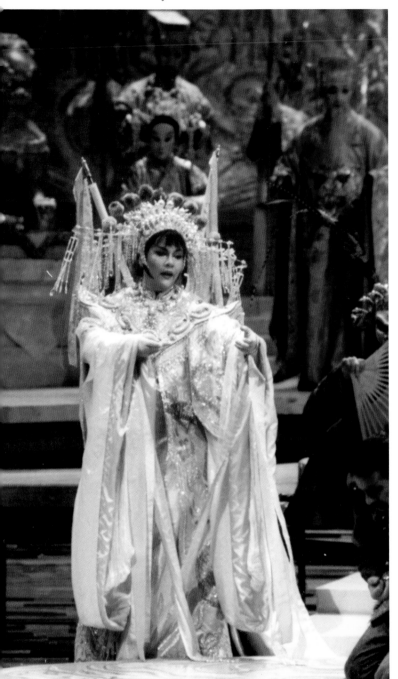

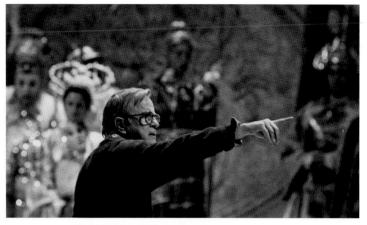

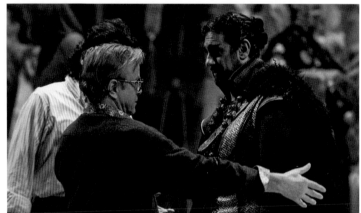

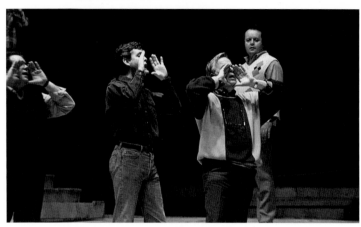

1987
MARCH 12

Conducts Franco Zeffirelli's new production
of Puccini's *Turandot,* with Eva Marton, Leona
Mitchell, Plácido Domingo, and Paul Plishka.

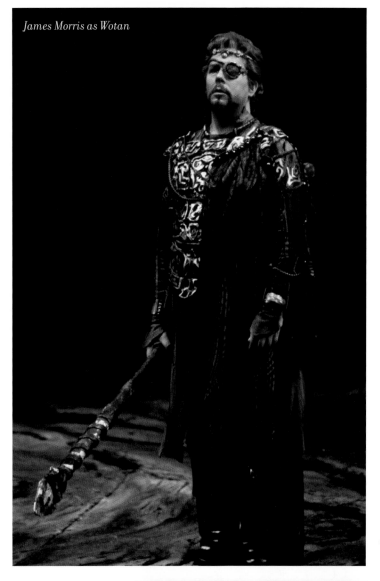

James Morris as Wotan

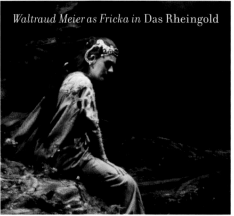

Waltraud Meier as Fricka in Das Rheingold

James Morris: The longest relationship I've had with anybody in the business is with Jim, and I feel very fortunate that it's with the most intelligent musician I know. We came to the Met the same year, and we have done hundreds of performances together, plus all the rehearsal time. I especially love that because it's where you build things. Jim is a big talker: 80 percent of rehearsal time is him talking, but it's fascinating because everything he says has a purpose, and he can open your eyes.

The really big step was when I started doing Wagner, and got to do it with the master. A huge turning point for my career was doing Wotan in the Met's *Ring.* In the beginning, it was very intimidating, but over the years, Jim and I settled into a wonderful, easy rapport. It took me a long time to get to *Meistersinger,* and as I was studying it over the years, my vocal score went flying across the room several times— too many words! One day, a lightbulb went on: *Meistersinger* was different from the other Wagner operas because it was a comedy—duh! To be able to do it with Jim is an incomparable experience. A lot of the role of Sachs is introverted, and Jim gives you the time to prepare mentally and to create your own inner character. If it hadn't been for him, I wouldn't have gotten as far as I have with *Meistersinger.* In fact, I don't know where my career would be today if it weren't for Jim.

APRIL 1987

Leads the Met in a return to the recording studio with *Die Walküre,* to be followed in subsequent years by the other parts of the *Ring* cycle, the company's first ongoing recording project since the 1950s.

OCTOBER 9

Continues the new *Ring* cycle with *Das Rheingold,* with James Morris singing his first Wotan and Waltraud Meier making her Met debut as Fricka.

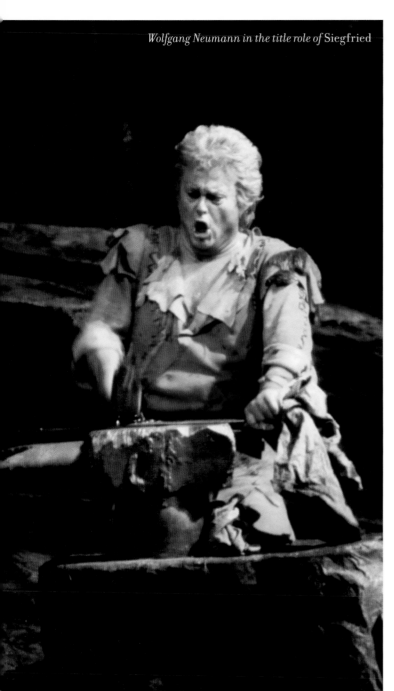

Wolfgang Neumann in the title role of Siegfried

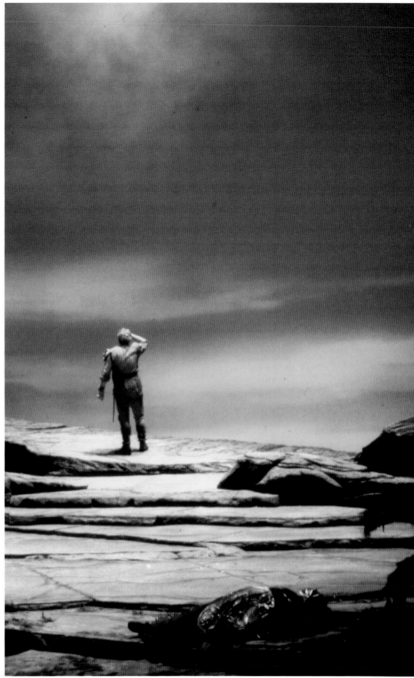

1988
FEBRUARY 12

Siegfried is added to the *Ring* cycle.

JL: I adore touring. At home you always play for the same audience, and you have all the problems and challenges of everything at once. On tour, you distill your work in front of new audiences, and it puts the company in touch with itself in a completely different way. Instead of going back and forth from home to work and work to home, we're together for that period, and invariably, some remarkable artistic development happens— and we have a very good time, too. I always look forward to going to Japan. I find the audience and the culture terrific.

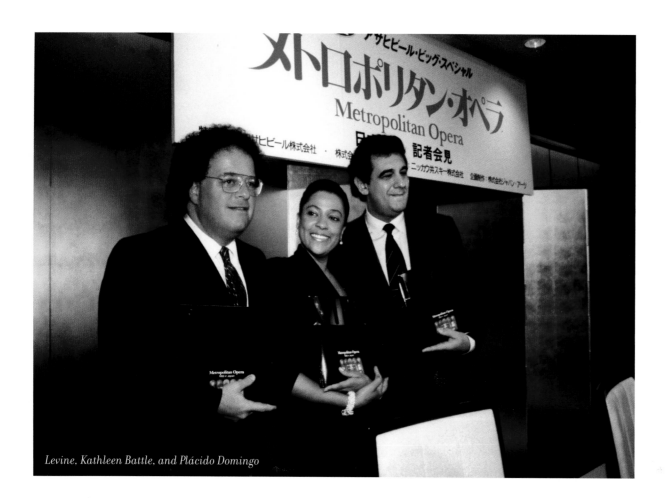

Levine, Kathleen Battle, and Plácido Domingo

MAY–JUNE 1988

Takes the company to Japan, conducting *Le Nozze di Figaro,* Offenbach's *Les Contes d'Hoffmann,* and a concert with Kathleen Battle and Plácido Domingo.

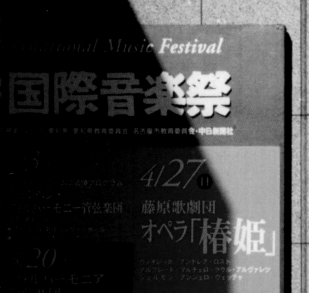
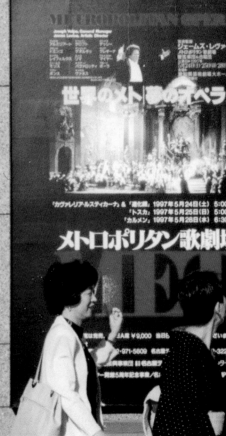
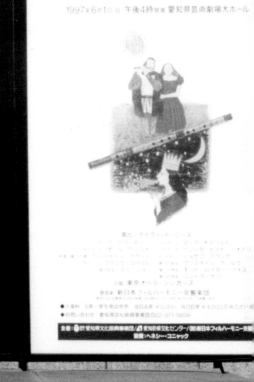

The Met's Japan Tour, 1997

JL: Hildegard was a terrific musician, very disciplined and well-schooled, but with the flair of personality and drama. Whatever it is you worked on, whatever you wanted, she was there; it didn't take a lot of words or repetition. Her technique had aspects which were not standard, but solid and effective for her. And she was very articulate about expressing any difficulty or wish. That's a point to make: every one of these artists who may appear to the public as a great *bête de théâtre,* a theater animal—every single one of them knew exactly what they were doing. The fact that they could impress you, the viewer and listener, with an effect of instinct would be useless without the control.

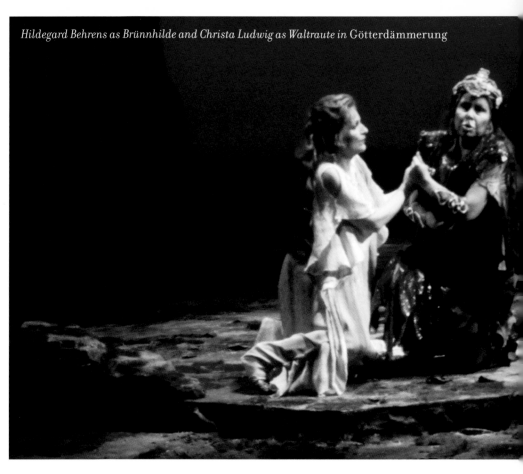

Hildegard Behrens as Brünnhilde and Christa Ludwig as Waltraute in Götterdämmerung

JL: Christa was an artist who had impressed me very much in my youth, and I subsequently got to work with her a lot, in opera and recitals and concerts. She was one of my favorites because she was one of those have-everything people: an absolutely glorious instrument, a wonderful technique from the very beginning, a great expressive power, and a big stylistic range.

OCTOBER 12

His 1089th performance, *Das Rheingold,* moves him past the previous Met record, held by Artur Bodanzky, of most performances by a conductor.

OCTOBER 21

Completes the new *Ring* cycle with *Götterdämmerung,* starring Hildegard Behrens, Christa Ludwig, Toni Krämer, and Matti Salminen.

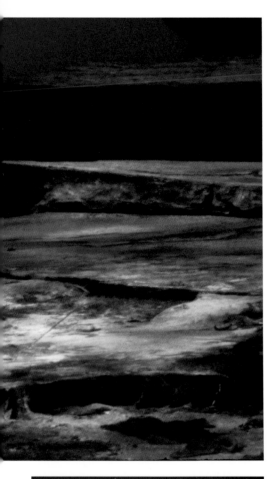

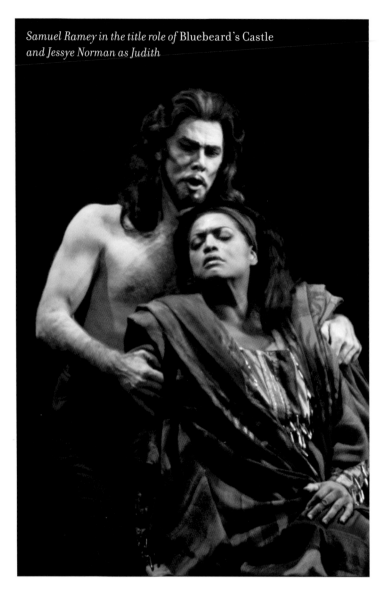

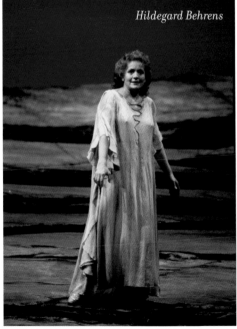

Hildegard Behrens

JL: *Bluebeard's Castle* was great with Jessye and Sam, and we did *Erwartung* along with it because we thought Jessye's artistry was unique enough that the public would go for it. It's very hard to find a context in a theater as big as the Met for one-acters. But I believe in these pieces as much as anything. They're both tremendously stage-worthy. *Erwartung* is often done in concert, but I've seen it on stage several times in different approaches, and it can be an extraordinary experience.

1989
JANUARY 16

Leads the Met premiere of Schoenberg's *Erwartung* with Jessye Norman, who also appears with Samuel Ramey in Bartók's *Bluebeard's Castle*.

JL: The first complete cycle that I conducted was the Met's. The better you know it, the more you do it, the more you are intrigued by trying to get the ideal proportions. Generally speaking, musical interpretation consists of solving a lot of paradoxes, and in the *Ring,* there are particularly tricky and significant ones. The more you work on things, the more things are revealed.

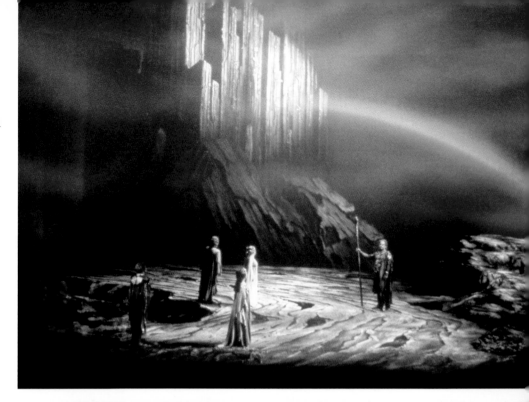

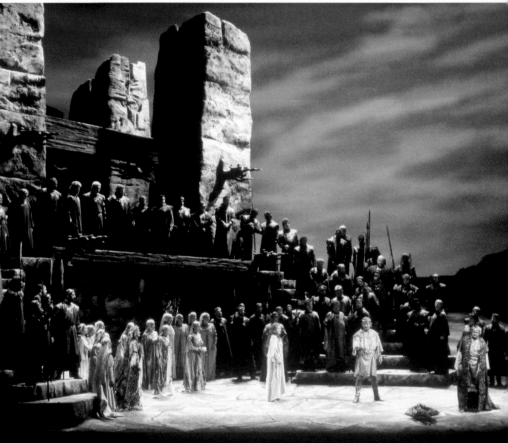

APRIL 1, 8, 15, 22

Conducts the first full cycle of Wagner's *Ring* in nearly 15 years. Two of the three cycles performed this spring take place over the course of a week, making it the first time since 1938–39 that the Met performed it according to Wagner's wishes.

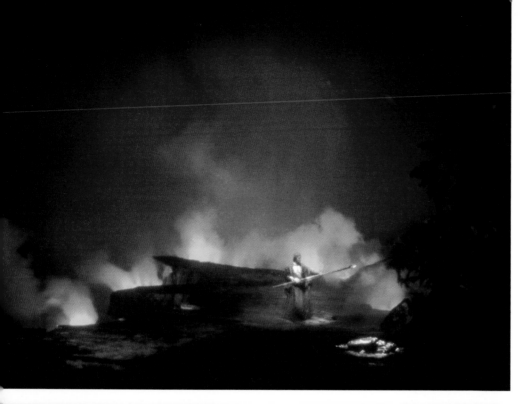

Otto Schenk's production of Der Ring
des Nibelungen *(clockwise from far left):*
Das Rheingold, Die Walküre, Siegfried,
and Götterdämmerung.

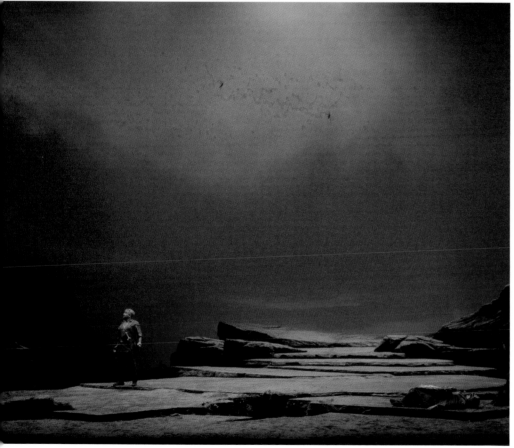

DECEMBER 11

Leads *Der Fliegende Holländer* in a new
production by August Everding, with James
Morris, Mechthild Gessendorf, Paul Plishka,
and Gary Lakes.

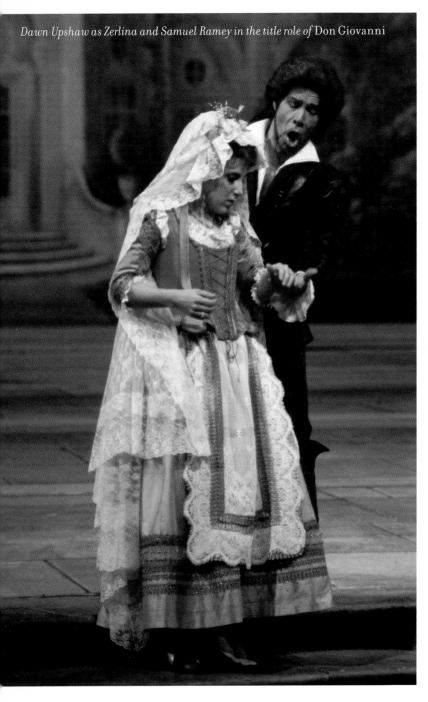

Dawn Upshaw as Zerlina and Samuel Ramey in the title role of Don Giovanni

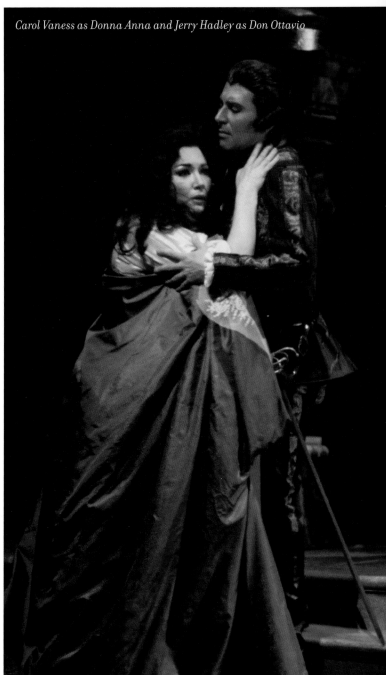

Carol Vaness as Donna Anna and Jerry Hadley as Don Ottavio

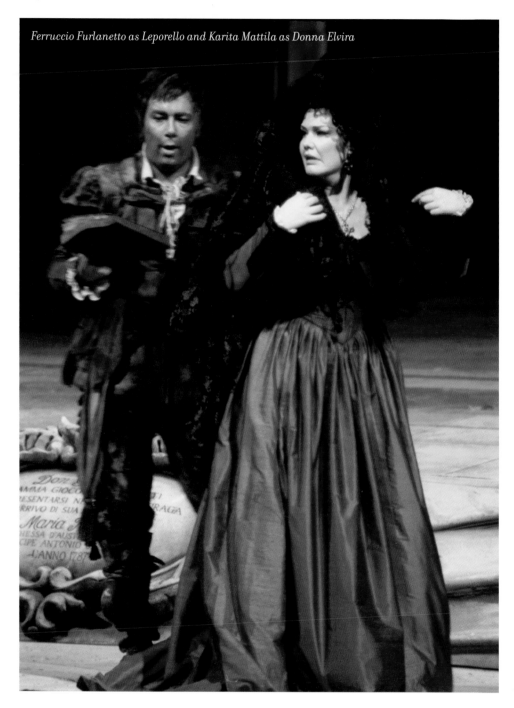

Ferruccio Furlanetto as Leporello and Karita Mattila as Donna Elvira

Ferruccio Furlanetto: I have always thought that Jimmy is the best conductor a singer could have. He knows everything inside out, which is a great advantage because his face, his eyes, and his smile are always with us onstage. It's so important to have a conductor who loves voices. He has created a sensational ensemble as an orchestra, so you feel sustained by this wall of sound that is coming toward you but is never overwhelming.

1990
MARCH 22

Anticipating the Mozart year, leads Franco Zeffirelli's production of *Don Giovanni*, starring Samuel Ramey, Carol Vaness, Jerry Hadley, Ferruccio Furlanetto, and Dawn Upshaw, with Karita Mattila making her Met debut as Donna Elvira.

JL: Jimmy Morris came to the Met just a little bit earlier than I did, and I always adored his work. You know, certain movie actors are very big with makeup and rubber features and making themselves look a certain way, and this gives them the distance that they need. But there's a certain kind of actor I call the Spencer Tracy kind— mostly he played part after part looking just like he looked, and whatever part it was, you believed every word he said. Jimmy's like that. He's not an actory actor. He's a guy who takes the part and absorbs something about the speed and the detail and the pace and the feeling. I always found him inhabiting the essential content of the part without being preoccupied with props or makeup or external effects. And, of course, it doesn't hurt that he's such a terrific singer! In the *Ring,* he has a great grasp of differentiating the three incarnations of his part. When he plays *Rheingold,* he reminds me of the kid in high school who's good at sports and grows up taller than the others and becomes a sort of natural leader type. And then, it turns out he's not clever, so he needs the help of some strange guys who have a lot of intellect but are not as appealing to everybody. And then, ultimately, he has a certain philosophical distance from it all. That's put into ludicrously simple terms, of course, but Jim delineates this very well. You are really sympathetic for him at the end of *Walküre* even though he hasn't stinted on being foolish in *Rheingold.*

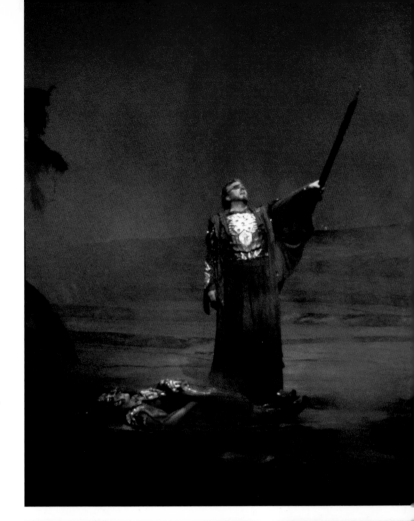

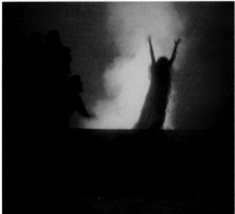

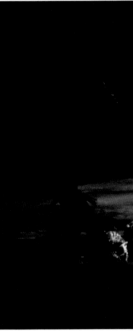

JUNE 18–21

The new *Ring* makes its screen debut on PBS on four successive evenings.

Images from the PBS telecast of the Ring *cycle*

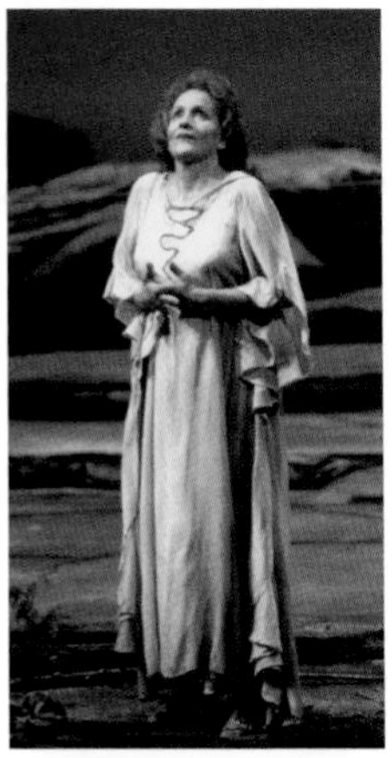

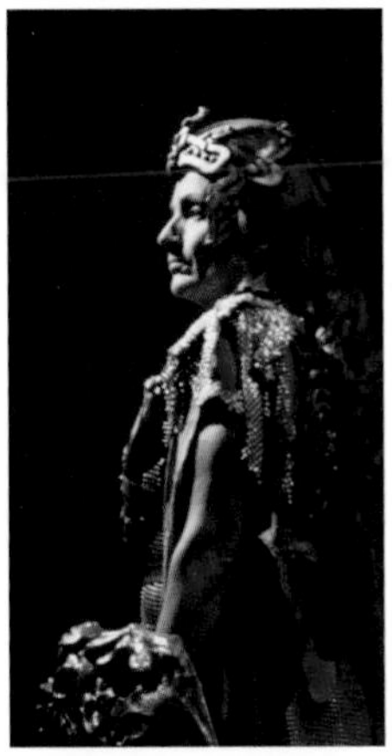

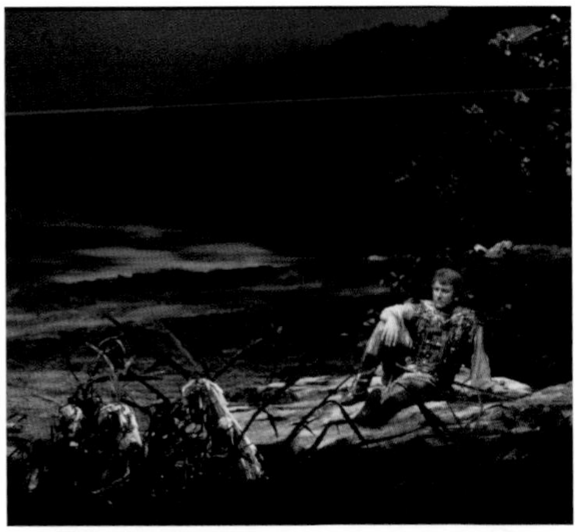

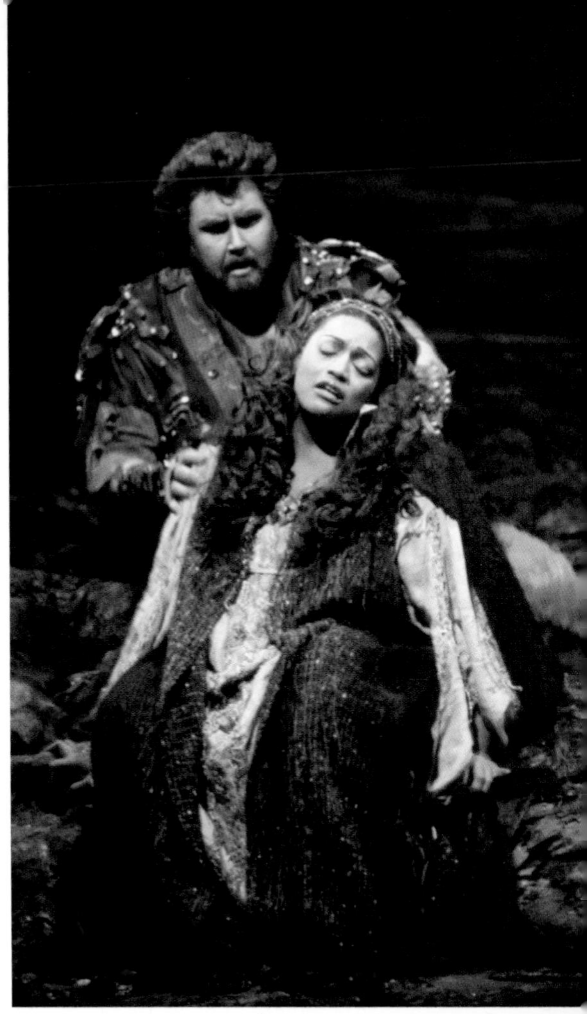

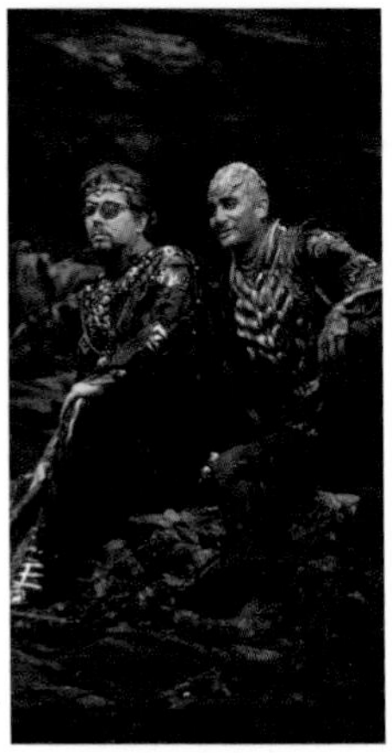

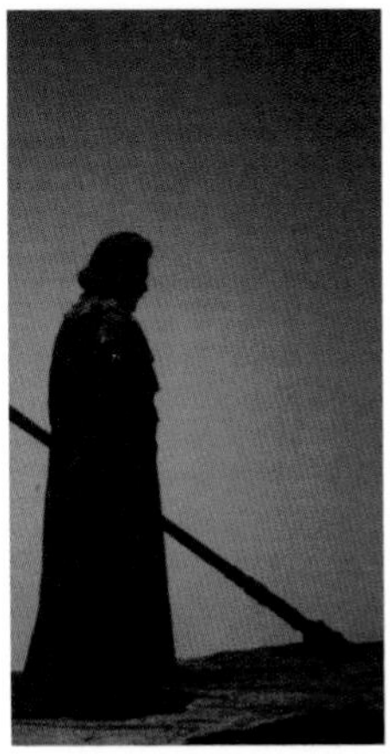

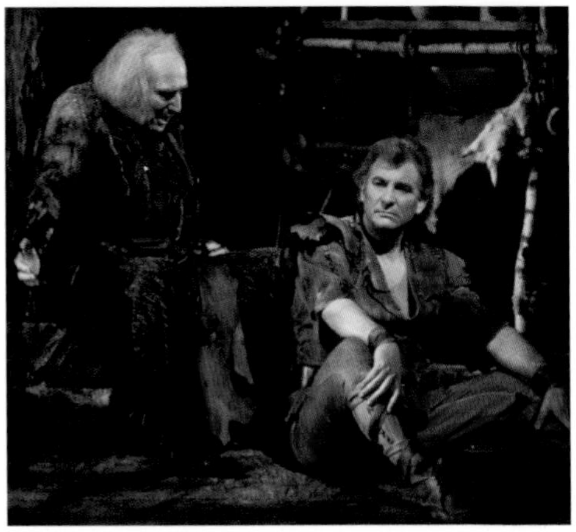

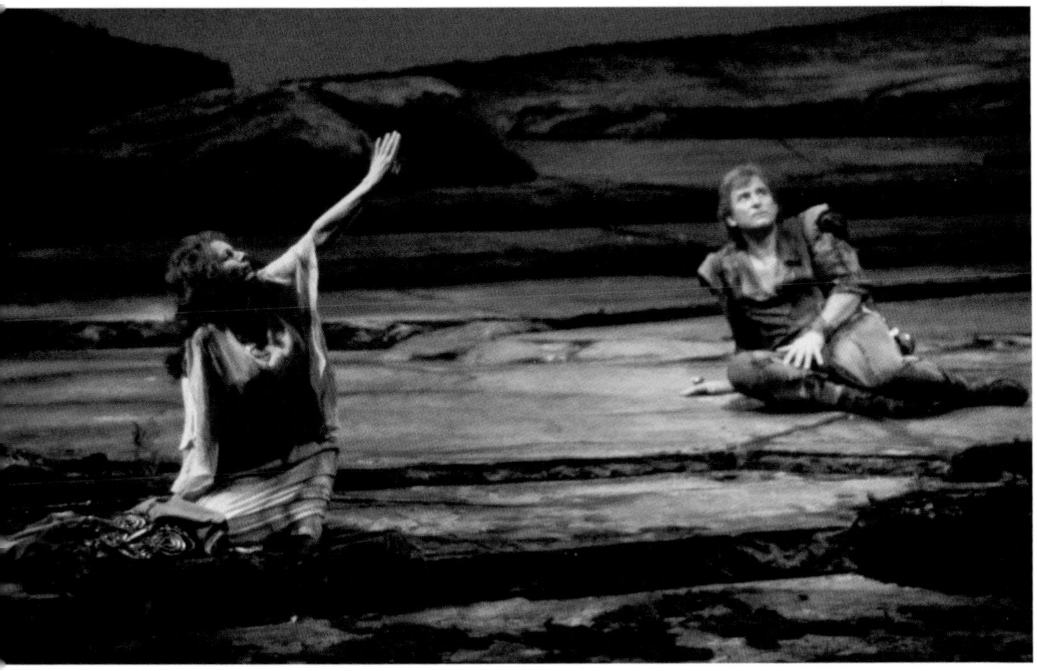

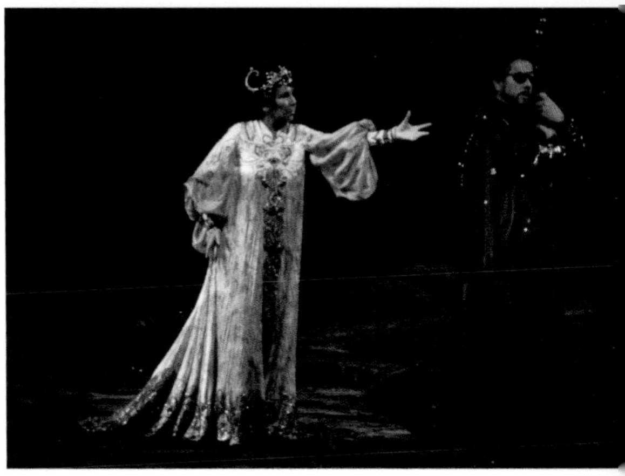

Building a Rapport: Levine's Orchestra

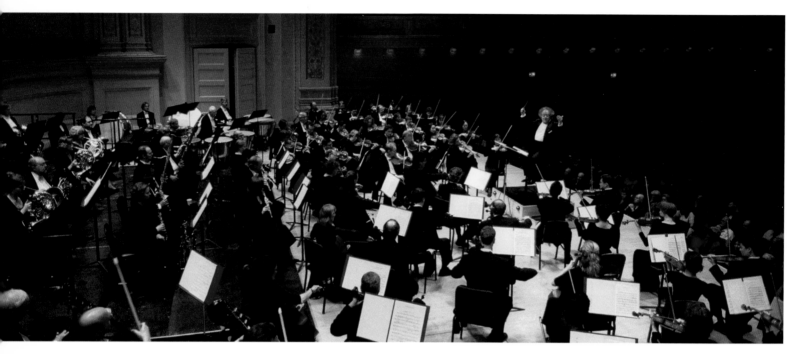

JL: If you take a frontal approach when you want a musician to change something, you run the risk of getting in the way of the unconscious process. If all a conductor had to do was stand up there and say, "That's out of tune, that's too slow, that's too loud"—any idiot could do that. The player has to feel it, hear it, and know to what degree to change it and how—it's a very big mistake to take that process away from the player. Or the singer—if I say, "I must have that phrase in one breath," I just guaranteed she'll never be able to do it. It will be completely different if I say, "It would be so beautiful to try to achieve this phrase in one unbroken arc." What you have to understand before you open your mouth is that one of the biggest components is confidence. People always say, "Well, they're not babies." I say, "No, they're artists. And they have nerves. They play with their nervous system, and it isn't fair that you want the product of their nervous system but then you don't want them ever to feel nervous."

From the beginning I built a rapport with the orchestra that was based on these people knowing I will not kick them when they're down. If they come from home, and they had a problem, and they're having a lousy day in rehearsal, that is not the day I say, "Hey, you're having a lousy day." That day we pass over. Because they need to know it's safe in there. And if they know that, then all kinds of by-products happen, and all kinds of things are possible to do under stress that wouldn't be possible

otherwise. Over these 40 years, our orchestra has become more dramatic, more lyric, more vocal, more consistent, more committed, more able to deal with pressure. There's a stability to the way we work that produces a different kind of result than you can get in a relationship which is more ad hoc.

I guess some conductors use an approach which is more like a coach or a teacher, and some people use an approach which is more gestural. I always found that if you insist you have to be able to do it with a gesture, you are automatically limited by what the group collectively can understand from the gesture, rather than all the things that you might be able to get out of it if you could in fact suit it to an explanation. The result, it must be said, is that I talk a lot in rehearsals. If you ask any orchestra musician, even the most dedicated ones, they hate it. I don't like it much myself. But the reason it's a necessity is that you want an entire group of musicians to do paradoxical things, all at the same time. You want them to play really short notes but not to accent them, or to play something really profoundly accented not because it's attacked hard, but because it comes from inside. You can gesture and make faces until you're blue in the face, and that will not make 32 violins all do the same thing. But you can get them to do the same thing if you repeat the passage four times, and gradually the paradoxes come out, and then they can feel them and repeat them.

Daniel Barenboim: For 15 summers, Jimmy and I had adjacent dressing rooms at the Bayreuth Festival. I went to his rehearsals and he went to mine, and we always had very open conversations and discussions afterwards. "Why do you do that like this?" Or "Oh, yes, I didn't think of it like this." From the very beginning, our friendship was based on a mutual musical respect of the highest order.

When I made my Met debut conducting *Tristan und Isolde* in 2008, I knew how well prepared the orchestra would be. At Bayreuth, what Jimmy was doing in orchestra rehearsals was training the musicians to listen to each other. Although they knew the pieces inside and out, he would show them connections that maybe they had not talked about, and it was amazing how quickly you could hear the results.

It sounds like a paradox, but when a music director has a very strong hand, an orchestra has more flexibility. So when I did the *Tristan,* I was able to feel all the work that Jimmy had done with the orchestra, on that piece in particular, but also in general: the homogeneity of the strings, the solo playing of the winds, the balancing, the sensitivity to different sounds. And yet, I was able to do what I wanted to do with the greatest ease.

But it was with Verdi recently that I saw just how remarkably the orchestra and Jimmy work together. I went to a rehearsal of *Simon Boccanegra,* and it was astonishing, how you felt that the orchestra was not so much following him—they knew what he was thinking and played according to that. This is how you make great music.

Most people with talent get by on sheer ease, but Jimmy is always interested in delving deeper into the music. This has showed itself, for the 40 years that I have known him, in the way he conducts pieces that he and everybody know very well, but also in his curiosity for new music. What he has done for contemporary American music, for instance, is really mind-boggling.

Raymond Gniewek: When Jimmy made his debut with *Tosca,* I had already been concertmaster for 14 years [Gniewek held the position from 1957–2000], and I told him, "That was the greatest debut since Karajan was here." He loved that, and he never forgot it.

Jimmy spent years refining and polishing the Met orchestra, or "chipping away," as he said. He made little improvements—a diminuendo, for instance, that does not get piano soon enough. It sounds like a minor detail, but it's what makes the difference. He would say, "Every phrase says something, whether it has a dynamic, or a specific accent or not. If it has nothing, it still must have shape." If he was going away for a stint, he would say about other conductors, "I'm going to let them drive my Rolls-Royce."

Once, during an orchestra reading the morning after a performance of a difficult opera, Jimmy stopped and said to one of the solo players, "Can I give you a little more time on that solo? Did I cramp you?" The player said, "Oh, no, Jimmy, I just cracked. It's my fault." Jimmy's approach gives players—especially those who had played under sterner, stricter conductors—confidence, that he is going to help you through a difficult spot, not challenge you.

One of Jimmy's incredible gifts is to verbalize solutions to problems, to articulate things to winds, brasses, everybody. Once when he did it with some string phrasing, I listened, smiling. He said, "Do you have any questions, Ray?" I said, "No. As a string player, I couldn't have said it better. I wish I had thought of that."

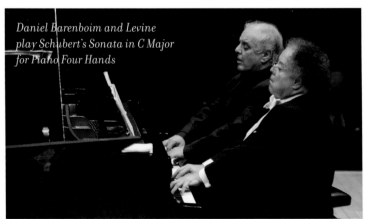

Daniel Barenboim and Levine play Schubert's Sonata in C Major for Piano Four Hands

Mark Gould: When I came to the Met as co-principal trumpet in 1974, the level of players throughout the orchestra was not nearly what it is now. What struck me at the first rehearsal I did with James Levine—*I Vespri Siciliani*—was his physical presence. He used his body almost like a force of nature. He was in total command. I went through some rough times in the beginning, just learning what to do, so he called a meeting with me. He was very encouraging and helpful. It wasn't his style to say anything confrontational or too specific. When you had a solo, he'd outline five different ways you could do it. He wouldn't say which he wanted, just let you think about it.

When it came to fixing one or two measures of music, there had never been anyone like him, for patience and meticulousness. He also had a very clear idea of what he wanted the orchestra to sound like, and he was relentless in developing that. New players kept coming in, and he got to the point where the people he really needed were in principal positions. And he was tireless: he could do a five-hour dress rehearsal of *Die Walküre* and then start rehearsing something else with the orchestra. He would actually pick up steam as the rehearsal went on—it was insanity!

And he never lost his temper. There were times when, if I were Levine, I would have killed someone. You could see when he was not happy with certain things, and he would take care of them later, but he never lost his cool.

At that first meeting I had with him, he said, "Well, Mark, I took this job in order to save opera in America." It stunned me, but he actually did it. He made this into a world-class ensemble, and he really invigorated the Met.

David Langlitz: Within the slide of a trombone is something called a lead pipe, and one day a few years ago I was experimenting with a new one. It was maybe an eighth of an inch longer than the old one, not much of a difference. We were rehearsing an act of *Don Carlo* that starts with a big trombone chorale. I've been here since 1974, and I've done *Don Carlo* with Jimmy many, many times, but on this occasion he looked over and said, "Can I hear the trombones again, please?" We played it again, then one more time, and then he let it go, but I could tell it wasn't exactly what he wanted. The next day I put the old piece in my trombone, and when we played the chorale Jimmy smiled at me and gave me a thumbs-up. He didn't know that I had replaced a lead pipe, but he knew there was something different. There are very few conductors on the face of the planet who have ears that sensitive.

He also has a kind of subterranean psychic ability. He listens to someone play, and in about 10 or 15 minutes he has a great sense of that person's strengths. And he has a way of enhancing and bringing out those strengths. He can be tremendously supportive if you have something difficult to play; he will sort of open the space for you to play with a certain amount of ease, almost like water flowing off a cliff.

He'll give a minimum of gesture, but you'll know exactly what he wants. Over time we have established a visual repertoire. I can tell if he's happy with something or if he wants to adjust it a certain way. I've seen him work slowly over a period of weeks, sometimes even months, looking for a particular sound, a particular interpretation, and just patiently going through it with a player. That's the way to build an orchestra: we feel as if what we're doing is valued.

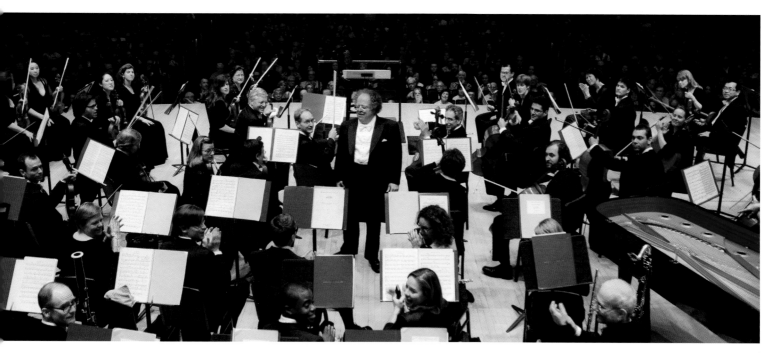

Ricardo Morales: I was only 21 when I joined the Metropolitan Opera Orchestra as principal clarinetist in 1993. My first day on the job, the minute we started playing, Jimmy gave this enthusiastic smile. That's something that I've always admired about him, his love for what he's doing and his positive intensity, the feeling of camaraderie.

He figures out where he can be demanding and squeeze the musical juice out of players, and where it might be a little excessive. He's very good about allowing for that space, musical and personal, to be able to do the things that he requests without painting you into a corner. Jimmy would work on things until they improved, then say, "Oh yes, this way it's a little perkier, there's more life to the sound. I like that," when what he could have said is, "I appreciate that now it's not flat."

I left the Met in 2004 and joined the Philadelphia Orchestra. Every day, as I play, I think about things that I learned from him: the way dynamics have to be in proportion to what else is going on, the way he balances power and delicacy… It makes you think about your approach to music—you have to have direction and fluidity, and it has to mean something.

Michael Ouzounian: I've been working with Jimmy since I was 16 years old, first as a student in Cleveland and then as a violist in the Met Orchestra. The most remarkable thing that I've seen, right from the start, is that he gives musicians a certain latitude for being temperamental, for being irrational or moody. I think he feels that his function is to get the best performance out of the forces, and not to be imposing, because he doesn't really believe you can impose. He grew up in a milieu where fear was a component of orchestra playing, but that doesn't suit his personality. He developed a way of getting great results without being autocratic. He makes allowances for people, and the upshot is that you can experiment a little bit more while you're playing, to try to get things better.

What I treasure is that Jim knows how to make every point vital. As an orchestra musician, you need to learn your part and get familiar with the music, but you also need it to sound spontaneous. He has taught us so many ways to draw out the vitality that's in the music and put ourselves in it as if it were for the first time. That's just an incredible boon for anybody who has been doing this job for so many years. When he does his umpteenth *Don Giovanni* it's like there's always more to get out of it, but you don't have to make it interesting by exaggerating or doing something that's out of character. That's the way it has always been with him: it's not James Levine, it's the music.

Expanding the Repertoire:
MET Orchestra at Carnegie Hall

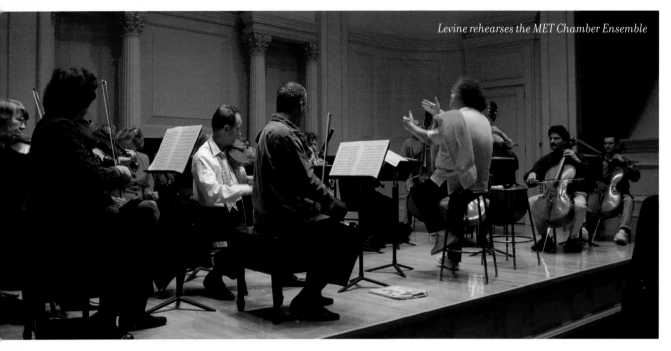

Levine rehearses the MET Chamber Ensemble

JL: It's a relatively modern phenomenon for a symphony orchestra not to play opera and an opera orchestra not to play symphonies and the rest of the repertoire. It was obvious to me that if we could make this development naturally, it would be very, very important for us artistically—if we could find a way to rehearse about three programs a year, and if we had an audience for them, that this would give the orchestra a crucial element in its artistic development that it would not get any other way. Usually, Carnegie Hall is the climactic stop on an orchestra's tour. But it's our hometown hall. Well, to say it worked out the way I dreamed it is putting it mildly. First of all, Carnegie was ready to work with the Met. Second, apparently the New York audience was interested enough in this orchestra to enjoy hearing them play some symphonic repertoire, with a sense of occasion and discovery.

It's the only access we have to a stylistic diversity that encompasses certain kinds of solo pieces for orchestra instruments, non-operatic music for singers, and symphonic challenges that are not related to opera, as well as the most important category, which is symphonic challenges that are related to opera in one way or another. Over the years now, we've played a remarkable depth and diversity of all kinds of symphonic repertoire. We've even commissioned composers for pieces! And it's been an altogether happy, stimulating, and fulfilling thing for us.

The Chamber Ensemble came about because it was very clear that this orchestra was going to lag behind the world in knowledge of contemporary music, contemporary techniques—and the stimulus and pleasure of the whole continuum from classical pieces to pieces where the ink isn't yet dry. The concerts we did in one of the small halls of Carnegie allowed us, sort of on our own initiative and with our own programming and counsel, to have a kind of unified diversity to this repertoire. And I think all these tools have been indispensable in building this instrument to the quality that it has.

William Bolcom: Jim has done quite a lot of my work, including two of my biggest symphonies, which he commissioned. The Seventh Symphony was for the Met at Carnegie Hall in 2002, and originally Jim had wanted to have a concerto for orchestra, because he had several people he wanted to feature. I decided that I wanted to have some kind of a plot going with it, so I turned it into a kind of play structure. It became twelve soloists and it was all, essentially, to show off what these musicians can do, because it's such a terrific orchestra. It's a very difficult piece, with lots of virtuoso passages for all kinds of instruments. How does an average orchestra deal with this? These days there is almost always a shortage of rehearsals, and usually the players get not much more time than they would for standard repertory that they've done since they were 12 years old. Of course, this isn't an average orchestra. What Jim does is to ask for parts months in advance and then he has them put into everybody's folders. When there's a spare five or ten minutes, he reads a bit of the piece with the orchestra. Over a period of weeks, they get some idea of what it's about and what some of the problems are, and the soloists have plenty of time to take home their parts and woodshed them. He's the only conductor I know who does this as a regular thing.

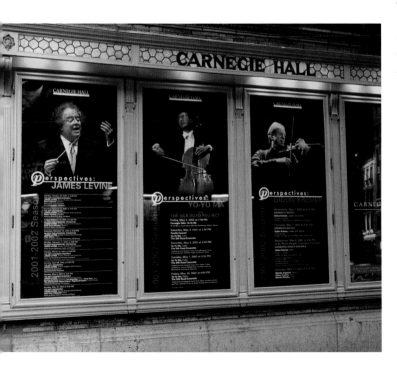

Pierre Boulez: It's astonishing to think that I have known Jimmy for more than 45 years. I first met him in 1965 in Cleveland, when he was about 22 and still the assistant conductor of The Cleveland Orchestra. Immediately there was a great sympathy between us, and we spent some evenings talking about music, about everything.

I admire him because it's extraordinary now for someone to remain with the same orchestra for 40 years. Jimmy has had the courage, and the force, to be there with this orchestra and to conduct a lot of performances. He didn't just do some premiere and then afterwards say, "Well, now they can do what they want." No, he was very obstinate, and it's this kind of obstinacy that has produced the quality of this orchestra. Having the orchestra play outside the pit, too, is a wonderful thing. An orchestra has pride. When they are on stage, they are the main event, seen and heard for what they are. They also have the chance to play pieces which are rarely performed. Jimmy has added to the repertoire in the opera house, too, and he has succeeded in that because he is convincing. He's convincing because he has convinced himself, and that's the secret.

In May 2010, I finally had the opportunity to conduct the MET Orchestra, for a concert of Bartók's *The Wooden Prince* and Schoenberg's *Erwartung* in Carnegie Hall. I worked with them with great pleasure. I did not need to explain many things. In fact, many things came normally, without any explanation at all. I was so happy with the work, in the rehearsals and at the performance, not only because the orchestra is highly professional, but because they are devoted to what they do. That is really so important, and so rare.

Joyce DiDonato: This concert was my first time working with the legendary Maestro of the Met. When I got the invitation, I couldn't believe it. No longer would I be the odd person out in the Met cafeteria as colleagues sang his praises and I had to nod politely, knowing that I was missing out on the artistic experience of a lifetime.

I have never arrived so early for a first rehearsal; I have never been so prepared, and I have never been so excited or nervous. And yet, it was the easiest, most organic, natural and vibrant first reading that I have ever known. He invited me to express, to celebrate the music, to give everything I had. He encouraged me to find the simplicity in the music, and in the simplicity there was depth.

He had programmed an arrangement of Rossini's *La Regata Veneziana,* which I had sung numerous times with piano, but never with orchestra. From the first rehearsal, it was clear how much fun he intended on having. He gently steered the players along the Venetian canal, evoking the anxiety and flirtatious qualities of all Rossini's markings, always encouraging the playful side of the work, which brought a sense of intoxication and liberation to my portrayal.

The real meat of the program was Mozart's "Ch'io mi scordi di te," which I had never sung. When he asked me if it would "be okay" if he tried playing the piano obbligato himself, I nearly wept. He conducted from the piano and led an unforgettable reading of this piece. Why is he so great? He bleeds musicality and sensitivity. He breathes with you and can feel what you need three measures before you yourself realize it. He smiles. He drinks in the phrases and the text and the arc of the piece. He knows the perfect tempo for your voice, and he knows how to make you feel perfectly safe so that you feel free to take risks, which is the thing we're all really after.

His eyes lit up, and he leaned in to me and said, "What if the audience is really happy? We should give them something else, right? What about some 'Non più mesta'?"

If ever there were a moment when a girl felt more like Cinderella, I don't know what it could be. This aria, from Rossini's *Cenerentola,* was the one with which I had auditioned for the Maestro six years before, and singing it with him was truly a dream come true. His outstretched left arm inviting me to celebrate and sing is an image that will always stay with me. He not only made me a better singer on that Sunday afternoon, he gave me that wondrous memory that I carry with me on every stage I stand on.

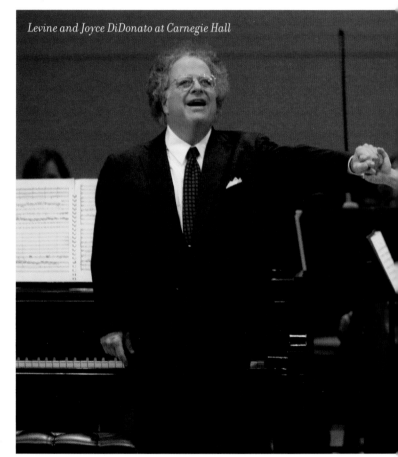

Levine and Joyce DiDonato at Carnegie Hall

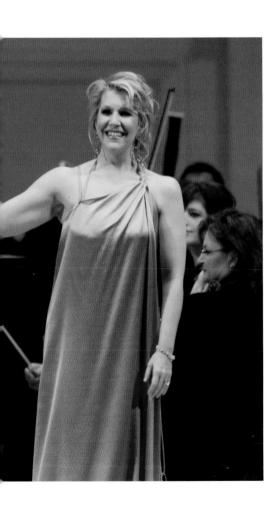

Gunther Schuller: Jimmy and I met and first worked together in 1966, when I conducted The Cleveland Orchestra, and he was the orchestra's pianist. I did five contemporary pieces, none of which the orchestra had ever played, and Jimmy was one of maybe a dozen musicians who were very excited by this program and very eager to face these challenges. The rest of the orchestra practically mutinied.

One of his greatest legacies is taking on all that music that almost nobody wanted to do—new music and neglected music and unheard-of music, even by famous composers from the past. He has done the whole Second Viennese School and American composers who wrote either 12-tone or atonal or highly chromatic music. He loves that music.

In 1995, when I sent him *Of Reminiscences and Reflections* for the MET Orchestra, he called me and asked highly intelligent, inquiring questions about some details which I think many conductors wouldn't have even noticed. It showed me how well he already knew the piece before he had conducted it. We talked over the phone, and I never worried because I knew that he would do the right thing. The way he comprehends a score, both vertically and horizontally, is amazing, and he understand it even more deeply through the years.

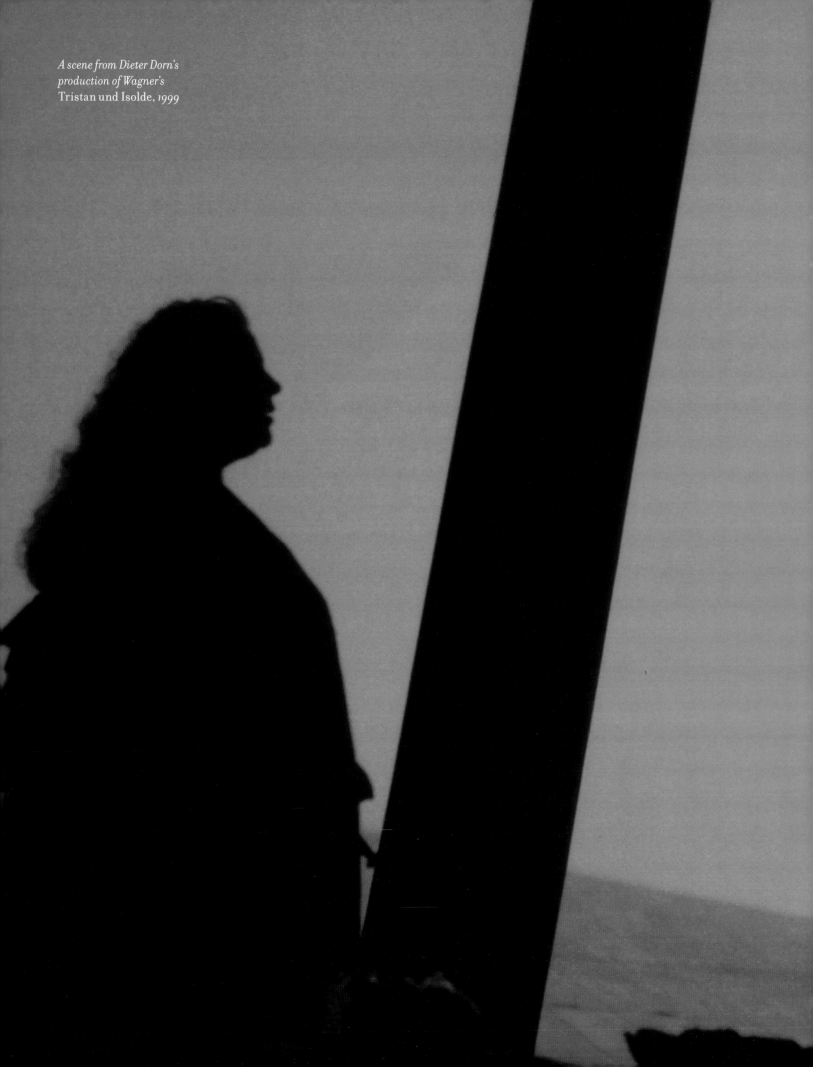

1990–2000

A Sustained Crescendo

PLÁCIDO DOMINGO

In November 1970, I arrived in San Francisco for some performances of *Tosca* and asked the company's director who the conductor was to be. He said that it was a 27-year-old named James Levine. I said, "I've never heard of him." I was only 29 at the time, but I already had worked with many well-known conductors. By the time we were a few minutes into our first rehearsal, I realized that this was an astonishing talent. Jimmy not only knew every detail of the score: he also had good taste, was thoroughly familiar with all the traditions, and had the rare ability to bring unity to an interpretation. I had sung *Tosca* 47 times, whereas Jimmy was conducting it for the first time, but we were completely together from start to finish. Not surprisingly, within a few months he had made his Met debut and was chosen as the principal conductor.

It is hard to believe that more than four decades have gone by since then. In the meantime, I have done far more repertoire, live performances, recordings, and radio and television broadcasts with Jimmy than with any other conductor. I don't know who is second on the list, but it's a very distant second! Jimmy and I often appeared together in operas that he was conducting for the first time or that I was singing for the first time, and I think that on those occasions the presence of the one gave extra support to the other. Among other important events in my life, Jimmy conducted my very first *Otello,* in Hamburg in 1975—and my first at the Met, on Opening Night in 1979. And still fresh in my memory are our performances of *Simon Boccanegra* in January 2010—the first time I sang a baritone role at the Met. To me, he is like a brother.

What amazed me about Jimmy from the start, and what continues to amaze me, is his ability to interpret so much music in so many different styles, and to do all of it so well. This is true not only in opera but also in the symphonic repertoire, not to mention when he plays the piano in chamber music or lieder performances. It doesn't matter if the piece is a comedy by Rossini, a tragedy by Verdi, or a vast drama by Wagner; whether it is a Baroque classic, a difficult work by Schoenberg or a new piece by Elliott Carter; no matter if it is a huge Mahler symphony or a simple Schubert song. Some performers become stale after they have rehearsed and performed a work 50 or 100 or 200 times, but with Jimmy there has been a sustained crescendo. There is also the unrivaled clarity of his baton technique, as well as the enthusiasm and the collaborative spirit that he communicates to everyone, whether it is a veteran star singer or a beginner, or a musician sitting at the back of a string section in the orchestra.

So many occasions come to mind. I remember when my wife Marta and I were staying at the same hotel in Bayreuth that Jimmy and his brother, Tom, were staying at—a very fine hotel with the best wines and excellent cuisine, and we would meet and have great meals together. Once, when we were on the same plane together, Tom would pass notes from Jimmy to me and Peter Hofstoetter, my assistant, would pass my comments back to Jimmy. We joked about how maybe I would do a Saturday matinee double-bill of *Cavalleria Rusticana* and *Pagliacci* and then an evening performance of *Otello.* I have quite a bit of stamina, but I think that would have been the end of me. But mostly what I think about are all the rehearsals—at the piano and with orchestra—and all the performances we've done together. The list is a very long one: so many Verdi operas plus *Les Troyens, Lohengrin,* and on and on! At this point, we've been part of a considerable portion of the history of the Metropolitan Opera, and I am proud to have been part of it with Jimmy.

During all these years, James Levine has been the Met's backbone and has guaranteed that the company maintains its extraordinarily high quality. For me, he is a wonderful colleague and a real friend. Long may he continue to be this great ensemble's guiding spirit!

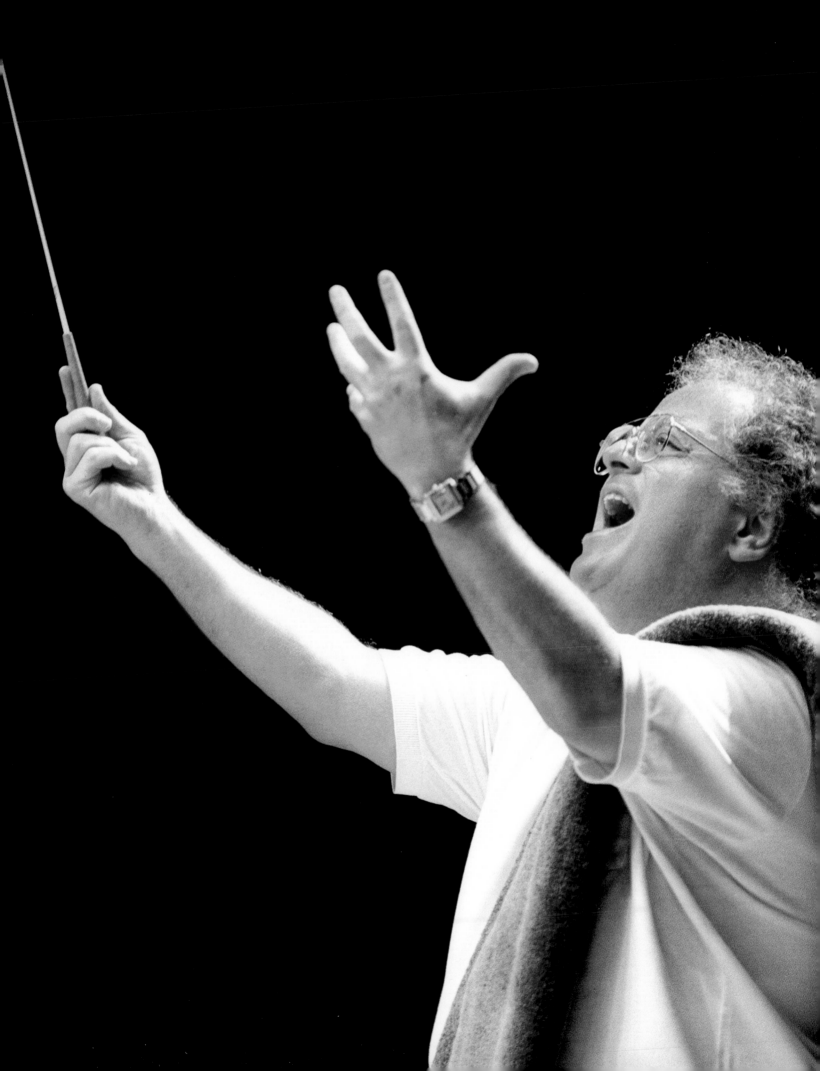

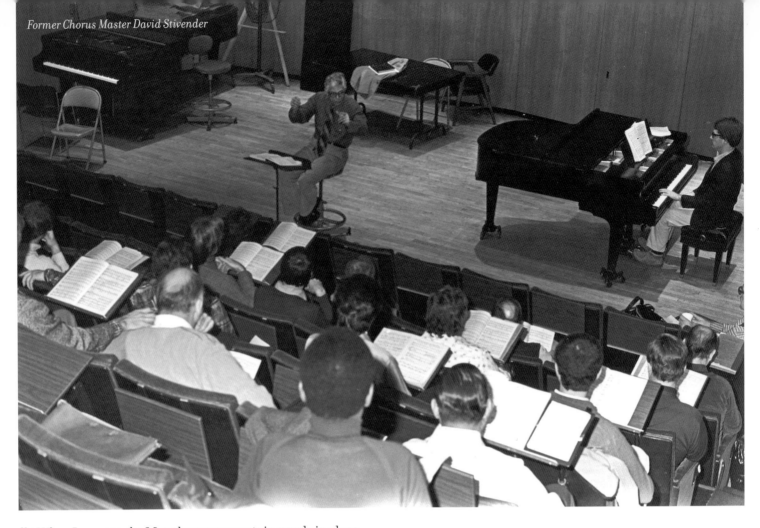

JL: When I came to the Met, there were certain people in place already, like David Stivender, who were real geniuses at what they did. He was the Associate Chorus Master, and at the request of the choristers he became the successor of Kurt Adler as the Chorus Master. He and I had a superb rapport. He was a great musician, a great Met person, a great teacher—a major inspiration for the chorus.

1990

SEPTEMBER 21

In a memorial concert for Chorus Master David Stivender, Levine leads the chorus in the "Hymn to the Sun" from Mascagni's *Iris*.

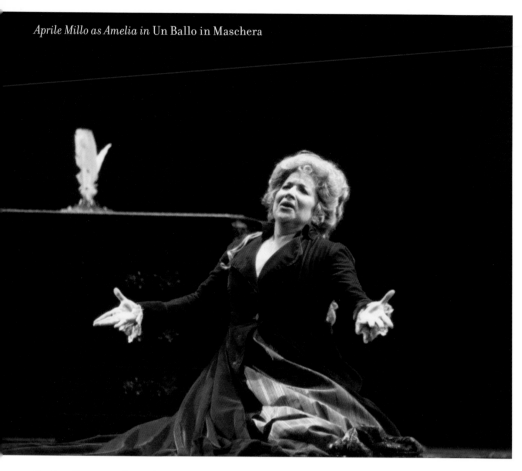

Aprile Millo as Amelia in Un Ballo in Maschera

JL: Aprile was a throwback to something that didn't exist anymore when she came along. She had not only a terrific voice, but an instinct for these Italian roles, a real feel for the phrase, the text, the style. She also had an instinct for the history of the style, the way these roles were meant to be done, which had gradually changed through the generations. There are a great many operas we would have been unable to do with any kind of stylistic pizzazz if she hadn't appeared. She was also a very good-humored and positive, enthusiastic character, always willing to work and give 100 percent. And she had an excellent relationship to the public—they understood who she was.

Aprile Millo: To know James Levine is to know firsthand a sunrise, the deep and profound colors of a day just starting, vivid and breathtaking, warm and full of promise. His beautiful sky-blue eyes have such life and carry enormous power. His world is awash in love and unlimited possibility. He creates an environment that begs the curious, invites the creative, and inspires the free and daring. I remember a 1990 *Aida* recording session in which the orchestra was playing the dance in the second-act Amneris salon, with its never-ending variations of rhythm and energy. With great pride, Jimmy lowered his baton, walked off the podium, and watched as the orchestra successfully "conducted" itself. At the final chord, he returned to the podium, a smile etched from ear to ear—not only on his face but on all those of the gifted men and women of his orchestra. During a performance he would do the same thing: smile. Excellence pleases him; it tickles him. For me, he will always be a point of reference and reverence, and a great and loyal friend.

OCTOBER 25

Adds Verdi's *Un Ballo in Maschera* to his Met repertoire in a new production starring Aprile Millo and Luciano Pavarotti.

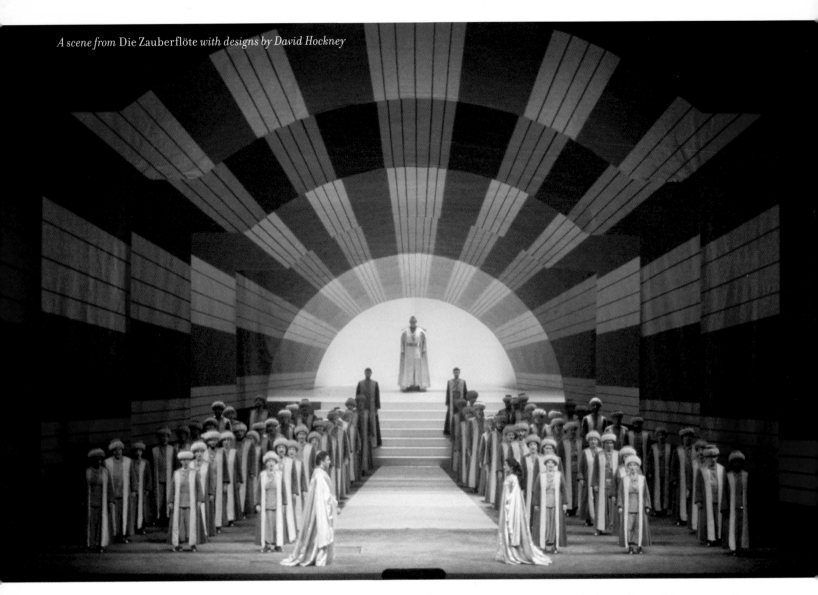

A scene from Die Zauberflöte *with designs by David Hockney*

JL: This *Magic Flute* was a wonderful kind of a substitute accident. We were supposed to do it with Ponnelle, and then he died. The next thing I thought to do was ask Werner Herzog to do it. Werner had a lot of good ideas, but I think he was dealing with a pretty neophyte designer, and [General Manager] Joe Volpe and [Technical Director] Joe Clark were very nervous about it. So they asked David [Hockney] whether he thought that the San Francisco incarnation of his old Glyndebourne *Flute* could be done at the Met, despite the size difference. David adapted it, and it was a real save. He is a great, great artist whose eyes and ears are very connected. He's brilliant and very funny, a guy whose creativity is closely tied to a lot of buoyancy.

1991
JANUARY 10

Conducts his first Met performance of Mozart's *Die Zauberflöte,* in a new production designed by David Hockney, with Kathleen Battle, Luciana Serra, Francisco Araiza, Manfred Hemm, and Kurt Moll.

JL: Kundry was a natural role for Jessye, the tessitura and timbre and conception. Plácido, with his beautiful Latin timbre, was different from the norm of German-style Parsifals, though the best ones have some version of Italianate radiance in the tone, too. But Plácido was always interested in everything, artistically. And you know what he uses to rehearse Wagner operas? A little book that has the German text in it—parallel to a literal Spanish translation. He remembers the music so quickly and so instinctively that he doesn't need to look at it very long; he only needs the German words. The audience wanted Plácido to sing these Wagner parts, and when he did, they were not disappointed. He put in a lot of hard work, and he was successful on stage as Lohengrin, Siegmund, and Parsifal.

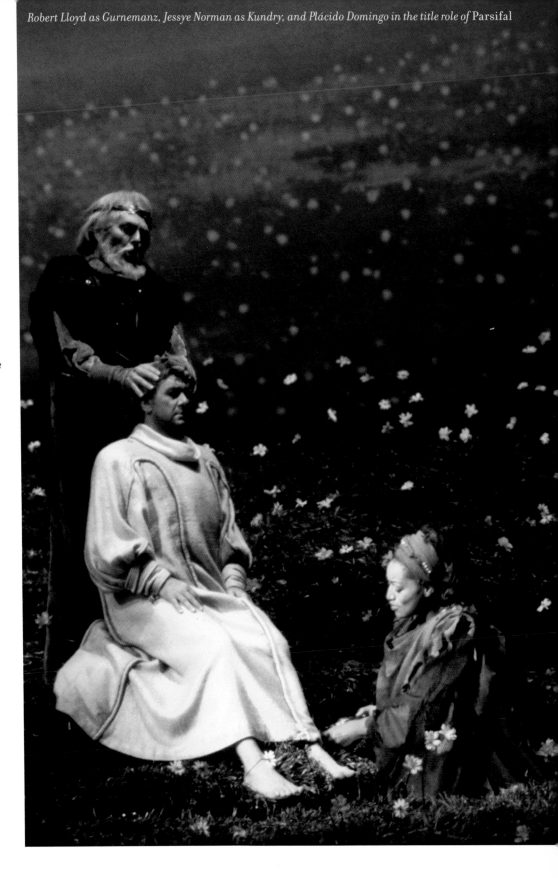

MARCH 14

Conducts Otto Schenk's new production of *Parsifal*, with Plácido Domingo, Jessye Norman, Ekkehard Wlaschiha, and Robert Lloyd.

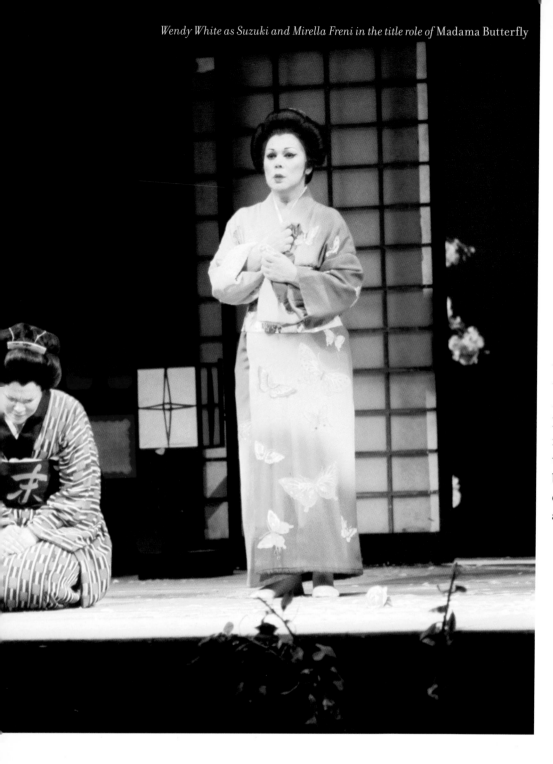

Wendy White as Suzuki and Mirella Freni in the title role of Madama Butterfly

JL: Mirella did something wonderful for me that day: it was the one and only time she sang an act of *Butterfly,* staged and in costume. She was always afraid to sing Angelica or Butterfly. She was afraid that the emotion would get to her, and she'd lose control on stage. And this, I understand—it's something that a sensitive artist always has to deal with on some level or the other. Mirella understood that her stock in trade depended on not harming the beauty of the instrument. She said, "If I do that, then whatever I have is not me anymore." There are some artists who recognize an almost opposite philosophy, who know their artistry is about flinging in and taking the risk, but she knew that her artistry was bound up in the beauty of her timbre. Her visits to the Met were never as frequent as I wanted them to be because she was based in Europe, but we still hit it off in our artistic collaboration—we were close right away and enjoyed everything we did.

MARCH 24

Conducts a gala celebrating the 25th Met anniversaries of Mirella Freni, Nicolai Ghiaurov, and Alfredo Kraus, with scenes from *Faust, Don Carlo,* and *Madama Butterfly.*

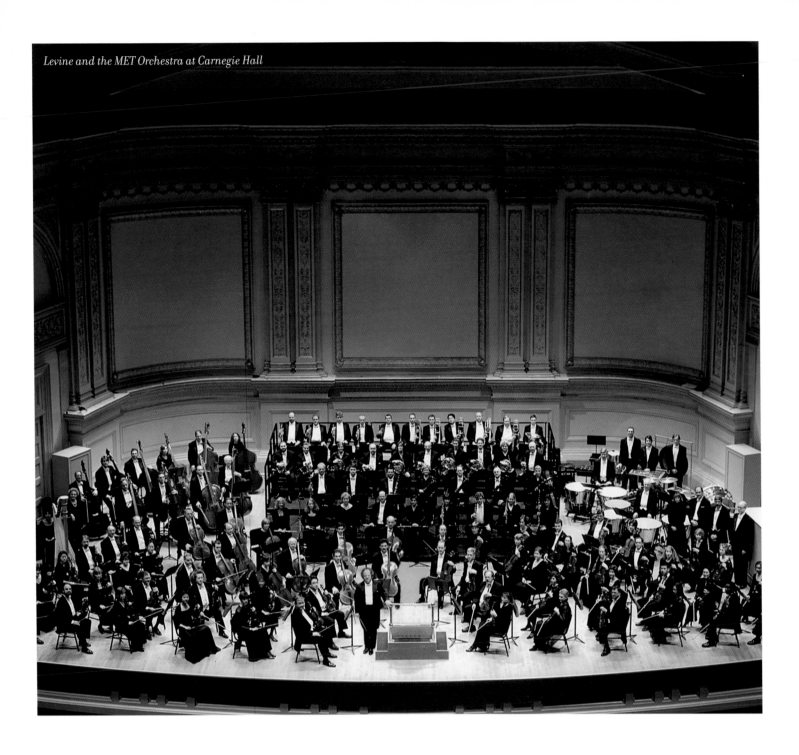

Levine and the MET Orchestra at Carnegie Hall

Takes the MET Orchestra on its first U.S. tour and leads a concert at Carnegie Hall, which launches the annual concert series.

SEPTEMBER 23

Conducts the gala celebrating the 25th anniversary of the Met at Lincoln Center, performing acts from *Rigoletto, Otello,* and *Die Fledermaus.*

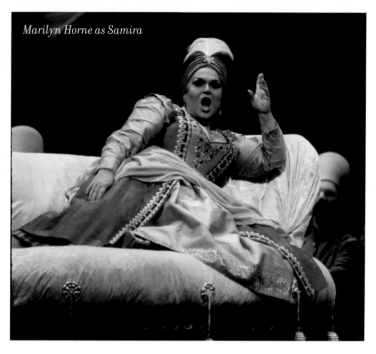

Marilyn Horne as Samira

Marilyn Horne: Jim is at home in every style and every period, and that's one of the reasons I adore him. When the Met commissioned John Corigliano's *The Ghosts of Versailles,* it was a really wonderful experience to be singing Samira, a role that was written for me. But when I was studying and learning her scene, I couldn't quite figure out how to do it. Jim and I sat down in a rehearsal room, and I said, "I need help with this, Jim. I haven't got my finger on it." And he gave it to me immediately, the key: he said, "She is a hugely extravagant, over-the-top kind of character."

Two of the things I most appreciate about him are his diplomacy and his positive attitude. Once, when we were rehearsing a recital, I knew that when I sang a particular note I was pressing on it vocally. Jim didn't say to me, "Jackie, that note is just awful." He just said, "Jackie, I don't think you would like that note!" That was diplomacy at its utmost, and he works that way with orchestras, too. A long time ago, before he was The Great James Levine, we did the *Rückert-Lieder* with the London Symphony. Those orchestras can be very tough on a youngish conductor, and there was one place where they were not playing together. Jim put the whole thing on himself by saying, "I'm trying to get this together." That's great psychology.

John Corigliano: *The Ghosts of Versailles* was the first opera the Met had commissioned since Samuel Barber's *Antony and Cleopatra* and Marvin David Levy's *Mourning Becomes Electra* in 1966 and 1967, and the first ever for Jimmy. It was such an enormous responsibility. When I would go to the gym on West 63rd Street, I would ride my bicycle over to Central Park West, because just seeing the Met would strike fear in my heart. When I finished the first act, I left it with Jimmy and anguished over whether he

DECEMBER 19

Conducts the world premiere of John Corigliano and William M. Hoffman's *The Ghosts of Versailles,* starring Teresa Stratas, Renée Fleming, Marilyn Horne, Graham Clark, Gino Quilico, and Håkan Hagegård.

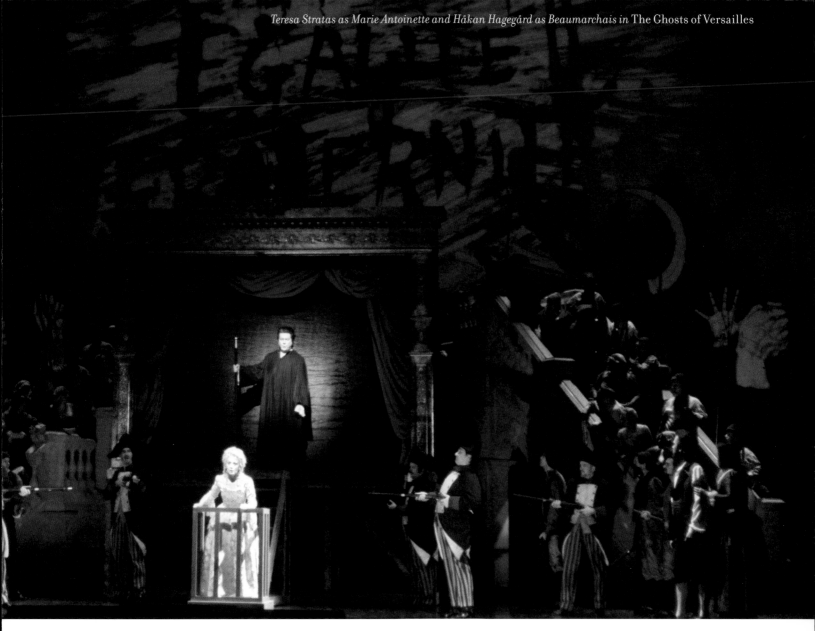

would like it. After a long time, he called me in, told me that it was fine and that I should go ahead with Act II. He said something interesting at one point: "You know, I don't understand parts of this libretto. They don't make sense to me, and I don't know how they're going to work theatrically, but that's my opinion. Do you think you can make it work theatrically?" After I said yes, he said, "Then go right ahead, because I would have said the same thing to Mozart about the *Magic Flute* libretto,

and look what happened." It was very generous and trusting of him. And when he finally saw it onstage, he said, "It plays gorgeously. I get it now."

One of the really important things that Jimmy did after we finished the piece was to let us make an audio tape for everyone to hear. It was a big project. We used young artists at the Met, and a synthesizer for all of the orchestra parts. In those days they didn't have sampling as they do now, and it was much more primitive. When we gave the tape to the

Met, everybody got very excited, because they could hear the opera. The director could do his timings, the singers could hear their lines, and they'd hear them with instruments that sounded more realistic than the piano would have. When the Met heard the tape they said, "This is terrific," and they put a lot of money into the production. Jimmy didn't need the tape to see *Ghosts* would work, but he understood that everybody else did.

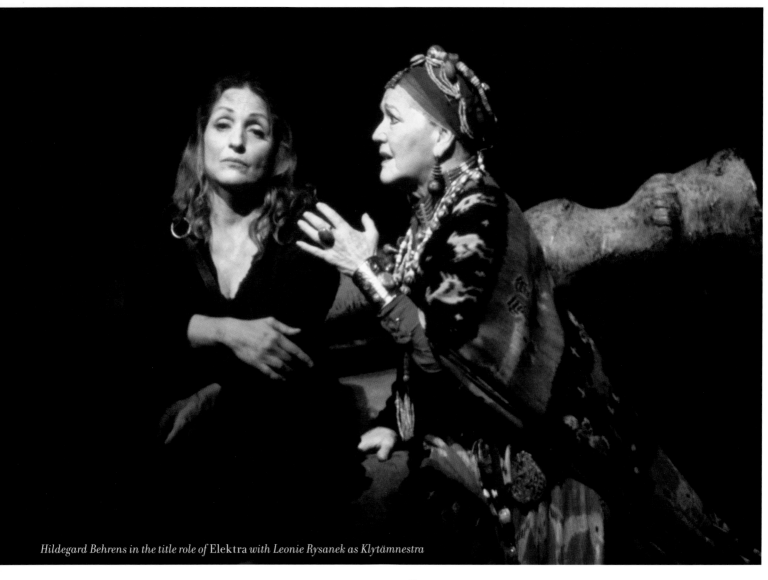

Hildegard Behrens in the title role of Elektra *with Leonie Rysanek as Klytämnestra*

JL: Hildegard used everything—her face, her body, her gestural language, the text, the music—to communicate this character. You were swept along and sucked into the world of her imagination as it merged with that of the composer and librettist. It was good to have a Chrysothemis with a different kind of timbre, to differentiate her since they sing in a similar register, and Debbie's voice was so bright and radiant. And Leonie, who had gone from singing Chrysothemis earlier in her career to singing Klytämnestra, was as always a unique and amazing performer.

1992
MARCH 26

Conducts a new production of *Elektra,*
directed by Otto Schenk, starring Hildegard
Behrens, Deborah Voigt, and Leonie Rysanek.

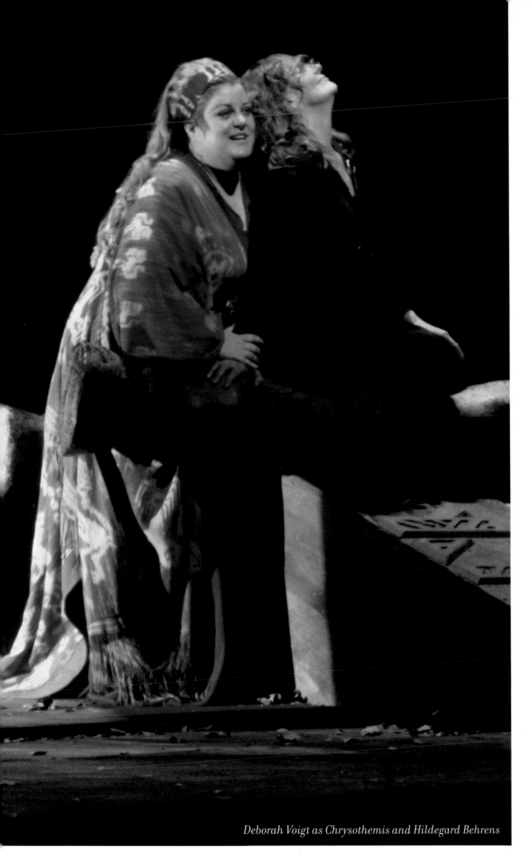

Deborah Voigt as Chrysothemis and Hildegard Behrens

JUNE 3

Takes the MET Orchestra to Europe
for Seville's Expo '92, the first of a number
of international tours for the orchestra.

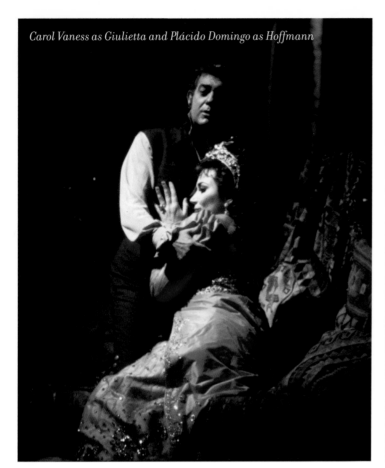

Carol Vaness as Giulietta and Plácido Domingo as Hoffmann

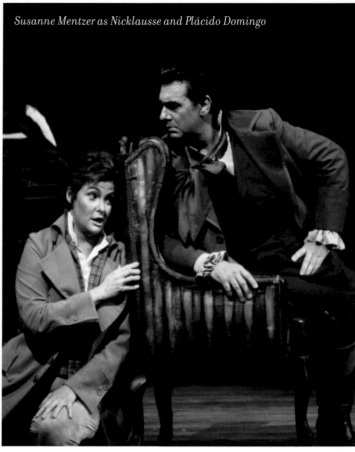

Susanne Mentzer as Nicklausse and Plácido Domingo

Rosalind Elias: This is absolutely true: Jimmy rejuvenated my whole life and my career. In the 1983–84 season, I was the Witch in *Hänsel und Gretel,* but after that I wasn't at the Met for many years. Florence Guarino, a beloved woman at the Met, passed away in 1990, and at her memorial service I sang "Must the winter come so soon?" from *Vanessa.* Jimmy was right in the first pew, and evidently, he spoke to some people about how young my voice still was and how much he enjoyed my singing. Soon there was an arrangement for me to meet with him in List Hall.

I was kind of frightened before that meeting, but then he sat at the piano and it was like old times. We went over some music, just the two of us, and we talked and sang some parts of different pieces. What struck me most was the care, and I will never forget it. He cared for me, and from that came my new career. On Opening Night in 1992, I was the Mother's Voice in *Les Contes d'Hoffmann*— the first in a whole series of character roles not just at the Met but elsewhere. Jimmy gave me my chance to sing my first Old Prioress in *Dialogues of the*

Carmelites, and many other things. When I was young and doing Cherubino and Dorabella, there was someone in me who wanted to do the character roles. I didn't care if I was on the stage singing for three minutes, so long as people said, "Wasn't that a wonderful characterization?"

Jimmy wants the best for everybody. He's wonderful to the young artists, but I am so grateful to him for the encouragement that he has given me even as an older artist.

SEPTEMBER 21

Opens the season with his first performance
of *Les Contes d'Hoffmann* in the house,
starring Plácido Domingo in the title role,
Carol Vaness as the four heroines, and Samuel
Ramey as the four villains.

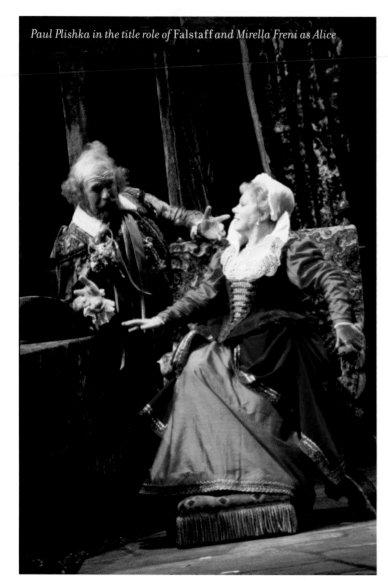

Paul Plishka in the title role of Falstaff *and Mirella Freni as Alice*

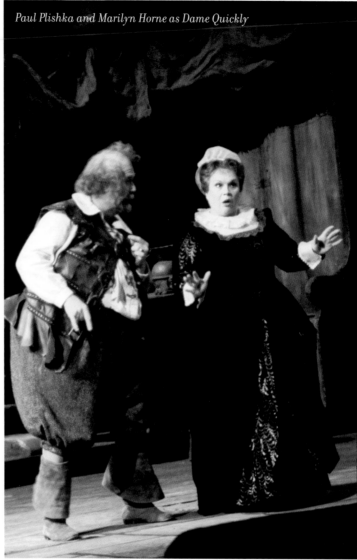

Paul Plishka and Marilyn Horne as Dame Quickly

JL: Doing that particular *Falstaff* meant a lot to me, because it was the piece I had stepped into for Bing, just before he retired. And we had a cast of similar quality—*Falstaff* is a quintessential great ensemble masterpiece, like the Mozart operas. I think nobody knew just how wonderful Paul was going to be in this opera because Falstaff is a very difficult and specialized part. It can be sung by bass-baritones like him, who have the right kind of technique and comedy, but it's also part of the Italian baritone tradition. Paul has sung everything, marvelous buffo parts and basso cantante parts. He was memorable in both comedies and serious drama, from big Verdi roles to Pimen in *Boris Godunov*—a wonderful artist and company member.

OCTOBER 14

Conducts Paul Plishka in the title role of *Falstaff*,
celebrating the singer's 25th Met anniversary,
with Mirella Freni, Heidi Grant Murphy,
Marilyn Horne, Stanford Olsen, and Bruno Pola.

Karita Mattila as Eva, Jan-Hendrik Rootering as Pogner, and Francisco Araiza as Walther in Die Meistersinger von Nürnberg

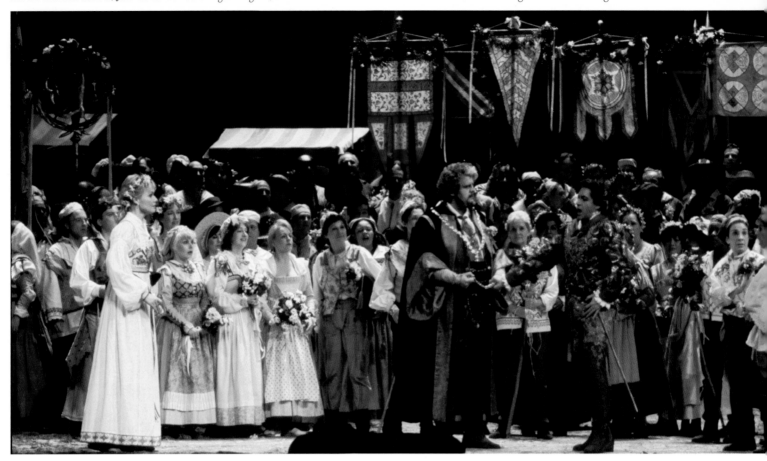

JL: Schenk and I work together with a kind of a telepathy, as you always do with the people who are best for you. You discuss things, but it's not in the discussion that stuff happens. It happens as you use your ears and your eyes with each other, and with other people, and gradually the priorities come out. I think the key has to do with bringing the best aspects of the people you're working with to the foreground rather than forcing them to imitate someone or take over a concept that's not organic for them. Schenk's approach comes from being a theater animal, an actor. I always love the way his results are so persuasive for the singers. It's especially fun for me to notice that in rehearsing certain scenes with them, he assumes the characterization of one part or another to some degree, depending on what the singers need. It's a very effective way of directing, and the singers get a lot out of it.

1993
JANUARY 14

Adds Wagner's *Die Meistersinger von Nürnberg* to his Met repertoire, in a new production by Otto Schenk, starring Karita Mattila, Francisco Araiza, Donald McIntyre, and Hermann Prey

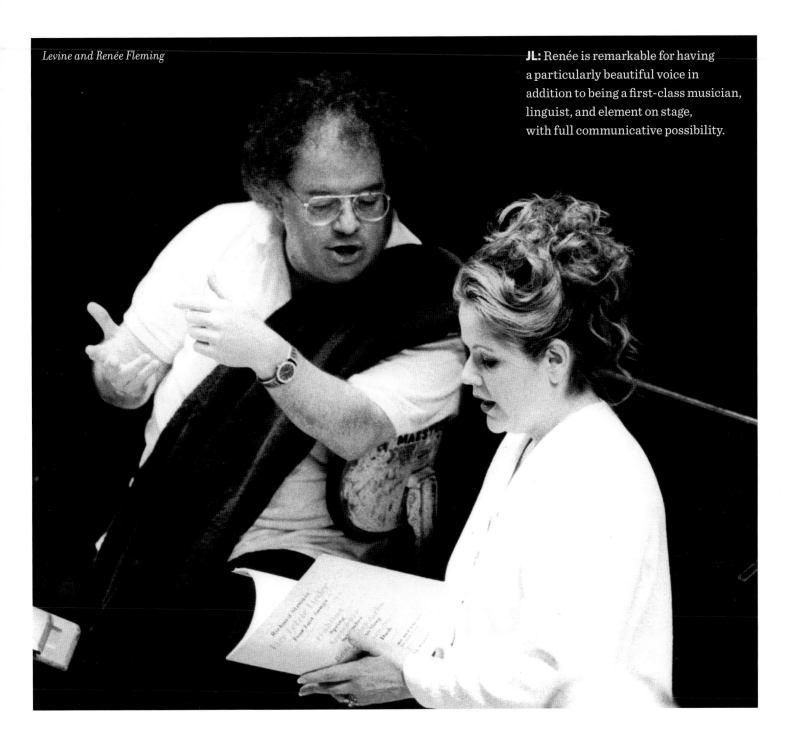

Levine and Renée Fleming

JL: Renée is remarkable for having a particularly beautiful voice in addition to being a first-class musician, linguist, and element on stage, with full communicative possibility.

MAY 9

Leads the MET Orchestra in a sold-out all-Berg concert at Carnegie Hall, with Itzhak Perlman and Renée Fleming as soloists.

JL: When *Time* magazine was doing an article about Plácido and Luciano, [Arts Editor] Martha [Duffy] called me and asked how I would describe the difference between these two guys. I said, "My God, that's not so easy. They can sing the same notes of certain pieces, but their best stuff is not the same." There was a long pause, and she said, "Like white wine and red wine?" I said, "Oh, you're good." I'll tell you one of the real nifty tributes. You know whose recordings Luciano used to listen to when he was learning a new role? The ones I'd made with Plácido. He knew their voices were completely different, but he knew that the recording would be musically completely sound in the details. It was a great thing for opera that the two of them had the kind of relationship they did, because they held down their repertoire virtually alone for many years. In their different ways, both Plácido and Luciano were as close to me as any human being could be. Each has, in every tricky situation, proven to be an even greater friend than you could ever imagine. Amazing guys.

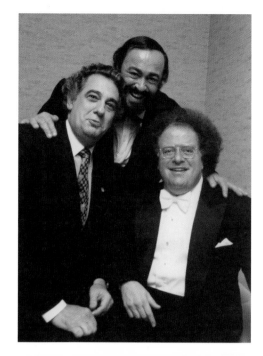

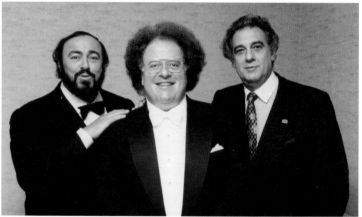

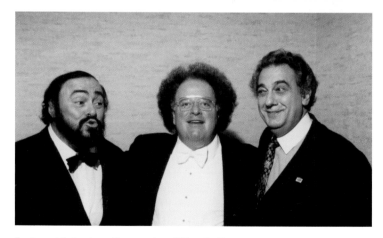

Levine with Luciano Pavarotti and Plácido Domingo

SEPTEMBER 27

His 16th Opening Night celebrates the 25th Met anniversaries of Plácido Domingo and Luciano Pavarotti, who perform in acts of *Die Walküre* and *Otello,* respectively, then share the role of Manrico in *Il Trovatore.*

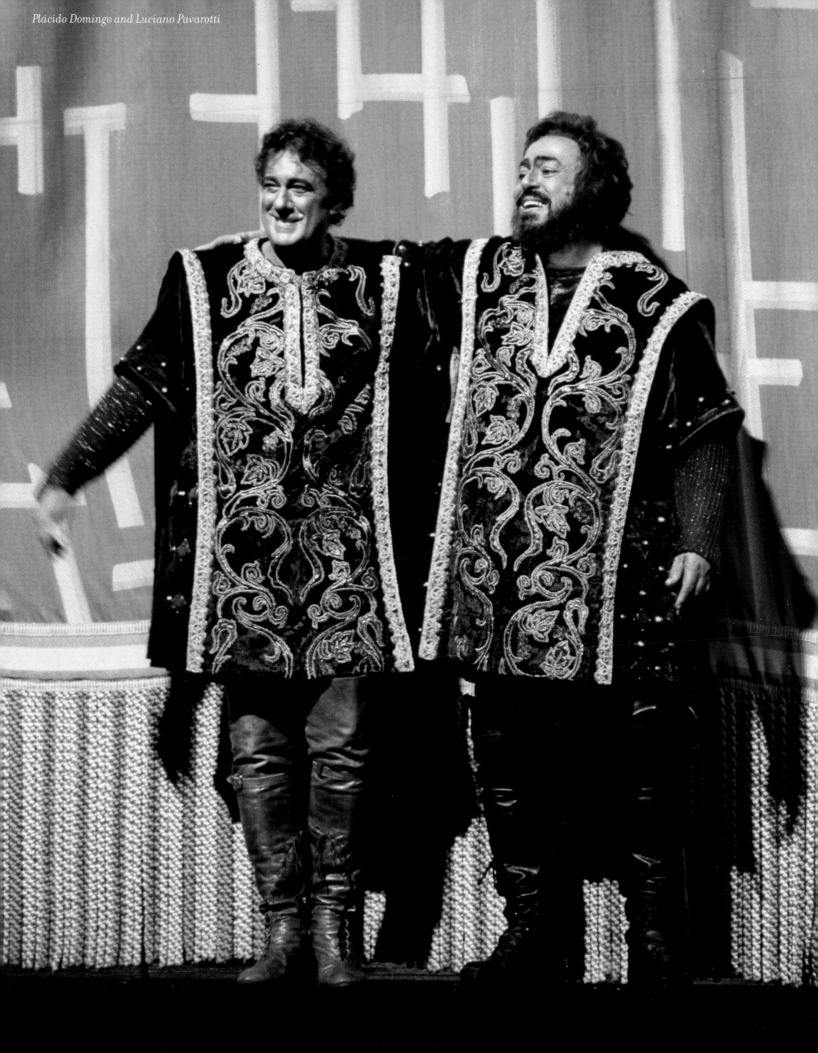

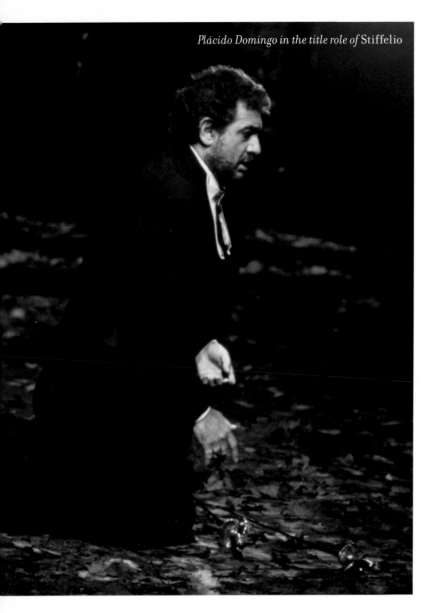

Plácido Domingo in the title role of Stiffelio

JL: That was a big anniversary year for Luciano and Plácido. I kept thinking about what we should do to celebrate these two guys who were making such an extraordinary contribution to the Met in their prime time. And I came up with a really neat and extravagant idea: "Let's do four new Verdi productions— two operas that we haven't got and two that we need to redo, and offer a pair to each of them." The new production that I wanted Luciano to do was *Forza del Destino.* It was an opera he hadn't done. And for the Met premiere, he suggested *Lombardi* because he had sung it a long time before. In the end, although he learned almost all of *Forza,* he wound up not doing it on the stage. Plácido's pair included a new *Otello.* He wanted one, anyway, that wasn't as big as the old one and had a different approach. And we decided the best opera to premiere that was a real tenor protagonist piece was *Stiffelio.* When it came to choosing whether I should do the new production or the new piece, we both felt I should do the new piece. Plácido had just done *Otello* somewhere with Valery Gergiev, so Valery made his Met debut with that. And *Stiffelio* turned out to be one of the most wonderful discoveries in my whole time at the Met. It's a missing link from that period of Verdi's writing. When I was growing up, the Verdi canon was carved up into parts, and what were called "the early pieces" were basically *Rigoletto, Traviata,* and *Trovatore.* They were all much closer to middle than early, and an interesting thing emerged: one of these pieces was completely misplaced. *Traviata* is a social commentary piece featuring a soprano in the title role, and *Rigoletto* is the same kind, with a baritone. But *Trovatore* is not similar at all, though it has a tenor title role—*Stiffelio* is! And restoring it meant we got a great masterpiece in our hands.

OCTOBER 21

Leads his second Verdi premiere at the Met:
Stiffelio, with Plácido Domingo in the title role.

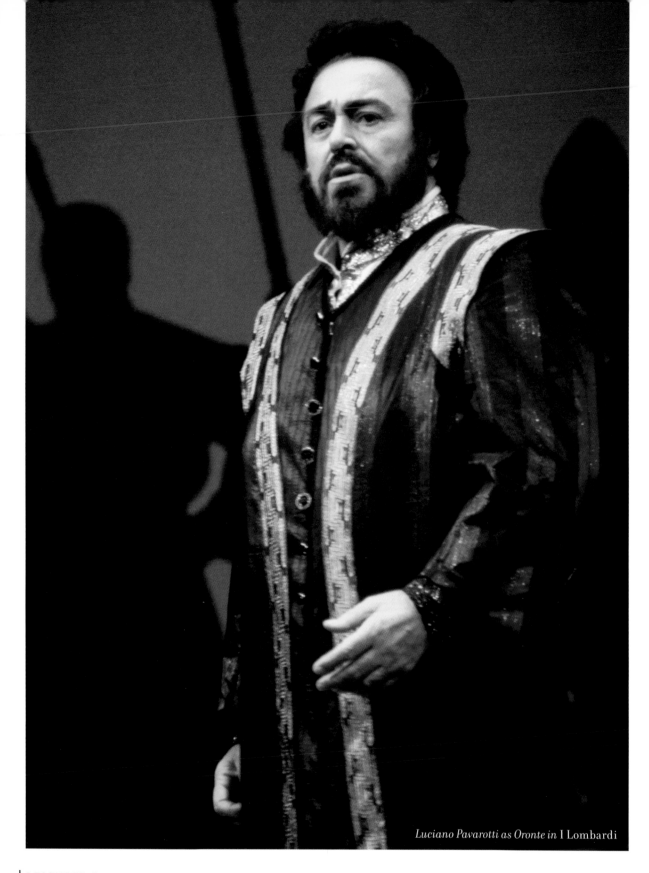

Luciano Pavarotti as Oronte in I Lombardi

Adds Verdi's *I Lombardi,* with Luciano
Pavarotti, to the Met repertoire.

JL: Ceci auditioned for me in Salzburg years before that, and I just wanted her to sing all day! I asked her what else she had, and she sang for an hour. Everything about it was absolutely sensational—the technique, the voice itself, the language, the style, the personality, the detail, you name it—it was just a mind-blowing time. The Met was never going to be her ideal venue because although her voice projects perfectly in the Met, and plenty of not-large voices have succeeded there, psychologically she was always going to be happier in smaller venues. She and I had a lot of fun in recitals and concerts. But she doesn't like to fly, so she came here less and less. It was a completely happy, wonderful thing, every time we got together. In fact, it's time we tried to do it again. She's fascinated by unusual repertoire, and since so many things about her are limitless, it's appropriate that she's not stuck with just what everybody else sings.

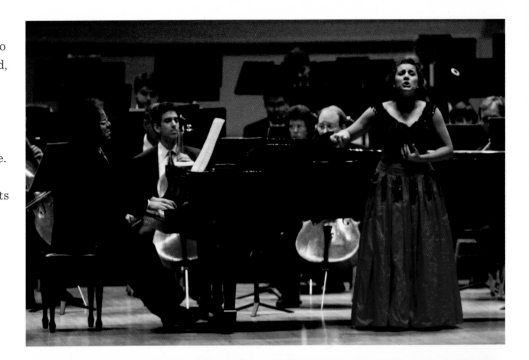

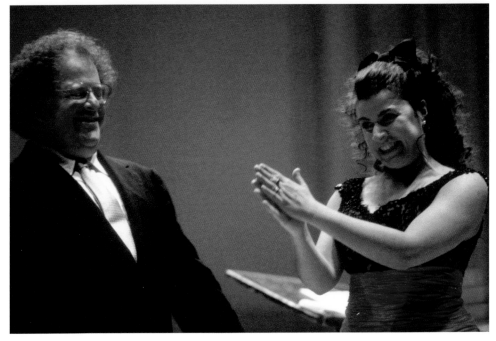

James Levine and Cecilia Bartoli at Carnegie Hall

1994

MAY 1

Conducts Cecilia Bartoli in her first appearance with the MET Orchestra at Carnegie Hall, prior to her Met stage debut.

MAY

Leads four concerts, including performances of *I Lombardi* and *Der Fliegende Holländer,* in Frankfurt on the Met's first visit to Germany.

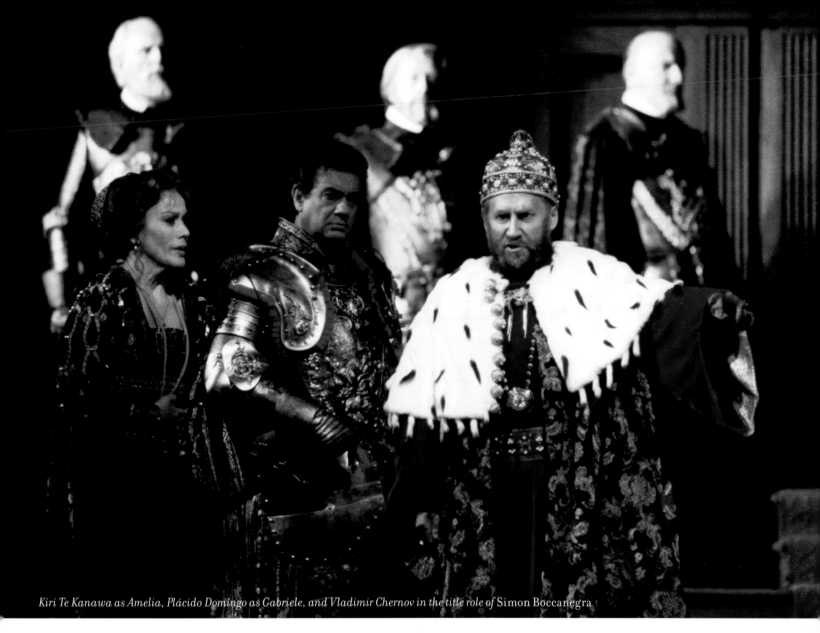

Kiri Te Kanawa as Amelia, Plácido Domingo as Gabriele, and Vladimir Chernov in the title role of Simon Boccanegra

JL: *Simon Boccanegra* has been particularly close to my heart for a very long time. It's a favorite of mine for every reason: the subject, the music, the tinta, and because of the particularly marvelous performance with Cornell MacNeil, Richard Tucker, Renata Tebaldi, and Ezio Flagello, in my first-ever performance in Cleveland in 1969. Verdi's original version was already a very good opera. But when Boito came up with the libretto for the Council Chamber scene, and Verdi made his revisions, it became an absolute masterpiece. I can never get enough of it.

1995
JANUARY 19

Conducts a new production of *Simon Boccanegra,* starring Vladimir Chernov, Kiri Te Kanawa, Plácido Domingo, and Robert Lloyd.

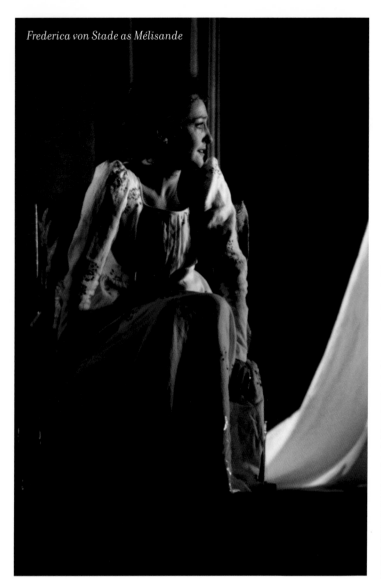
Frederica von Stade as Mélisande

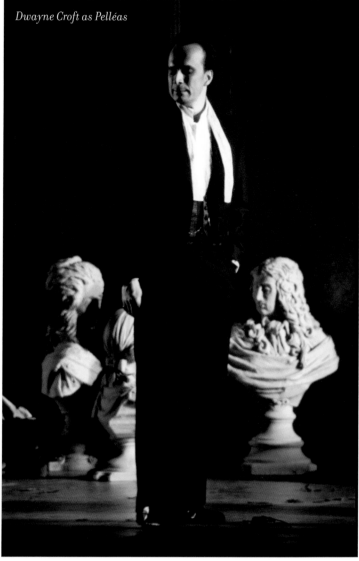
Dwayne Croft as Pelléas

JL: *Pelléas* has a special place in people's hearts when they get a chance to know it. And over the years, I've tried to revive it fairly regularly, so it would draw in a broader spectrum of people. We've had many wonderful casts, and this one was special because it represented a partnership of Flicka, the most experienced, successful Mélisande of our time, and Dwayne Croft, with his fabulous, beautiful voice, who worked on the part from the ground up to do it with us.

JANUARY–MAY

Conducts 13 MET Orchestra concerts at Carnegie Hall and on tour to Washington, D.C., Chicago, San Francisco, and other cities.

MARCH 23

Conducts a new production of *Pelléas et Mélisande,* directed by Jonathan Miller, that celebrates Frederica von Stade's 25th Met anniversary.

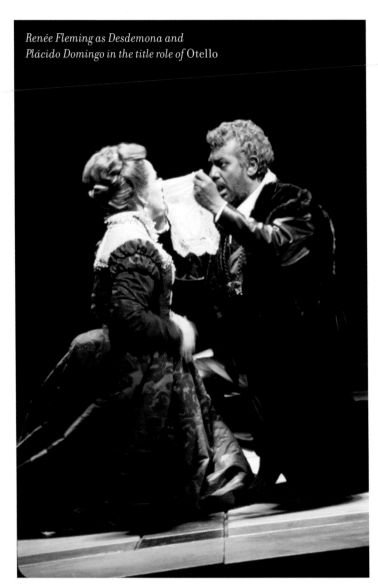

Renée Fleming as Desdemona and Plácido Domingo in the title role of Otello

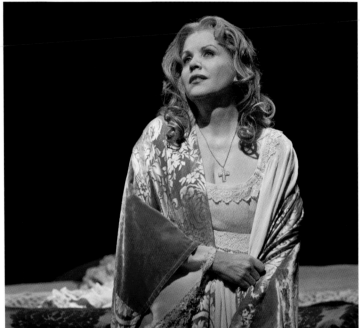

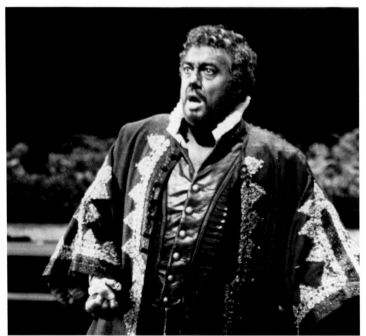

The Opening Night *Otello*, starring Renée
Fleming and Plácido Domingo, marks Levine's
1,500th opera performance at the Met.

Carol Vaness: You can always recognize James Levine's Mozart because all the singers are free and individual, but when they come together they're very secure in ensemble. I discovered this right away: I did five Mozart roles with him, beginning with Vitellia in *La Clemenza di Tito,* right after I arrived at the Met. He encouraged me to sing with my full voice all the time; he didn't make me try to be a floaty little Mozart singer. He insisted that the more human and vibrant the sound, the more the audience could understand the character's situation, and the more Mozart would have loved it. In *Figaro,* for instance, they could really get that the Countess was disappointed but still hopeful. Another thing about his Mozart is that even the slowest music has an insistence; the engine never stops. There are a lot of people who can go really, really slowly in Fiordiligi's aria "Per pietà," but Jimmy kept it moving, even the horn solo. Who else in the world is capable of taking care of the horn and the soprano at the same time? And there was never a time when he wasn't 100 percent with the recitative. You can't imagine how often, when you're singing so many secco [unorchestrated] recitatives, the conductor is waiting for the cue, as if he's saying, "Okay, I'll be right back as soon as the music starts." But Jimmy considered them all part of the music, which they are.

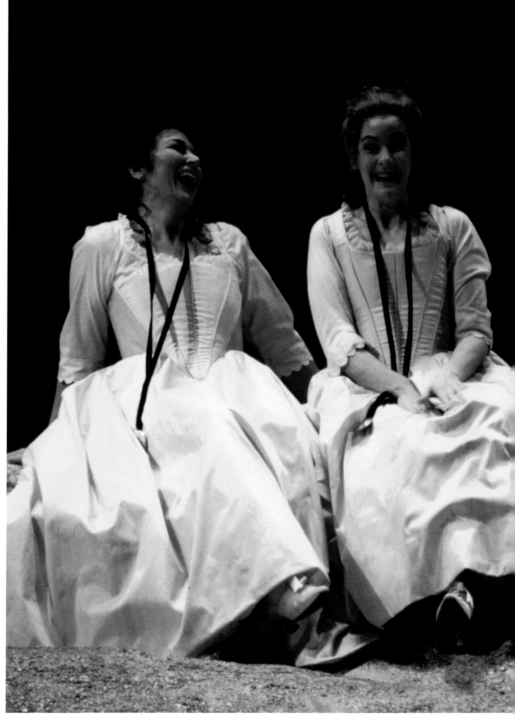

Carol Vaness as Fiordiligi and Susanne Mentzer as Dorabella in Così fan tutte

1996
FEBRUARY 8

Leads a new production of *Così fan tutte,* with Carol Vaness, Susanne Mentzer, Jerry Hadley, Dwayne Croft, Thomas Allen, and Cecilia Bartoli making her Met stage debut as Despina.

Levine with Carol Vaness, Dwayne Croft, Cecilia Bartoli, Thomas Allen, Susanne Mentzer, and Jerry Hadley

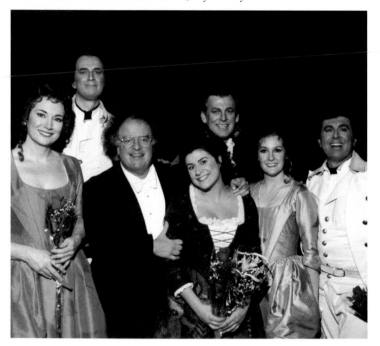

Dwayne Croft: One of the most important moments in my career is probably just a blip on Jimmy's radar screen. It was a music rehearsal for the new production of *Così fan tutte.* I was in awe of everyone in the cast, who had done their roles hundreds of times, it seemed. I was just out of the young artists' program, had never sung Guglielmo, and felt insecure. We got to the point in the story where I watch my love go off with my best friend. I didn't feel the moment, and I did it kind of caricature-like, "Oh, poor me, woe is me." Jimmy stopped. He was kind of stern with me, as if he were disappointed. He is extremely conscious of our egos and our need to feel good about ourselves, so it's very rare that he will come out and just say, "That was awful." My eyes welled up, and Jimmy said, "Do it again." Suddenly, I had the exact emotion that I needed. I sang it, feeling like I was going to cry, just as Guglielmo would be feeling. When it was over, Jimmy hugged me, and everybody said, "That was amazing, what happened just now." From then on, I sang that moment with frustration and anger and heartbreak, so it was real. That was an incredible lesson from him. When you're singing with Jimmy, there's no coasting. That's why I've had my best moments with him.

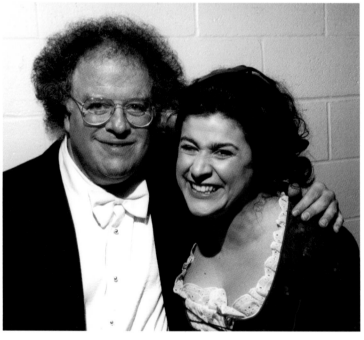

Levine and Cecilia Bartoli

FEBRUARY 10

Conducts a Saturday double-header of Verdi's two final masterpieces, *Otello* and *Falstaff,* one of 49 times he has led two performances at the Met in one day.

A scene from Giancarlo del Monaco's production of La Forza del Destino

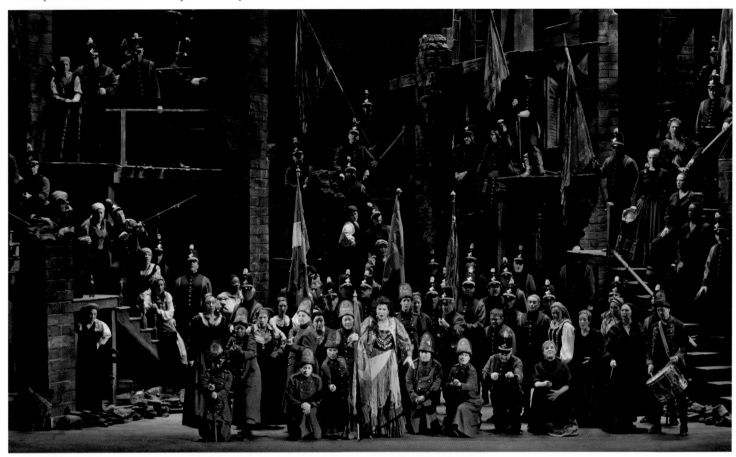

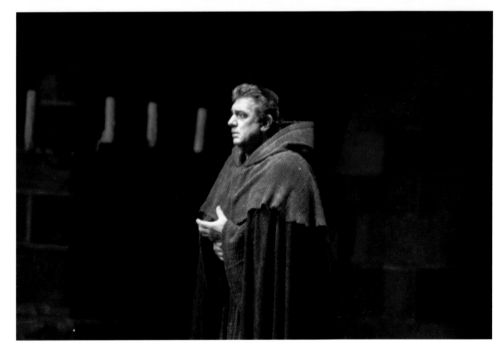

Plácido Domingo as Don Alvaro

FEBRUARY 29

**Conducts a new production of *La Forza
del Destino,* starring Sharon Sweet,
Plácido Domingo, Vladimir Chernov,
and Roberto Scandiuzzi.**

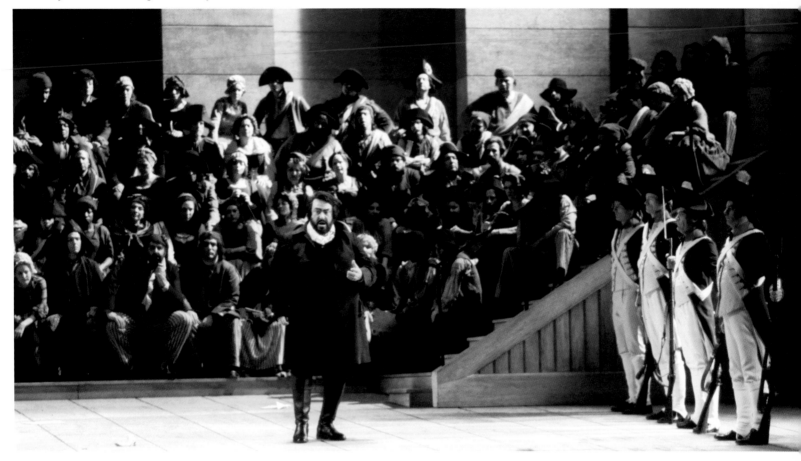

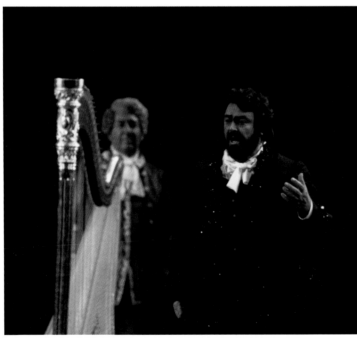

JL: Luciano was phenomenally generous, anxious to give and give and give. But as he got older, there were more nights when he felt unwell. That's when you really need the technique, and Luciano was an example of a famous singer who, among other things, had a superb technique. He was a great advertisement for knowing how to sing. He was unusually conscious of technical issues for a singer who was that generous a personality and who became that well-known.

Luciano Pavarotti in the title role of Andrea Chénier

APRIL 6

Conducts Luciano Pavarotti in a new production of Giordano's *Andrea Chénier*, opposite Aprile Millo and Juan Pons.

JL: That was one of the most amazing occasions I was ever involved in. So many artists came and sang, or wrote to me, and the atmosphere was unbelievable. As insane as 40 years sounds, 25 was already about the maximum anyone had ever done in a job like mine. The people who performed that night were an array of all types, generations, characteristics, styles, careers, people who flew in just to do something short, people who made more than one appearance... The difficulty is with all those little bits and pieces, how do you rehearse at moments when people can come? You need an orchestra and chorus and a company that have a lot of repertoire at their fingertips and are ready to make it work without having the extra luxury of cushiony time. And the real reason I wound up conducting that whole program myself was that we were unable to find a pragmatic way to carve up the rehearsal time that matched the availability of the singers into any kind of logical groupings.

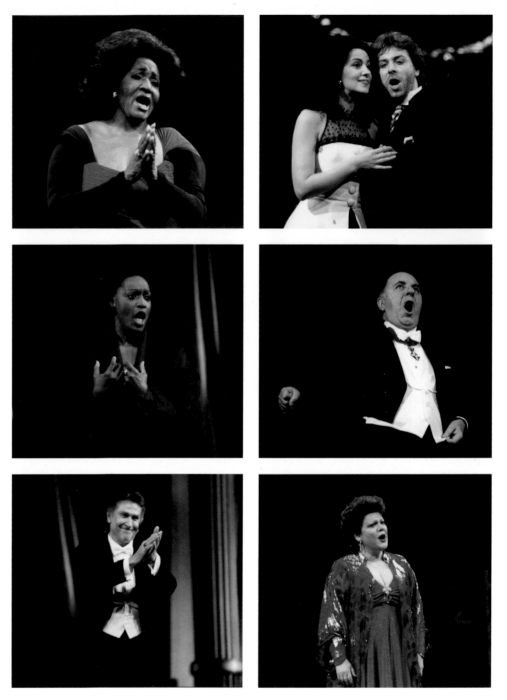

(clockwise from top left) Grace Bumbry, Angela Gheorghiu and Roberto Alagna, Carlo Bergonzi, Dolora Zajick, Sherrill Milnes, Jessye Norman

APRIL 27

Celebrates his 25th anniversary with the Met leading a gala performance of more than 50 Met stars in more than 35 different works.

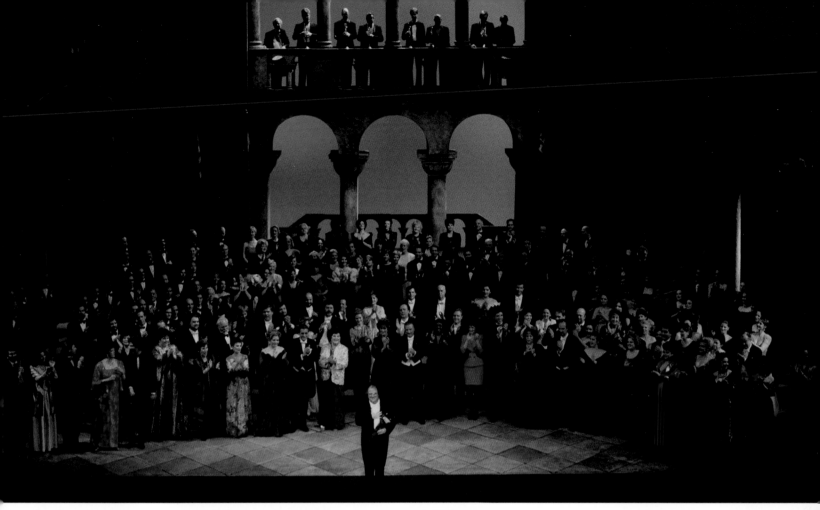

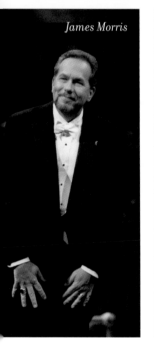

James Morris

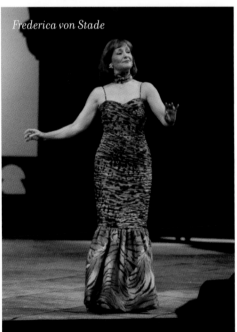

Frederica von Stade

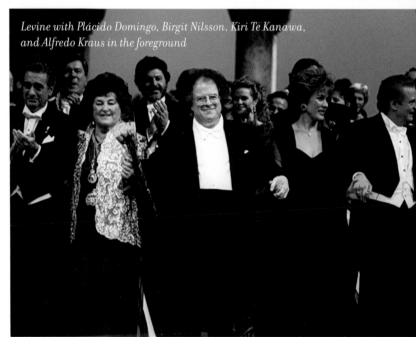

Levine with Plácido Domingo, Birgit Nilsson, Kiri Te Kanawa, and Alfredo Kraus in the foreground

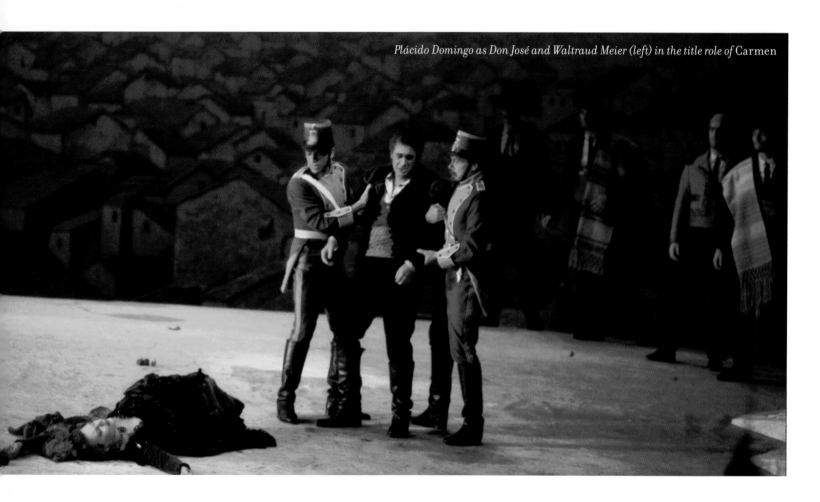

Plácido Domingo as Don José and Waltraud Meier (left) in the title role of Carmen

OCTOBER 31

FEBRUARY 10

Conducts Waltraud Meier, Angela Gheorghiu, Plácido Domingo, and Sergei Leiferkus in a new production of *Carmen* directed by Franco Zeffirelli.

Conducts a new production of *Wozzeck,* with Falk Struckmann in the title role.

JL: *Cenerentola* was a very happy experience because it's one of my favorite pieces, and the kind of piece I very rarely get the chance to do. I was so tickled, and we had a very good cast. It was altogether one of the most fun things we did.

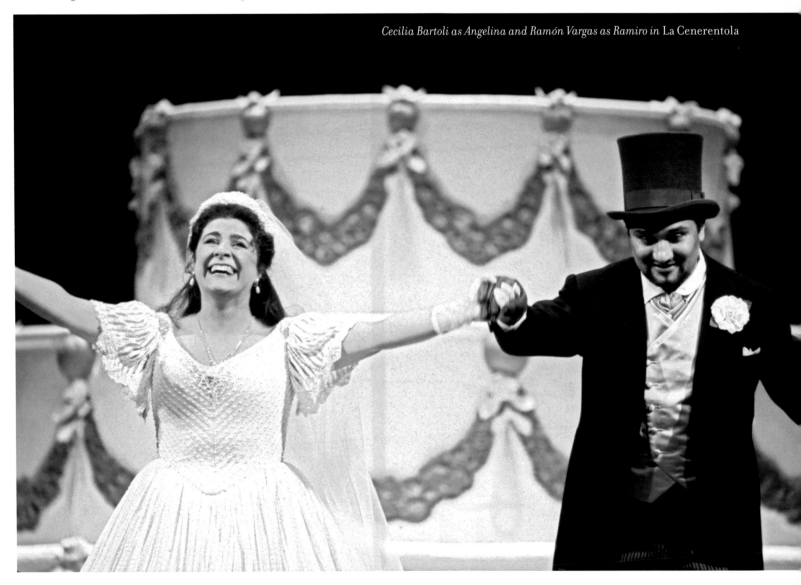

Cecilia Bartoli as Angelina and Ramón Vargas as Ramiro in La Cenerentola

OCTOBER 16

Conducts the Met premiere of Rossini's
La Cenerentola, starring Cecilia Bartoli
and Ramón Vargas.

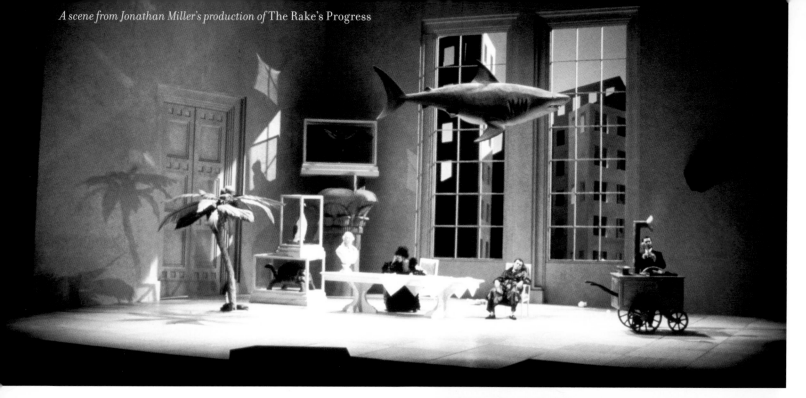

JL: It was important to me to do a new production of this opera in my time. There had been one shortly after the piece was written, which had excellent casting and excellent conducting, and the opera hadn't come back since those years. It plays better in smaller venues because they allow for brighter articulation. But it's a great and delightful opera, and its initial run at the Met had been quite successful, so it was always clear to me that it should have its chance again. Having certain kinds of singers who really wanted to sing it helped—we had a particularly stylish and committed group. Dawn, in particular, adores the role of Anne Trulove. Dawn is a completely unique communicator—what she understands about voice and technique and stagecraft and interpretation. As a student, she never really pictured herself as a major opera artist— she studied a lot of new music, recital repertoire, and oratorio repertoire. The first gigs I did with her were in that direction. But she responded to the things that I suggested she do operatically because even though I knew it wasn't where she was going to live, I felt the experience was going to really be important. And she was always so interested in everything. This performance as Anne was very moving, ideal, one of my favorites.

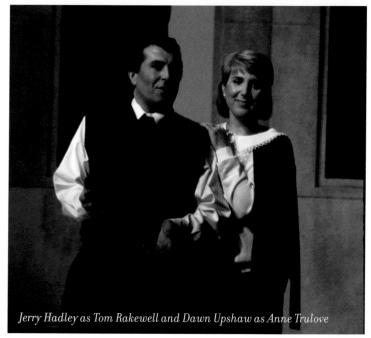

Jerry Hadley as Tom Rakewell and Dawn Upshaw as Anne Trulove

1998

NOVEMBER 20

MARCH 1

Stravinsky's *The Rake's Progress* enters his Met repertoire and marks the second new production that year of a 20th-century masterpiece.

Leads the inaugural concert of the MET Chamber Ensemble.

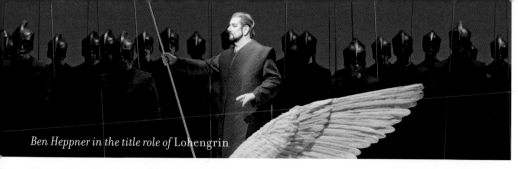

Ben Heppner in the title role of Lohengrin

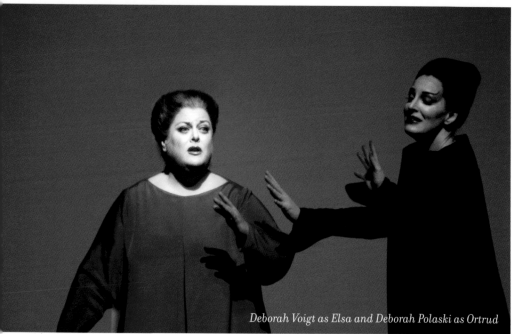

Deborah Voigt as Elsa and Deborah Polaski as Ortrud

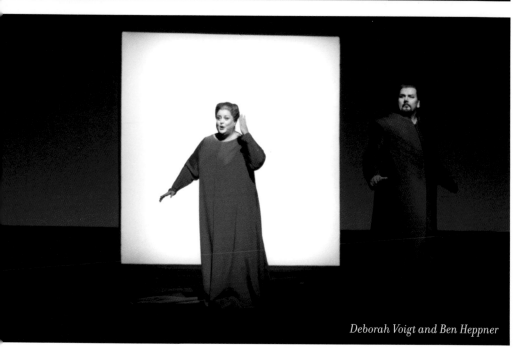

Deborah Voigt and Ben Heppner

JL: Ben's voice in this role was so classic, so romantic and beautiful, and so full of expression—an absolutely miraculous effect. And we had Debbie [Voigt], too, with a voice like a force of nature, just radiant. But with a new production, there's a tradition for our audience to have a kind of opening-night snap judgment. This one was booed. But the opening night of the first revival, it got nothing but yeas. I insisted on a few changes for that revival, allowing the singers to free their faces so they could release their voices, while holding the body positions and postures that Bob [Robert Wilson] wanted.

MARCH 9

Conducts the Met debut production of Robert Wilson, *Lohengrin*, starring Ben Heppner, Deborah Voigt, Deborah Polaski, Hans-Joachim Ketelsen, and Eric Halfvarson.

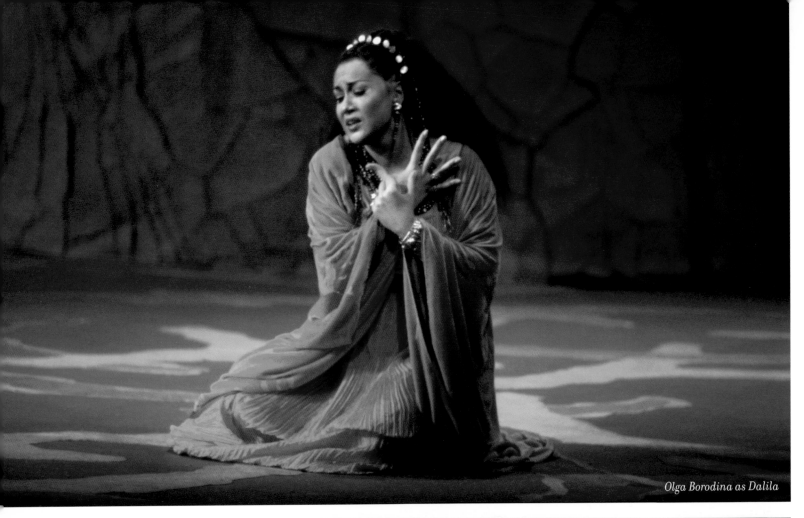

Olga Borodina as Dalila

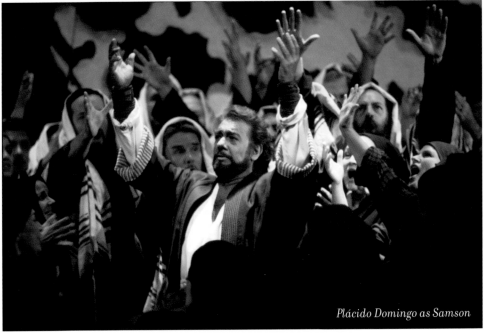

Plácido Domingo as Samson

SEPTEMBER 28

Conducts Saint-Saëns's *Samson et Dalila* on
Opening Night, celebrating Plácido Domingo's
30th anniversary with the company.

Renée Fleming: Years ago, I went through a period of really crippling stage fright, and it was at its worst right when I was the Countess in this new production of *Figaro*. Jimmy knew I was struggling, but he always gives you the sense of, "I'll get you through this. Don't worry." There's such a psychological element to what we do, and such risk. You need someone in the pit who's creating an environment where risk is okay. Jimmy did that for me in *Figaro*, especially with my aria "Dove sono." He said, "You can do it. Take more time. Take a long pause." He really encouraged me, even in the direst moment of stage fright, to push myself beyond my safety zone. The beauty of Jimmy is that because he's so natural and there's no anxiety, there's an understanding that you will perform at your best. He has guided me stylistically through the years—preferences about vibrato, wanting a fully colorful, engaged voice at all times. His ability to grasp the entirety of a piece, to grasp not only the whole but the details, is off the charts. Jimmy is really living and working on another plane.

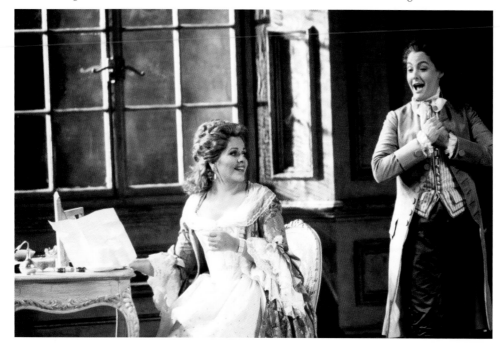

Renée Fleming as the Countess and Susanne Mentzer as Cherubino in Le Nozze di Figaro

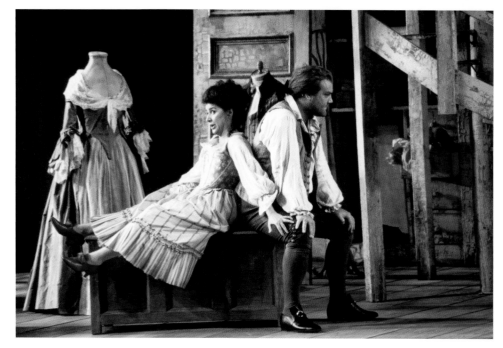

Cecilia Bartoli as Susanna and Bryn Terfel as Figaro

OCTOBER 29

Conducts a new production of *Le Nozze di Figaro,* directed by Jonathan Miller, with Bryn Terfel, Renée Fleming, Cecilia Bartoli, Susanne Mentzer, and Dwayne Croft.

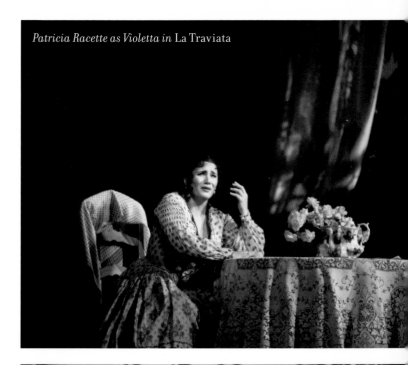

Patricia Racette as Violetta in La Traviata

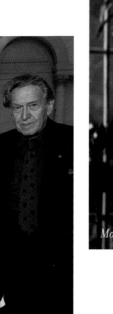

Levine with Charles Wuorinen, Elliott Carter, Milton Babbitt, and Leon Kirchner

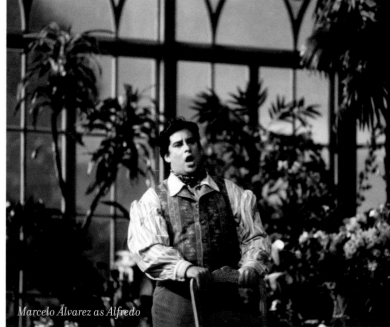

Marcelo Álvarez as Alfredo

NOVEMBER 15

Conducts the MET Orchestra in the world premiere of Milton Babbitt's Piano Concerto No. 2 at Carnegie Hall, one of numerous orchestra or chamber works commissioned by him, including pieces by Charles Wuorinen, Elliott Carter, and Leon Kirchner.

NOVEMBER 23

Conducts Franco Zeffirelli's new production of *La Traviata,* with Patricia Racette and Marcelo Álvarez in his Met debut.

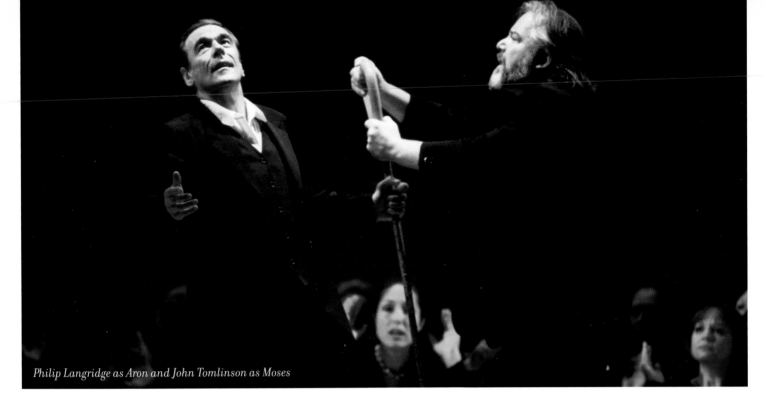

Philip Langridge as Aron and John Tomlinson as Moses

JL: I remember one time, Philip got on the Met stage and performed Loge [in *Das Rheingold*] with me without our having done a note of it together before—and we didn't get off track once. Loge and Aron are similar roles, both written for a kind of suave, sinuous, lyrical, persuasive, high tenor. Philip was the best, and he did all the *Moses und Aron*s I did. He was one of those people who used his whole artistic quality, so you could follow the line of instinct and thought right from the beginning. Tomlinson is another such artist, with a very different element and voice range, but a similar aesthetic.

Elliott Carter, composer: To do verbal justice to James Levine, once a child prodigy and now an adult prodigy, one of the most remarkable musicians I've ever encountered, is impossible. He is a musician who has thrown a shining light on every aspect of the musical world. The Metropolitan Opera Orchestra has become, under his 40-year leadership, one of our leading orchestras. The more than 2,000 performances of operas that he has brought to life is truly astonishing; he has grasped with great conviction each style and made each speak to us. For an outsider it is hard to imagine the planning that went into these: choosing which operas to present, finding the appropriate singers, stage designers and directors, sometimes far in advance; then having to deal with staging problems, like those of Arnold Schoenberg's *Moses und Aron,* which asks for 70 elders and 4 naked virgins and has all those on stage tearing off all their clothes! Jim prepared and performed this opera with such devotion that its ending—when Moses half sings, "Oh word, thou word that I lack"—is deeply moving and truly unforgettable. For myself, I lack the words to express the immense gratitude that I feel for his numerous commissions, for the vibrant understanding he brings to their interpretation, and for his deeply convincing performances of so many of my works.

1999
FEBRUARY 8

Brings Schoenberg's *Moses und Aron* to the Met for the first time, with John Tomlinson and Philip Langridge in the title roles.

Katarina Dalayman as Brangäne, Jane Eaglen as Isolde, René Pape as King Marke, and Ben Heppner as Tristan

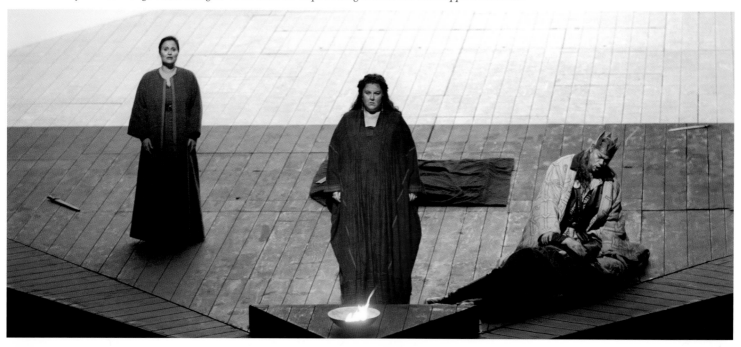

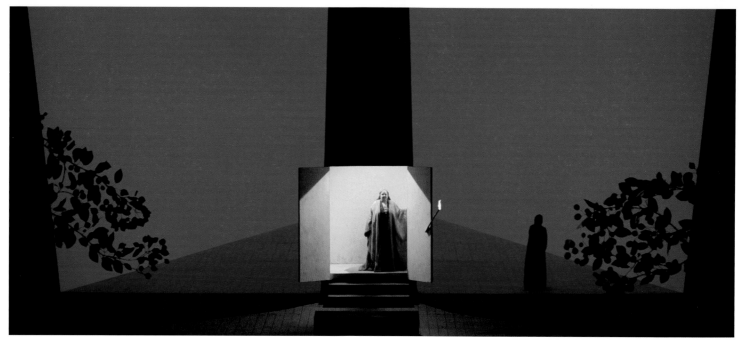

A scene from Dieter Dorn's production of Tristan und Isolde

NOVEMBER 22

Leads Dieter Dorn's new production of
Tristan und Isolde, starring Ben Heppner
and Jane Eaglen in the title roles, with
Katarina Dalayman as Brangäne and René
Pape as King Marke.

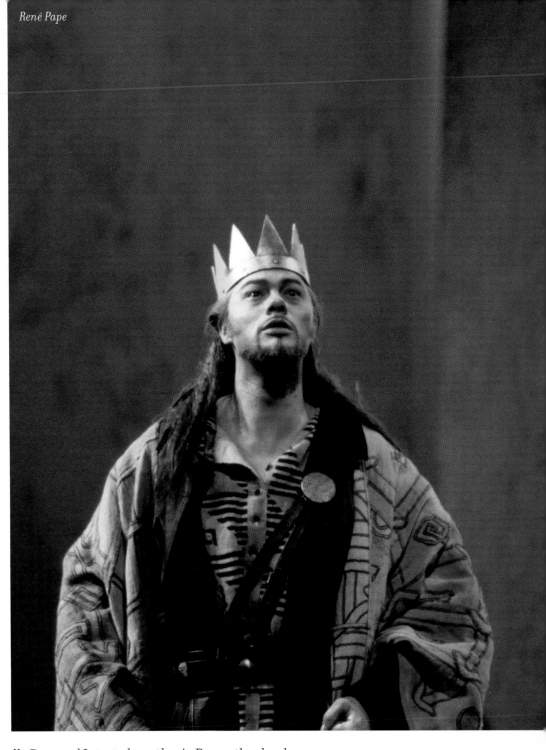

René Pape: I made my Met debut as the Speaker in *Die Zauberflöte,* and two days later I was the Night Watchman in *Die Meistersinger,* which Jimmy conducted. I was coming from East Germany, and the Metropolitan Opera was heaven for me. It still is. They flew me in just to sing small roles when they could easily have asked singers from around the corner. Later, I realized what a big favor it was from Jimmy. He gave me the opportunity to have a career in the States, not just in Europe, starting with small, but fine roles.

From the very beginning, Jimmy and I were very close in our musical visions. We always know what the other is doing and thinking. In *Tristan,* especially, I felt something magical. I had sung King Marke a couple of times in Europe, but Jimmy had been conducting it a lot longer than I had been singing it. I was very young, but nowhere is it written how old the king was. Adding my little experiences to the genius of Jimmy, everything came together and we created a Marke who was very human. For me, it was also a breakthrough, getting better known by the New York audience.

Jimmy does something that no other conductor does. When he's in the pit, and you're onstage and he likes things, he gives you a thumbs-up. He is so typically American! You get happy on stage, because Maestro is happy. He won't laugh during something like *Tristan* or *Macbeth,* but if he likes musical phrases, or something is well done, he smiles—it doesn't matter how hard the piece is, or how dramatic it is.

JL: Pape and I started together in Bayreuth, when he was Fasolt in the *Ring.* It was a remarkable voice and element to come along, and I think he's gone from strength to strength. But the King Marke was especially good.

JL: In addition to the gala, the Met asked me how I wanted to celebrate my 25th anniversary. I said, "What I'd really like is for the company to commission a new opera." They agreed immediately, and I knew I wanted it to be from John Harbison. John is a wonderful composer, and he doesn't write in a limited systemic container; he writes using whatever harmony and whatever instrumentation and structure he needs for the work. Plus, he has a very thorough knowledge of vocal music and opera. John suggested *Gatsby*, if we could get the rights. I thought it was a good idea, and it bore out very well: it was manageable in terms of time and characterization, and it transferred successfully from one medium to another. John wrote one of the greatest scores I have seen in recent years, and we had a wonderful cast. There could hardly be three more convincing female leads than we had. Dawn brought such tremendous truth of detail to her characterization of Daisy. Lorraine [Hunt Lieberson]—that's a phenomenon. And Susan [Graham] is a genuine, authentic artist that digs deep in a lot of styles.

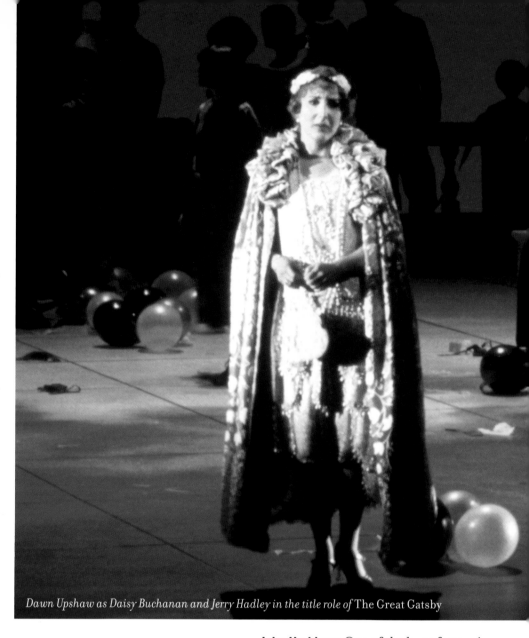

Dawn Upshaw as Daisy Buchanan and Jerry Hadley in the title role of The Great Gatsby

John Harbison: One of the huge factors in my writing *The Great Gatsby* was knowing that Jim was going to conduct. It's a very challenging opera, particularly in terms of pacing and in the general sculpting of the scenes. I banked on him and on the quality of the orchestra—their savvy about how to pick up balance, what sort of color the scene is really about, the character of the scene. What I particularly noticed in rehearsals is that for Jim, opera exists fundamentally at the musical level.

You do have to be willing to adjust.

DECEMBER 20

Conducts the world premiere of John Harbison's *The Great Gatsby*, **commissioned by the Met to commemorate his 25th anniversary, starring Jerry Hadley and Dawn Upshaw.**

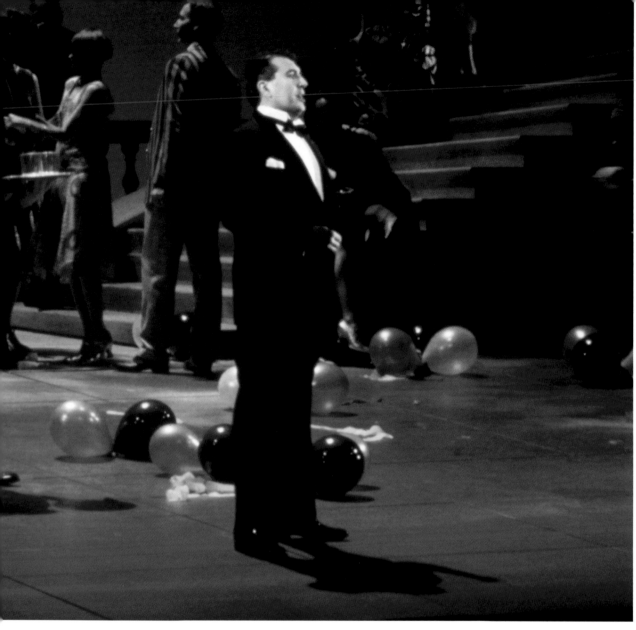

With *Gatsby,* I knew that if places bothered my stomach the first time I heard it all the way through, something should happen. Usually I make little excisions. But Jim was very protective of those musical structures and constantly advised me to be critical of the urge to cut. He was definitely an advocate for the piece, and his injunction to me was not to jump fast, and go with whatever the inner signals are. That's great advice.

People still come up to me on the bus with criticisms of *Great Gatsby,*
ten years after they saw it. Opera is a medium where people remember that well and all think they have a contribution to make. That's probably the great virtue of the opera audience—there's a different level of engagement, and I think that's something that Jim has always been aware of, too.

I think we need conductors to do the things that they believe in. There's no point in them doing something out of duty, but if they really care about something that's happening in the
present, then their conviction is more valuable to it than anything else could be. There are very few conductors who are as avid for new music as Jim is, and he has another rare quality, which is that he will stick with a new piece; he'll come back to it just as he does with the old pieces. He never seems to regard any performance as his final station—it's always part of a process.

At the Piano

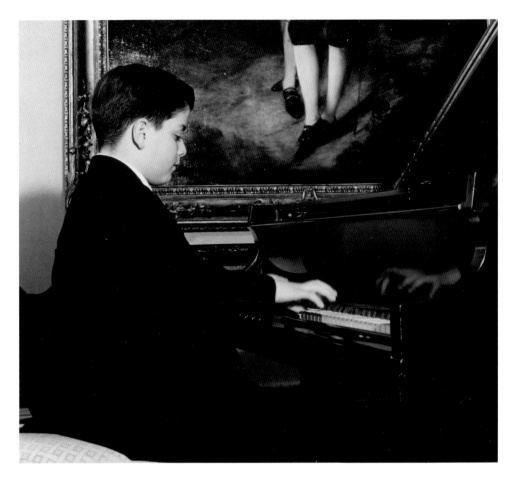

JL: When I was four, I had a speech impediment, and the doctor asked my parents what I was interested in. My mother said, "Well, when he passes the piano he reaches up and bangs on it and makes us crazy." So he suggested piano lessons, and I became a marathon talker. I made my debut playing with the Cincinnati Symphony when I was 10, but I knew deep down that I didn't want to run around the world playing on strange pianos by myself. I loved ensemble music, where people made music with each other. And being very drawn to the dramatic and lyric element in singing, I found myself gravitating toward vocal music as a kind of center. And I have never regretted it for a moment.

When I started conducting, I realized that the singers wouldn't have enough time to get oriented to my gesture if I played my own rehearsals. Also, when playing an opera score, it's tempting to try to make the piano sound like an orchestra, but that's a waste of concentration because you need to listen to the singer, not to your own symphonic piano playing. So, I got someone else to play. The people who play for me are driven nuts, I'm sure, by the way I'm always asking them to give less, so that the singer doesn't hear an impetus from the piano, which they will never hear from the pit.

Working on a piece that was written for piano—chamber music or songs or whatever—is a completely different process, though, and I have always had enough work to be able to stay in shape. The touch, from one pianist to another, is something that's incredibly personal, which people don't often realize because they look at the piano as a sort of machine. I try to bring to bear the same things on the piano that I exhort from the orchestra and singers when there is no piano.

Daniel Barenboim: If I have one wish to express on the occasion of Jimmy's 40th anniversary at the Met, it is that he take the time to practice and play a piano recital. We have talked about this very often. He even told me what pieces he would play in such a recital: the Schubert B-flat Sonata and the Schumann *Carnaval*. I think it would be wonderful if he would find more time for the piano.

Kurt Moll: Jimmy plays the piano incredibly well, especially German lieder, which he loves. He would often ask me to work on *Winterreise* with him, and it was wonderful because every one of the 24 songs is a little opera. We were just two people doing these little operas, and it was fantastic.

William Bolcom: Jim has always wanted me to give him lessons on how to play [my piano rag] *The Graceful Ghost*. He plays it very well, but he wants a particular swing or something. I was really struck when he played it at a special concert at Carnegie Hall the week after 9/11.

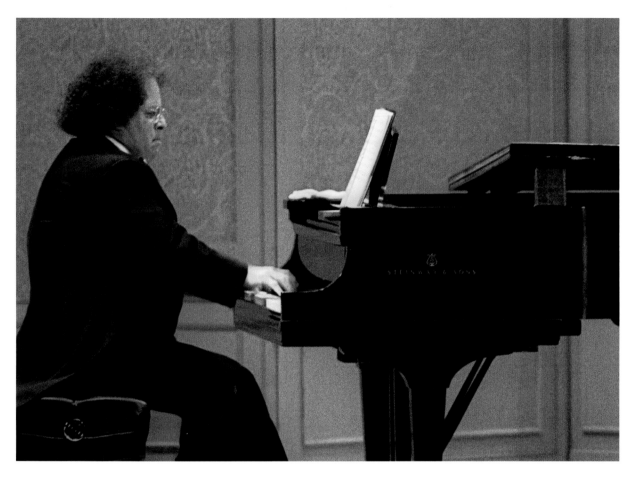

Marilyn Horne: His piano playing for singers is really special. His touch and the quality of what comes out of the 88 keys is astounding. He's one of those rare birds who knows how to lead and follow at the same time. I think that's the secret of accompanying.

Christa Ludwig: Of all the things I sang with Jimmy, the most impressive for me were the recitals because it was just the two of us. When we did Schubert's *Winterreise* at the Met, it didn't matter that it was a huge space. I sang it for myself, I sang it for Jimmy and the piano and the music.

Sherrill Milnes: I remember going to a memorial service when Jimmy and Frederica von Stade did the Schubert "Ave Maria," something we all know well. As I listened to them, I felt as though I'd never heard it before. It was a whole new level of musical existence that just elevated my soul. Jim plays two instruments—the orchestra and the piano—as well as anybody ever has.

Evgeny Kissin: From the very first time we worked together, it was clear to me that we understand and feel music in the same way. We have worked together on lots of repertoire, concertos and even some four-hand chamber music by Schubert. We always find the common language straight

away. He is equally great in music of different styles and times, both as a conductor and as a chamber music pianist. There are great conductors who are not such wonderful accompanists, and there are some truly remarkable accompanists who are not such great interpreters. Levine is one of those rare conductors who combine both qualities. It is always a wonderful experience for me when he is on the podium. Knowing what a fine pianist he is gives me the best possible background, the best opportunity to do anything that I want to do, and it inspires me to do my best. Having spent a good deal of time with him, I know that this man really lives in music. He doesn't trumpet about it, but this is really the way he lives.

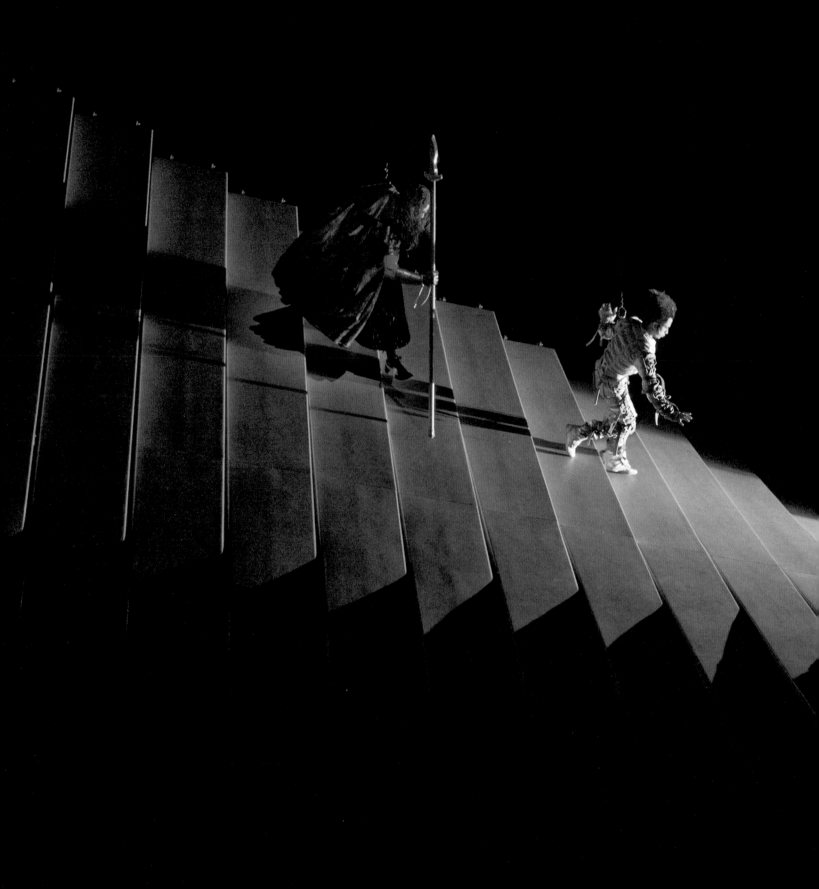

The descent into Nibelheim in Robert Lepage's production of Wagner's Das Rheingold

2000–2010

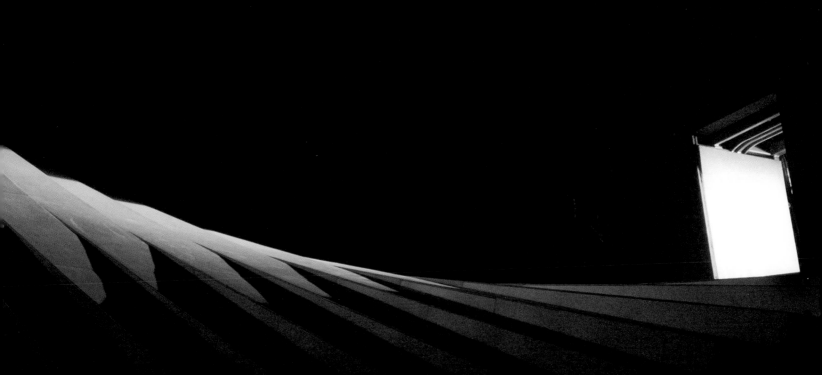

The Rewards of the Long View

ARA GUZELIMIAN

There's a lovely story about the composer Carl Ruggles, one of the more craggy and highly individual characters even among American maverick artists. One of his fellow innovators, the composer Henry Cowell, came calling on Ruggles at his Vermont farm, only to find him holed up in his studio, noisily at work at the piano. Cowell, not wanting to interrupt, waited patiently outside. It became immediately apparent that Ruggles was playing the same harshly dissonant chord over and over again. After a seemingly eternal wait, Cowell couldn't bear it any more and burst in, asking Ruggles just what the hell he was doing. "Giving it the test of time," replied the famously laconic Ruggles.

James Levine's extraordinary 40-year tenure at the Metropolitan Opera is a remarkable triumph of "the test of time." In a world of immediate gratification and instant value judgments, the conductor's infinitely patient long view of the process of music-making is testimony to far more profound artistic values. Exploring a great opera is a lifetime's work, full of boundless possibilities, deepening over time.

At the mention of even just a few of the many iconic Levine/Met operas—say *Parsifal, Wozzeck, Don Carlo, Pelléas et Mélisande,* or *Elektra,* for starters—one's memory begins to overflow with the riches of how performances of these works have evolved, grown, shed new light, and come to life anew with each revival or new production. For Levine, each performance is an opportunity to look deeper, to examine anew, to get one more detail in clearer light. A backstage visitor after a Levine performance generally finds him in good spirits, energized by the performance but almost immediately focusing on a detail, a balance, a transition that he would like to get better at the next performance. This isn't some sort of neurotic self-criticism—there is always a sense of aspiration, an excitement about what more remains to be done, a movingly optimistic sense of the continued work to "get it right."

Levine's generously long view has had especially memorable results in creating a house tradition or style in repertoire where none had existed before. A major but not much heralded part of Levine's broad view has been to build a deep understanding of a composer's vocabulary over time. The first Levine/Met

performances of Berg's *Lulu* or *Wozzeck* in the 1970s were already notable achievements. But then starting in the 1990s came a carefully planned series of concerts by the MET Orchestra and the MET Chamber Ensemble of so many of Berg's orchestral and chamber works at Carnegie Hall—the Three Pieces for Orchestra, the *Seven Early Songs,* the Chamber Concerto, the Four Pieces for Clarinet and Piano, etc. The musical style began to be built into the artistic DNA of the casts and orchestral musicians over time, and the result has been an unmatched depth of understanding in Berg's operas. The two operas have returned to the repertoire with welcome regularity, bringing a succession of memorable casts. There is no opera house or orchestra in the world which plays this breadth of Berg's music with such profound understanding. A similarly comprehensive view of Berlioz over many seasons culminated in unforgettable performances of *Les Troyens* and *Benvenuto Cellini* in 2003, the bicentennial of the composer's birth. That's the rich reward of the Levine long view.

My own first encounter with the conductor at the Met came in a searing performance of Verdi's *Otello* with a cast led by Jon Vickers in December 1972. I have heard him conduct the opera five or six times in the years since, each time hearing something new—an unexpected sonority, a line given just an infinitesimally greater weight or more time, a long arc building deliberately to an overpowering climax.

In a recent conversation, the conductor gave a telling glimpse of his working process. He acknowledged that when he returns to an opera after an absence of some time, he begins his study with a fresh, unmarked score. He is happiest when he is studying the score—any conversation with him circles back to his sense of wonder at the riches to be found in the score.

Although he readily recalls great casts and colleagues from his many years at the Met, there is no time spent on nostalgia—he talks happily about what could be done better the next time. For James Levine, the long view leads to tomorrow's performance.

Ara Guzelimian is Provost and Dean of The Juilliard School. He was Senior Director and Artistic Advisor of Carnegie Hall from 1998 to 2006.

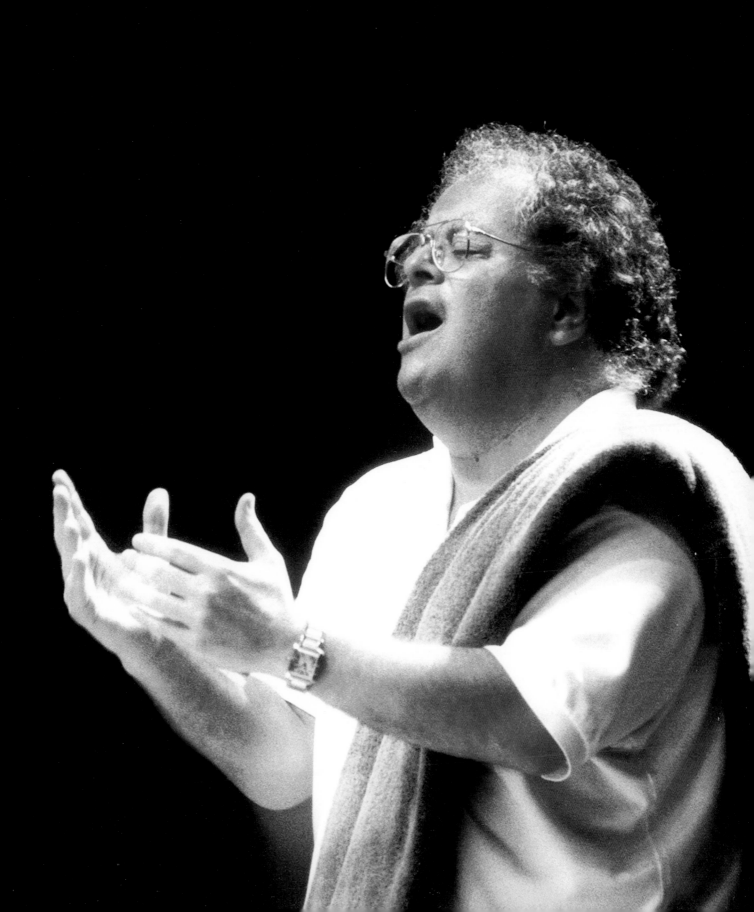

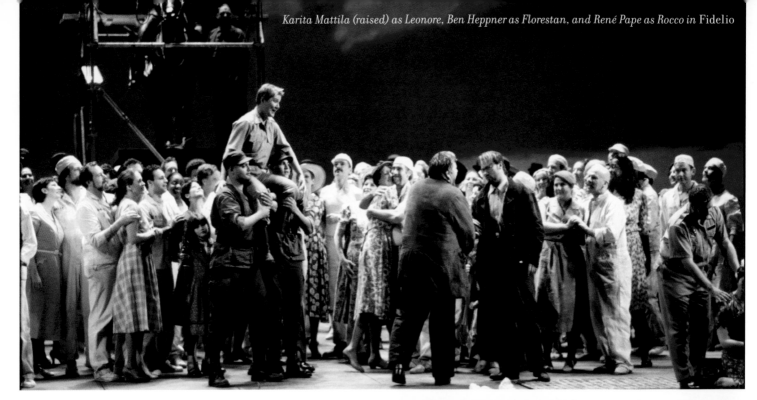

Karita Mattila (raised) as Leonore, Ben Heppner as Florestan, and René Pape as Rocco in Fidelio

JL: This was an effective, lively approach to *Fidelio*. I had a little bit of nostalgia when we replaced the old one, because it had been one of Schenk's first, with remarkable scenery by Boris Aronson. But this new production and cast were very, very good. Karita is a remarkable artist who really immerses herself in her roles. I had waited to do *Fidelio* at the Met until I had a situation where there was enough time and I could make it work with the artists. It was not an opera I was ready to approach in a random revival, because the details don't come out as well, and nothing is worse in *Fidelio* than not having everyone focused on the details together.

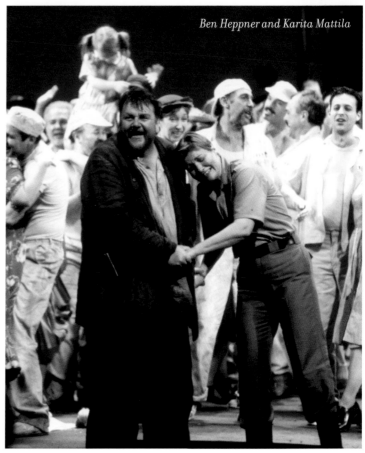

Ben Heppner and Karita Mattila

2000
OCTOBER 13

Adds Beethoven's *Fidelio* to his Met repertoire, in a new production directed by Jürgen Flimm, starring Karita Mattila and Ben Heppner, Falk Struckmann, and René Pape.

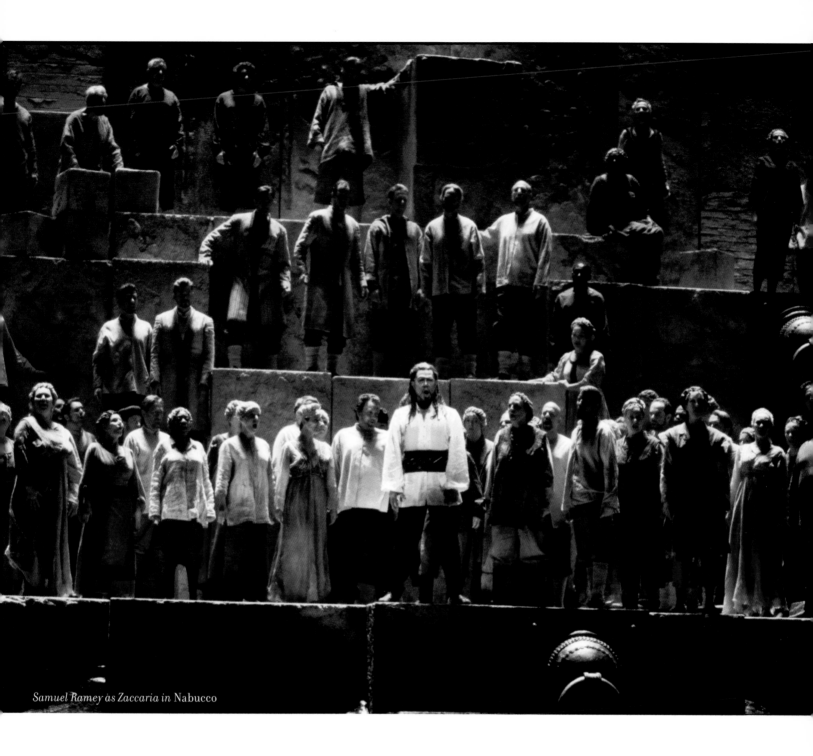

Samuel Ramey as Zaccaria in Nabucco

2001

MARCH 8

Adds Verdi's *Nabucco* to his Met repertoire,
the opera's second Met production, with Juan
Pons, Maria Guleghina, and Samuel Ramey in
the leading roles.

MAY 6

Performs Schoenberg's *Gurrelieder*
with the MET Orchestra at Carnegie Hall,
a first for the company.

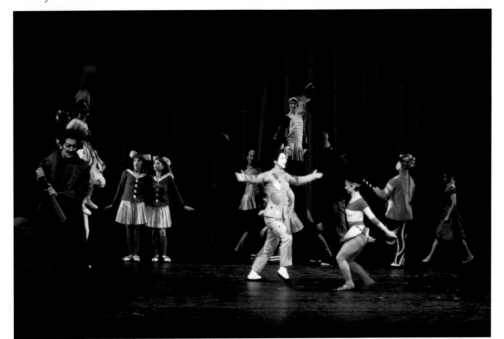

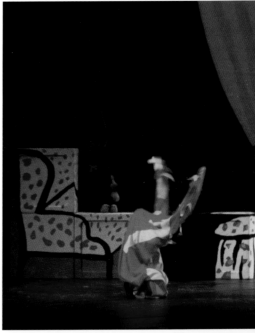

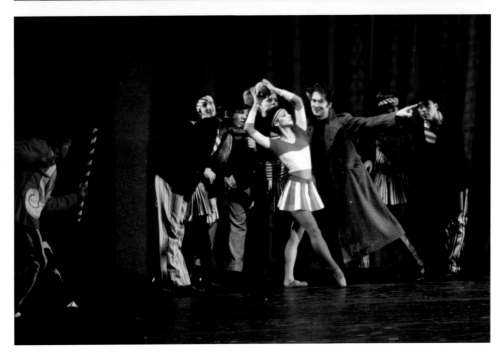

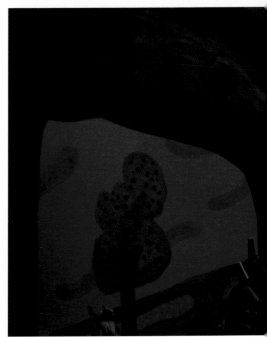

2002

OCTOBER 26

Brings *Luisa Miller* back to the repertoire
in a new production by Elijah Moshinsky,
with Marina Mescheriakova, Neil Shicoff,
and Nikolai Putilin.

MARCH 4

Adds the *Parade* triple bill—Satie's *Parade*,
Poulenc's *Les Mamelles de Tirésias*,
and Ravel's *L'Enfant et les Sortilèges*—
to his Met repertoire.

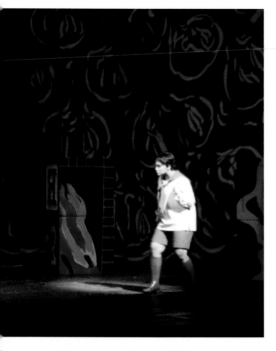

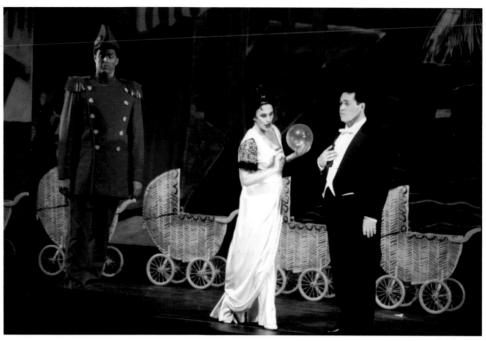

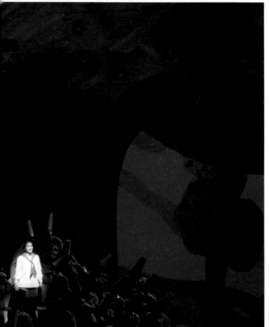

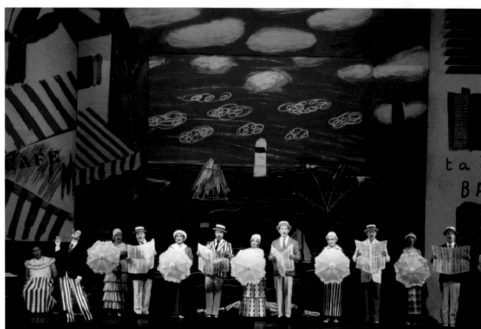

JL: These three pieces work together brilliantly. The reason I didn't conduct the production when it was new, in 1981, was we had an ideal conductor in Manuel Rosenthal, who had an authentic knowledge of this repertoire, having been a Ravel protégé, among other things. But I always wanted to do it at some point, because I believe *L'Enfant et les Sortilèges* is one of the great masterpieces, and the other two are marvelous, too. I think Hockney's design resulted in one of the most beautiful productions we ever had on the stage. The moment when it went from the child's room to the garden in *L'Enfant* was breathtaking in a way that very few things are and remains a really palpable, memorable effect.

Jay David Saks, Music Producer: "Wait until we get to Berlioz!"

This was a comment James Levine made to me in the late 1970s. I was one of his recording producers during those years before I came to the Met. He had been recording Mahler symphonies, and at a point mid-session during a playback in the control room, I mentioned to him how deeply affecting these Mahlers were to me in his hands... whereupon he looked up and made that statement about Berlioz, as if there was utter certainty in his mind that there would soon be major Berlioz recordings from him.

What I could not have anticipated back then was that it would happen, at least regarding my own involvement, not in the recording studio, but rather live in performance at the Met, first with *Les Troyens* in the 1980s and again in a new production in 2003, then the following season *Benvenuto Cellini,* and most recently *La Damnation de Faust.* The experience of broadcasting and recording live staged performances of masterworks such as these was by then far more electric and exciting to me than the artistically odd process of working in the dissection room of the formal recording studio, where every moment requires both artist and producer to evaluate, weigh, and decide—all while watching the clock of expense—whether the whole and parts are of sufficient standard for permanent documents. In live performance, the artists start, and sometimes it's great, and no one is thinking "hmm, let's stop and do that again" (well, maybe just for a moment here and there). The entirety, the whole, IS the goal.

This is why I treasure each time we put out microphones for James Levine's Met performances. At the Met, I have a video monitor in front of me that's trained on the conductor, for logistical purposes, and when Levine conducts I have a habit of watching it more closely than at other performances. It's wonderful to see the connection he brings to the music with his gestures, expressions, and contact with the musicians and stage performers... but occasionally, there's more required. At one particular rehearsal I observed that he was not satisfied with the playing in a particularly complex passage, even after repeating it... whereupon he stopped and simply said to the orchestra, "Watch me, please," then proceeded to conduct the passage again, but this time leading them with an astonishing show of multifaceted gestures that indicated every single subtle point of shape, nuance, tempo, and articulation, well beyond the normal sweep of his more typical larger-picture conducting. This time, every point he sought was reproduced brilliantly by the orchestra. He stopped again, praised them for their latest effort, then went back and played that same passage and continued on, but this time with his original unfussy gestures, and the results were again perfect. Problem solved, lesson taught. It illuminated to me that while he abhors the kind of over-conducting that one occasionally sees in others, that sometimes diminishes the whole of a performance by flailing, he was nonetheless technically equipped beyond reproach to give a lesson employing a conducting style of super detail when it served a true purpose. It's the house, not the nails, of course, that makes for great architecture, and no one knows it better than Levine, but this time he needed to hammer a few nails into place, and the result was that the house was the better for his having done it.

In my years at the Met and making many recordings with him, I've been ever reminded that this gentle genius enriches us not only by his extraordinary musicianship but also in the way he delights in bringing his experience to all of us.

2003

FEBRUARY 10

Premieres a new production of *Les Troyens,*
with Deborah Voigt, Lorraine Hunt Lieberson,
and Ben Heppner in the leading roles.

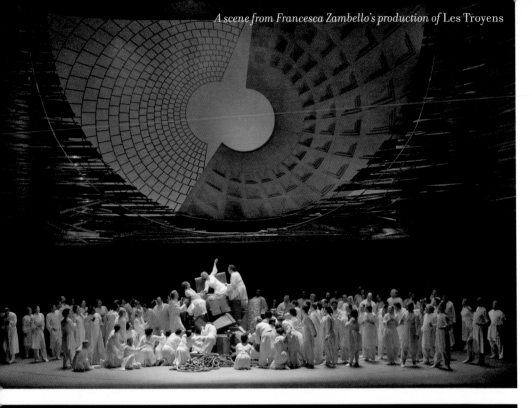

A scene from Francesca Zambello's production of Les Troyens

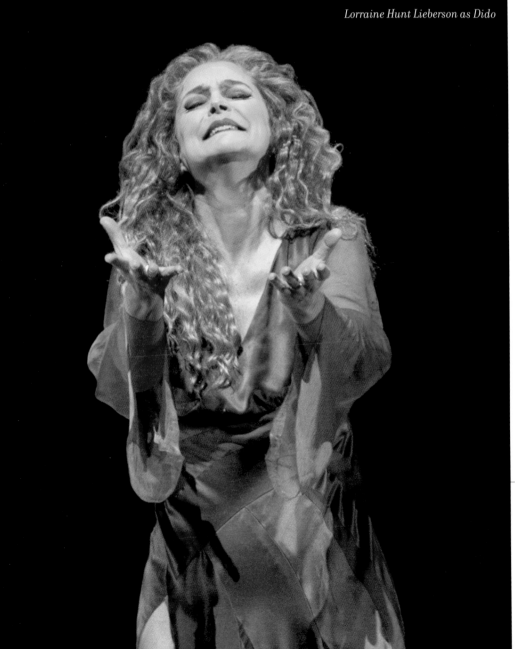

Lorraine Hunt Lieberson as Dido

JL: Lorraine was one of a kind—the instrument itself and its expressive range, her quality of expression, detail, discipline, freedom... When she would bring me a piece we were going to do, a symphonic piece or whatever, she had worked through all the possibilities, in order to have them in her arsenal ahead of time and be ready for whatever I was going to ask her for. When artists get the kind of results she got, people always believe it's instinct, but the ones who have the instinct have the instinct to work hard. That's Lorraine. If I had asked her to do another version of almost anything she ever brought me, she could've done it like that. Fortunately, her own imagination was so strong that I could just encourage her to do the things she wanted to do, and that gave them her own personal conviction.

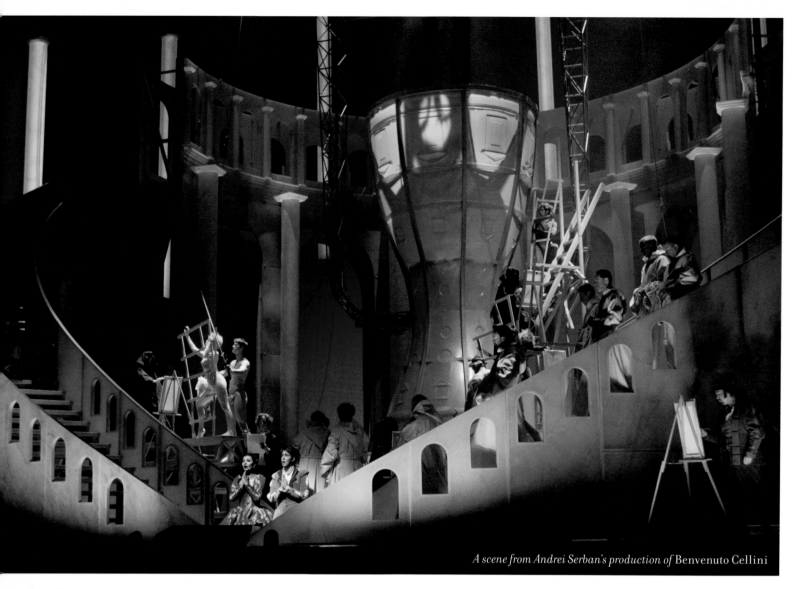

A scene from Andrei Serban's production of Benvenuto Cellini

JL: Berlioz is one of my favorite composers, brilliant and innovative—and the things that are striking about his work differ from piece to piece. I've always loved *Cellini,* an unusually energetic and exciting opera, but it's extremely hard to do. There are a couple of very difficult roles, a large cast of important characters, intricate ensemble writing, a great deal of action... and you want to bring the right tone to it. Our company thrived on the challenges of it, and it was a lot of fun for the audience.

DECEMBER 4

Adds Berlioz's *Benvenuto Cellini* to the
Met repertoire, starring Marcello Giordani
in the title role, with Isabel Bayrakdarian
and John Del Carlo.

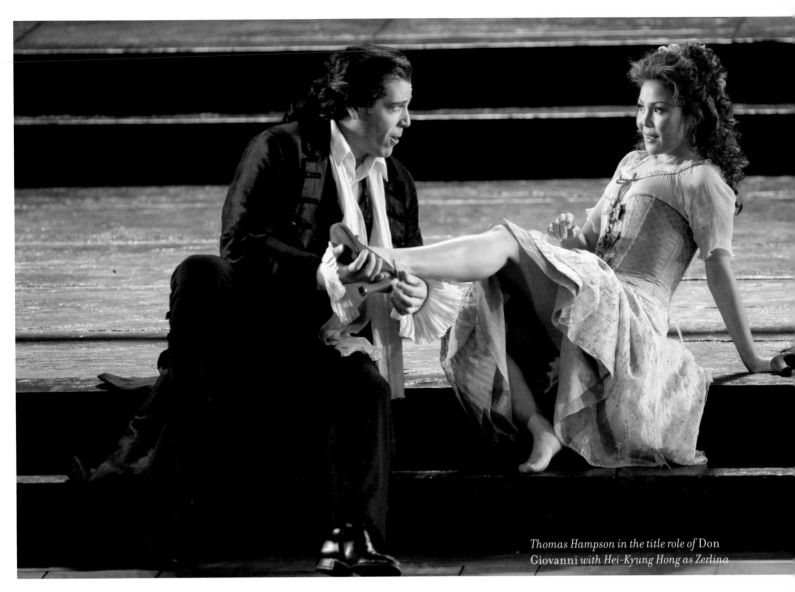

Thomas Hampson in the title role of Don Giovanni *with Hei-Kyung Hong as Zerlina*

JL: I remember when Tom first sang for me, in Salzburg. He sang a couple of standard arias, and it was wonderful. The first operas I did with him were auspicious because he was one of the later-generation singers who worked with Jean-Pierre [Ponnelle], as Don Giovanni and as the Count. He's extremely responsive, both musically and dramatically, and very versatile.

2004
MARCH 1

Conducts a new *Don Giovanni* with Thomas Hampson in the title role, Anja Harteros, Christine Goerke, Hei-Kyung Hong, Gregory Turay, René Pape, and Ildar Abdrazakov in his Met debut.

Joseph Volpe, former General Manager: It was June 5, 1971, and we were doing *Tosca.* I was the Met's master carpenter at the time, and I said to myself, "Who's the curly-headed kid on the podium? Is he adjusting the light? Is he an electrician?" It wasn't until he started waving his arms around that I realized that he was the conductor. It was James Levine, who was making his debut.

We didn't have much contact over the next few years, until he became Music Director and I was Technical Director. After I became General Manager, that prior relationship was an enormous help, especially when there were difficult decisions to make. We never really had disagreements. If a question arose, I would give my opinion and Jim would give his. His, of course, was more eloquent, longer by far, and more well-informed. If he convinced me, we would agree to go his way; if not, I would give my opinion again, and we would come to some understanding. Jim is very special in that he knows how to lead, and many times the way you lead or get people to follow is by getting them to understand your point of view. You don't beat them over the head. Jimmy is a peacemaker and can always find a way to get the most out of everyone. He obviously got the most out of me.

We used to meet regularly to discuss future planning, and any time there was a major decision, even if it didn't pertain to his area of music, I wanted his counsel and judgment. We discussed board members, union problems, personnel— everything. I think the relationship that developed was unique, very strong and trusting. We did some incredible things in the 16 years that we worked so closely together, including 26 premieres. We wanted a varied repertoire to reach a wider audience, and to educate people and bring to their attention something they might not be aware of. There was a benefit for the company, too, because it's great to have new challenges.

The Met is paradise for workaholics and, of course, Jim is at the top of the list. He's the only one who would come in, do a rehearsal, race around and study in the afternoon, be supposed to take a nap which he didn't, come back, conduct, and then go out for dinner. An orchestra musician told me that at the end of a *Parsifal* performance, Jim went striding out, and a trombonist looked at him and said, "You know, Jim, we're exhausted." And he said, "Really? I could do it again." And they believed him because he was so wound up about it. That's Jim.

He is also a great judge of other people's stamina. At one performance of *Tosca,* Luciano Pavarotti had finished the third-act aria, "E lucevan le stelle," and all of a sudden you heard the clarinet and realized that Jimmy was doing the aria again. Luciano sang it, but at the curtain call he said to Jimmy, "Are you mad?" Jimmy said, "Oh, I knew you could do it." And he did. He knew exactly how much energy Luciano had.

There is no end to what Jim has done and continues to do for the Met, but I think that the most important might be what he has done with the orchestra and chorus. He built them into one of the finest ensembles in the world. That's what Jimmy does. He is a builder, and I guess I'm a builder, too, which made working with him so rewarding.

JL: There had long been a policy forbidding encores of solo arias because they had gotten gradually undisciplined and completely out of hand—so there had not been a solo encore at the Met in many, many decades. But I had begun to think it would be fascinating to find out what it might be like if, in certain circumstances, the audience's reaction could provoke an encore.

On this particular Halloween night [in 1994], when we performed *Tosca,* I was feeling exceptionally mischievous. As usual the audience applauded vociferously and at great length after Luciano's third-act aria. Spontaneously, I thought, "What a great opportunity!" and whispered to the orchestra to play the opening bars of the aria once again. The audience realized what I was doing, but Luciano looked at me with a really marvelous surprised and perplexed look on his face... and then he sang the aria again, even more beautifully than he had the first time—with an incredibly light, romantic sound and tremendous expression.

When the opera was over, he said, "At first I didn't know what you were doing, since we don't do encores at the Met! And I had given so much the first time that I can't imagine how you knew I could do it a second time." I told him that I could tell that he would do it wonderfully, and besides, it was Halloween. I said, "I may have 'tricked' you, but what a spectacular 'treat' you gave us all!"

At the next performance of *Tosca,* the audience applauded and applauded. But I just smiled and shook my head, and we went on with the performance. But we did establish the possibility of occasional encores again in modern times.

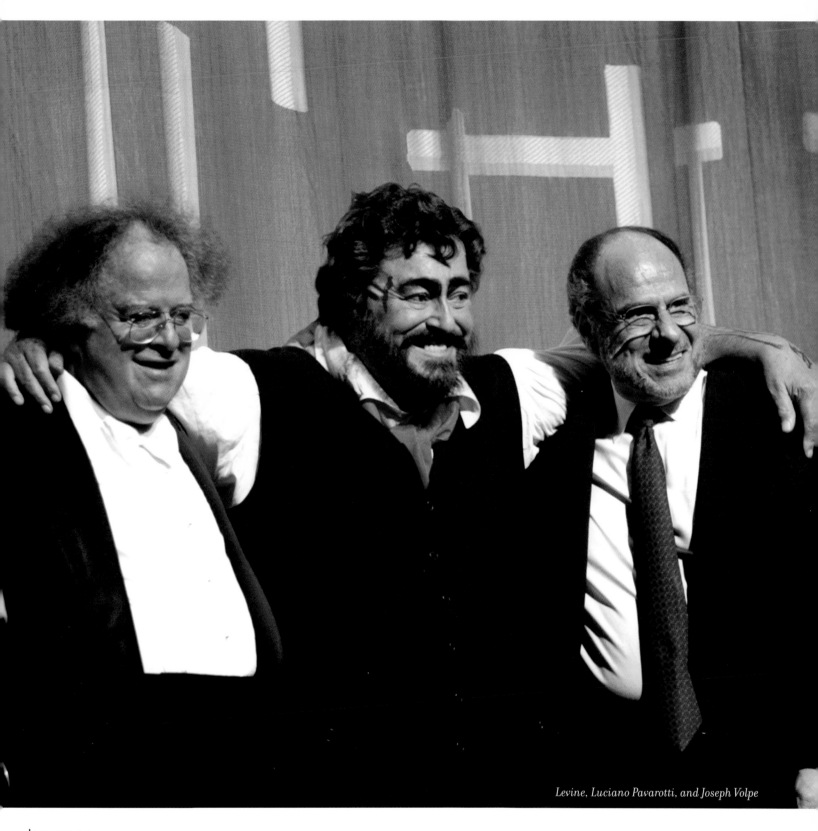

Levine, Luciano Pavarotti, and Joseph Volpe

Conducts Luciano Pavarotti's farewell
performance in *Tosca*.

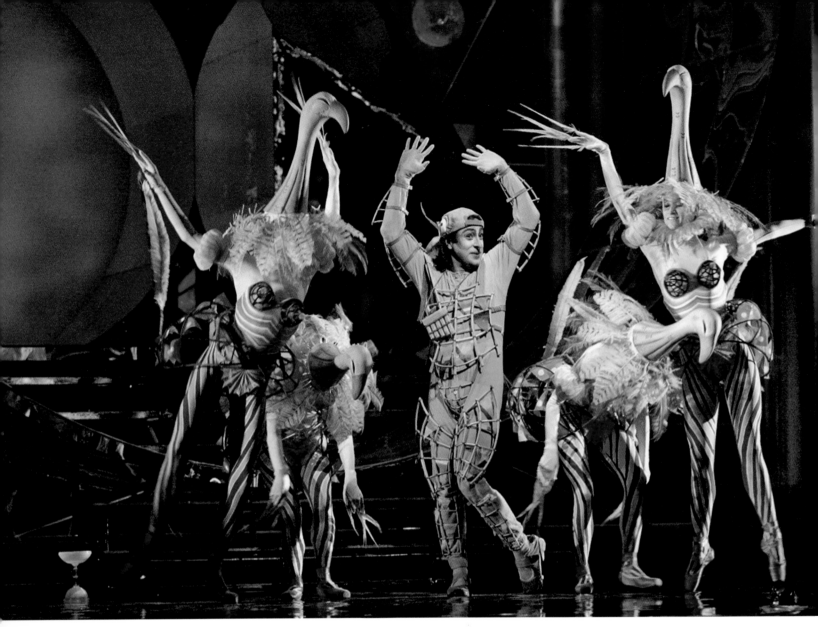

Rodion Pogossov as Papageno in Die Zauberflöte

JL: I think it's remarkable and fascinating that when I was growing up we had a Chagall design for *Magic Flute,* and then we subsequently had a Hockney design, and then we got this production. This means the Met has had a persuasive and diverse way with this piece at each incarnation. There's a large fantasy element to Taymor's production which is very good with the piece.

OCTOBER 8

Leads Julie Taymor's new production of *Die Zauberflöte,* with Dorothea Röschmann, L'ubica Vargicová, Matthew Polenzani, Rodion Pogossov, and Kwangchul Youn.

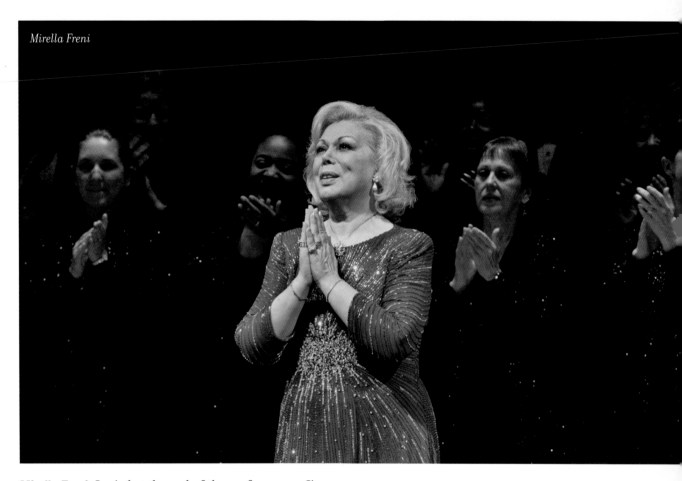

Mirella Freni: I cried at the end of the performance. Jimmy came to my dressing room and gave me a ring. I never expected it, or anything like it. Someone had given it to him for good luck, and he gave it to me. I love him for that, and I love and respect him for everything we did on stage. Jimmy and I were friends from the very beginning. It was as if we had always known each other. The first opera we did together at the Met was *Don Carlo*. I was nervous because you never know if a conductor is going to do something that is the opposite of what you know, but that didn't happen with Jimmy. He was so nice, and what I remember most is the fine colors he wanted. He conducts with such humanity. I always respected the questions he asked me, about how I wanted to do a role. When he and I were together at the piano, he would ask, "Do you prefer this or that?" When you work like that, you can create something really good.

2005

MAY 15

Conducts the farewell of Mirella Freni, celebrating the 50th anniversary of her operatic debut and the 40th anniversary of her Met debut.

APRIL 21

Conducts Gounod's *Faust* for the first time at the Met, in a new production featuring Roberto Alagna, Soile Isokoski, Dmitri Hvorostovsky, and René Pape.

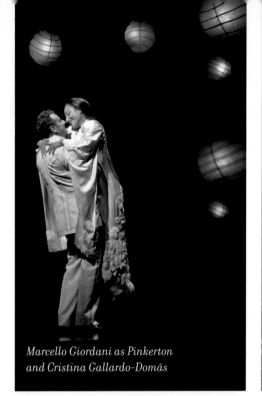

Marcello Giordani as Pinkerton and Cristina Gallardo-Domâs

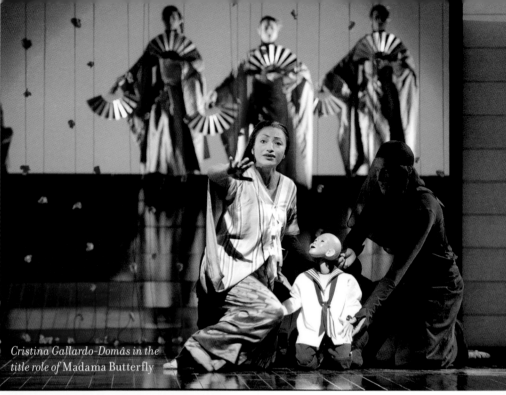

Cristina Gallardo-Domâs in the title role of Madama Butterfly

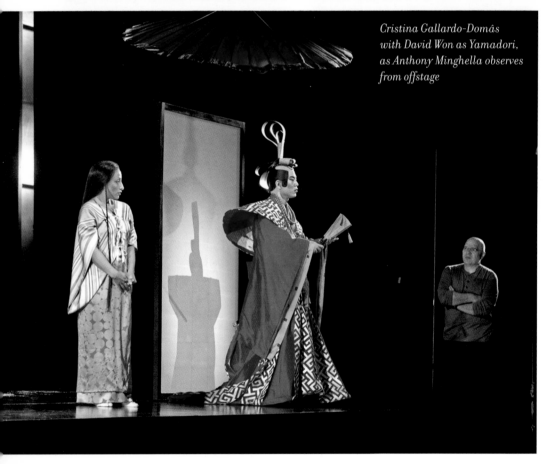

Cristina Gallardo-Domâs with David Won as Yamadori, as Anthony Minghella observes from offstage

JL: I'm a big fan of this production. It has such beauty of atmosphere, and I was fascinated and persuaded by the use of the puppet. Anthony was an amazing, sensitive man with a wonderful eye for this opera.

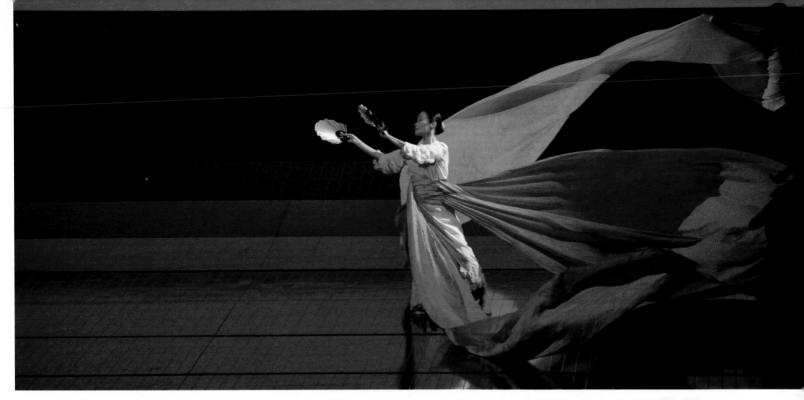

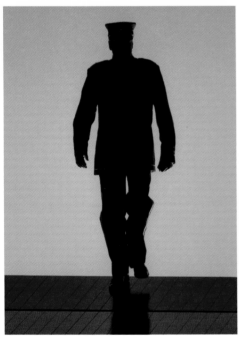

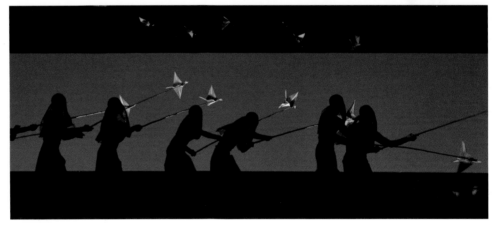

Scenes from Anthony Minghella's production of Madama Butterfly, *with sets by Michael Levine and costumes by Han Feng*

JL: When we started on Sirius, with its mix of very old and more recent broadcasts, as well as live ones, I was worried that there might be odious comparisons from one sound recording era to another. But there isn't—your ear makes the jump with no problem, and it's been marvelous. I was also worried that there might be a market glut. But the loyal fan base is remarkable, and new people are coming.

2006
SEPTEMBER 25

A new production of Puccini's *Madama Butterfly,* directed by Anthony Minghella, opens Peter Gelb's first season as General Manager. The performance marks the first live broadcast on Metropolitan Opera Radio on SIRIUS (now SIRIUS XM) and the first Opening Night transmission in Times Square.

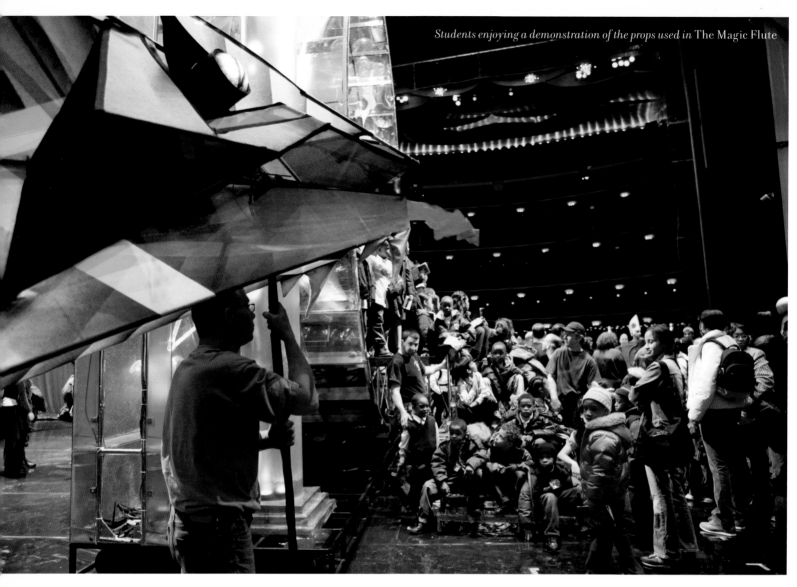

JL: On a broadcast day, I do feel excited by the increased size of the public. And I'm conscious of a sort of heightened awareness and energy from everyone, because more people will see and hear the performance, and therefore it's more important to have that one go right. On the other hand, one needs to let the energy flow and not get clenched, because otherwise you try to make it pop, and then you miss.

DECEMBER 30

Reaches new audiences of all ages with a special holiday version of *The Magic Flute,* abridged and sung in English, that launches *The Met: Live in HD,* the company's series of live performance transmissions to movie theaters around the world.

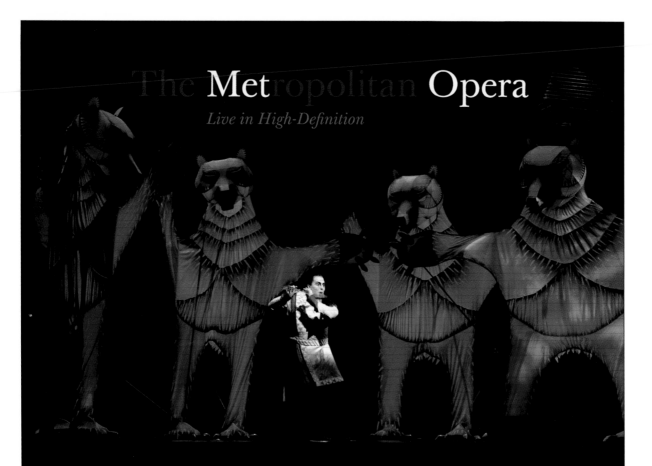

The Metropolitan Opera
Live in High-Definition

Live in HD
On the Big Screen

Via Satellite from New York City

1:30 PM ET / 10:30 AM PT

Visit **CINEPLEX**.com for ticket and location details

DECEMBER 30, 2006	JANUARY 6, 2007
Mozart The **Magic Flute** Directed by Julie Taymor	*Bellini* I Puritani Starring Anna Netrebko

JANUARY 13, 2007	FEBRUARY 24, 2007
Tan Dun The First Emperor Starring Plácido Domingo	*Tchaikovsky* Eugene Onegin Starring Renée Fleming

MARCH 24, 2007	APRIL 28, 2007
Rossini Il Barbiere di Siviglia Directed by Bartlett Sher	*Puccini* Il Trittico Conductor James Levine

cineplex
entertainment

In association with PBS, the HD broadcasts are made possible by Toll Brothers, America's luxury home builder

® Cineplex Entertainment LP or used under license

Tickets for the entire series must be purchased by December 29 at participating cinemas box office locations only (no on-line sales)

JL: I was very happy. Jack is a wonderful director for a piece like this. The cast responded very well because he got into the essence of it. He understood what you must do to make verismo pieces work on our stage; you can't make a symbolic-style production when the details are composed into the piece at the rate they are in *Trittico.*

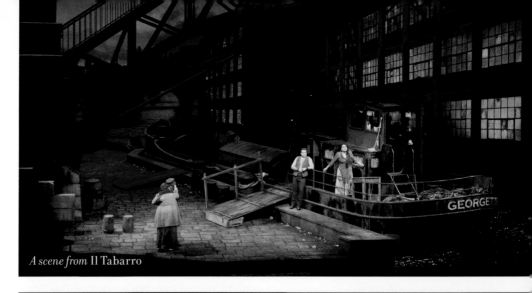

A scene from Il Tabarro

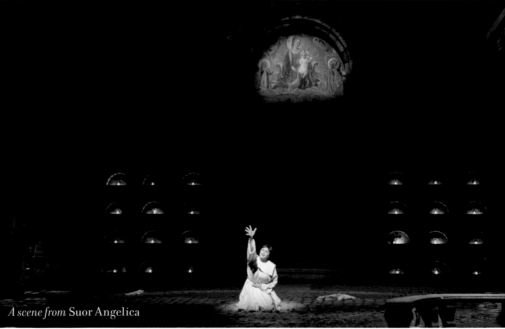

A scene from Suor Angelica

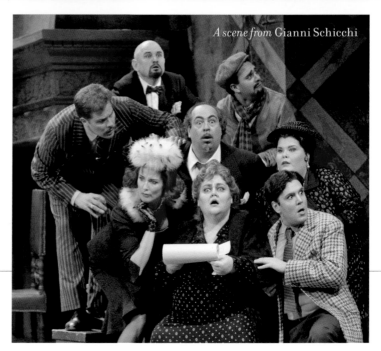

A scene from Gianni Schicchi

2007
APRIL 20

Il Trittico, starring Maria Guleghina, Barbara Frittoli, Stephanie Blythe, Salvatore Licitra, and Alessandro Corbelli, and directed by Jack O'Brien, is the first of four new productions Levine conducts this year.

JL: This is one of my favorite operas, one of the best pieces there is. And fortunately, it gave me a chance to collaborate with Mark Morris, which I've always wanted to do, because I love his work. I adored this experience, and I thought the characterization of the chorus in the production was wonderful.

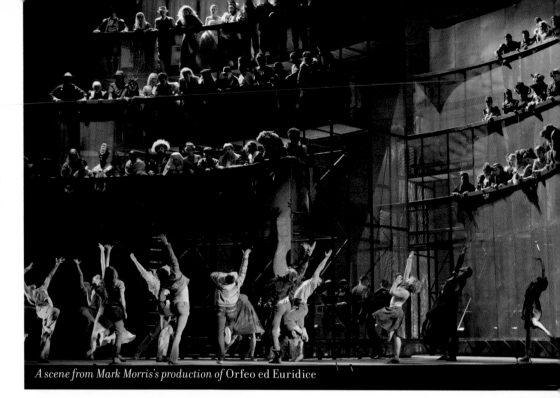

A scene from Mark Morris's production of Orfeo ed Euridice

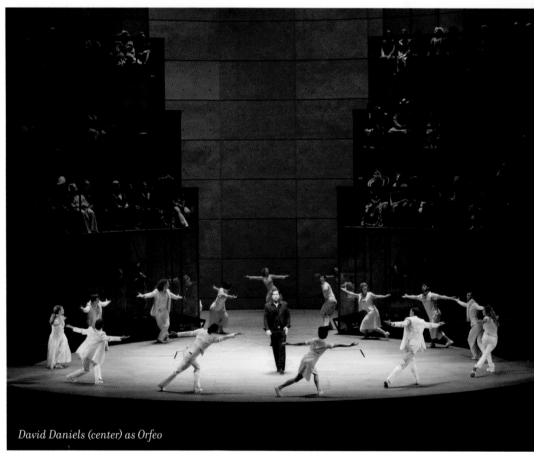

David Daniels (center) as Orfeo

MAY 2

Leads his first Gluck opera with the Met, Mark Morris's new staging of *Orfeo ed Euridice,* with countertenor David Daniels and Maija Kovalevska in the title roles.

Natalie Dessay: When we did *Lucia di Lammermoor,* Jimmy had never conducted it before. After so many years he could have said, "Okay, *Lucia* is not for me," but he had curiosity, which is something I like very much about him. It's a role that I know particularly well, yet he helped me find more and more precision, especially in the first aria, so that we were always together, even if I was moving around on stage. Jimmy reminds me all the time that we are here to make music, and not only to play or to mess around on stage. I have a tendency to do that, and to forget that I'm also here to sing. He brings me back.

The first time I worked with Jimmy was in *Ariadne auf Naxos* in 1997. I was young, insecure, and very impressed with him—so I was afraid. But I learned to trust that if I'm here, it's because he chose me. I was very glad that I had another opportunity to do Zerbinetta with him a few years later. I knew by then that I had to propose something very clear and very personal—he likes that. He can add things and drive you somewhere else if he wants, but when you know exactly what you want and what you need, then he's a wonderful accompanist. He helps you to fly away, to develop your ideas and your vision of the character and the music. I think he likes to be surprised— not by just anything, but when it's good, a new idea, a new phrasing or proposition of the cadenza, he laughs. He's ready for everything, for the trip, the trouble,

and the adventure of every performance. He may be very precise in his rehearsals, but I think he secretly likes that things can change from one performance to another. The more prepared you come, the more you can improvise. There's a paradox: you feel remote-controlled by him and very free at the same time.

With Jimmy, opera is alive. So many times, opera can be dead, obsolete or old-fashioned, like something from a museum. We are here to bring it to life,

again and again, and he helps us to do that. The most rewarding thing for me is when he seems to be pleased by something I'm doing, and he has a smile on his face. I'm the only one who can see that smile, and I have the impression that it is only for me. And one more thing: I love that we have the same favorite sandwich, a BLT! It's almost impossible to get one in France. The next time I'm in New York, I will invite Jimmy to have one with me.

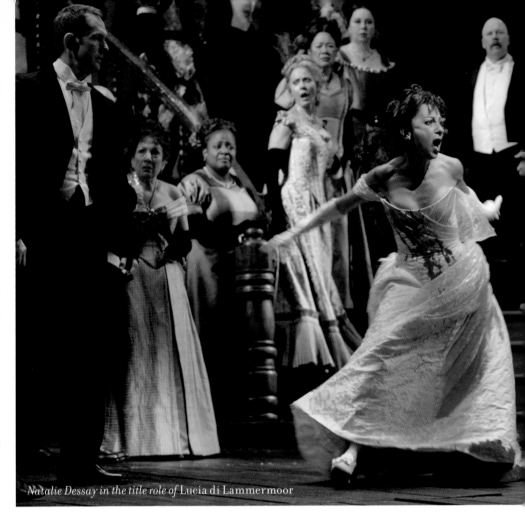

Natalie Dessay in the title role of Lucia di Lammermoor

SEPTEMBER 24

Opens the season with Mary Zimmerman's new production of Donizetti's *Lucia di Lammermoor,* his first with the company, starring Natalie Dessay, Marcello Giordani, and Mariusz Kwiecien.

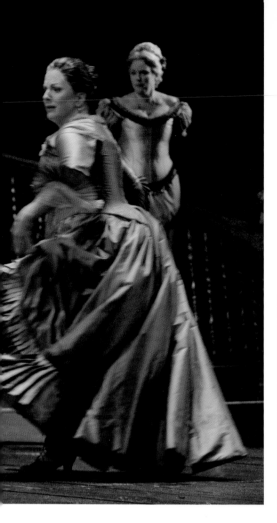

JL: Natalie is great fun to work with because she enters a role from its dramatic side. She wants to find a way to do what she imagines visually while she sings. And her results show this ambition. If you watch her during a performance as Zerbinetta, for example, it's absolutely astonishing, the way she sings it like a top but without one dramatic compromise—and this is hard stuff. Part of it is intense concentration, but it also comes from a conscious decision about her talents, her work, what she's trying to solve. If I ever point out anything musical that's getting lost in the physical motion, she understands it, converts it, and does it immediately. She wants to have everything.

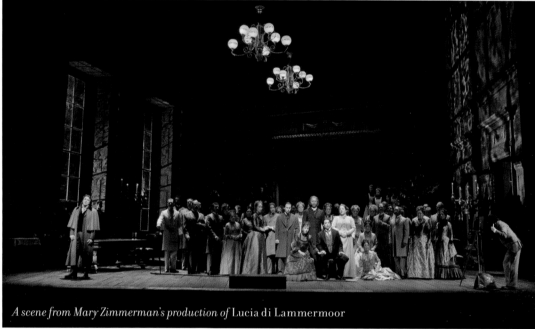

A scene from Mary Zimmerman's production of Lucia di Lammermoor

JL: There's always been a misconception that "Jimmy doesn't like bel canto." I adore bel canto! I haven't gotten to do so much of it because we have to do big operas for our big house, and it's my responsibility to lead large company pieces. But *Lucia* is a piece I would gladly have done long before, under the right circumstances. We had a very, very good time. And I have to say, I know a lot of people didn't like the staging of the sextet, with the formal photograph being taken, but I did. I thought that it was chillingly real in that situation, and the very alienation of it was disturbing in a way that was appropriate. It was considered pretty disturbing years ago when Lucia appeared on the stairs with a bloody knife in a bloody dress, instead of having a decorous mad scene.

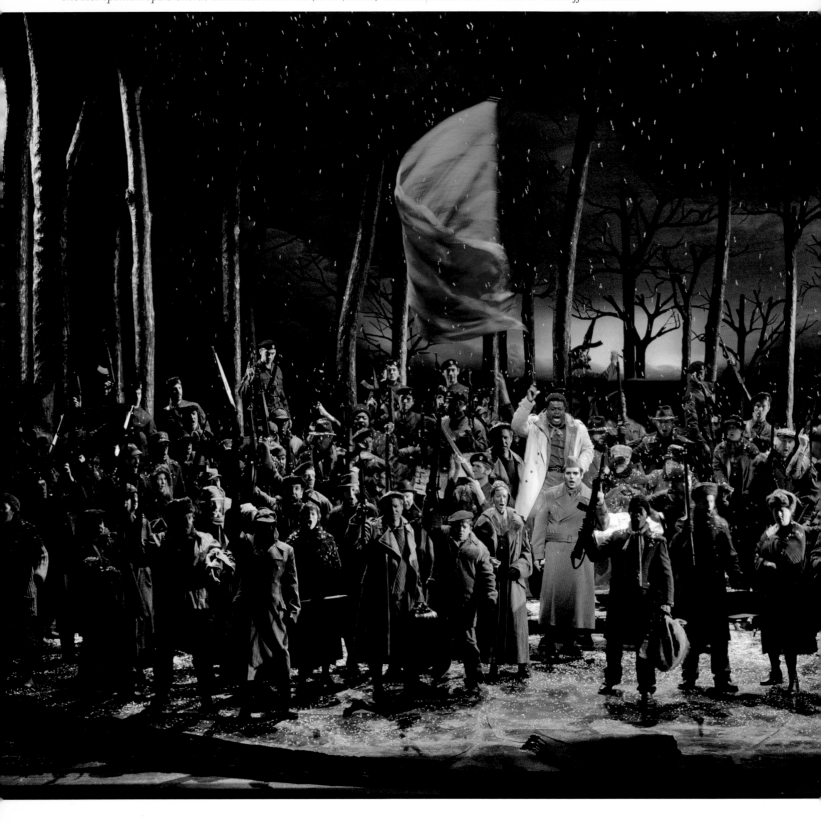

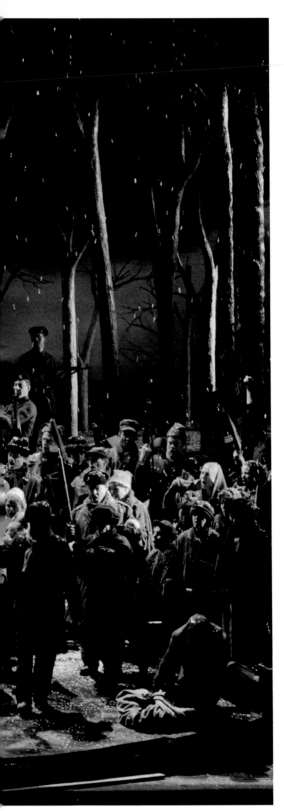

Donald Palumbo, Chorus Master: Our relationship is in the process. Basically, I prepare the piece the way I think he would want it prepared, and then sometimes we pull Maestro into List Hall, where the chorus rehearses. We go through the piece section by section. Sometimes he'll whisper things to me while I'm conducting, or we'll stop and have a little chat and try something else. Occasionally I'll say, "Maestro, why don't you conduct it for them so that they can get used to you?" It's very free and unstructured. We'll sit there with our scores, with the luxury of having the chorus right there, to hear what our ideas actually sound like. Sometimes when you're studying a score, you have to conceptualize what the sound produced is going to be, but in a situation like that, you can actually experiment and play around with things. And that's one of the joys of working with Maestro—he's flexible. He doesn't come in and say, "No, it has to be like this." I could see the choristers looking at us and wondering, "Gee, which one is in charge?" And sometimes I felt the same thing. I'd say, "Don't you want to jump in here?" We established this great relationship—it's a total sharing experience.

Maestro is always intent on making the words expressive in the context of the music. For example, sometimes when you're singing softly, the text can get indistinct. With the big, explosive passages, there's a lot of bite in the text, but it can get a little flabby when the dynamic drops down to *piano*. And so he's very insistent on making sure the text is brighter and more present when you sing softly. It's a technique that works, for example, with the witches in *Macbeth*.

He has an uncanny knack for hitting the right tempo. There's a term in Italian called *tempo giusto,* "the right tempo." Sometimes it's dictated by the orchestration, the rhythmic structure, the amount of text involved, the length of the phrase, all sorts of aspects. For a chorus, it's extremely important to get the right tempo, because you've got to get all 80 people on the same wavelength, the same train. With a soloist, there's a little bit of play and freedom. But 80 people have to know what the correct tempo is at any given moment, and that is one of Maestro's incredible strengths. You never sense, "Oh, this is awkward to phrase at this tempo." Everything feels right. When we take a breath, it's because we should breathe at that particular moment, not because we're put in a position that we have to or we're not going to make it. He's the perfect blend of the conductors that favor rhythmic impulse and accuracy and then conductors that favor long lines, blended sounds, and a bit of a dark, languorous approach to lyrical phrases.

He's insistent about the chorus being in favorable acoustic positions for the sound to get out to the house. I know that drives some stage directors crazy because Maestro will say, "Excuse me. Keep coming down further. We need more sound here. Come down, come down." He's very concerned that the aural impact of the opera is just as strong as the visual, dramatic impact, and he will not back down on points like that. I'm certainly in support of that all the time!

OCTOBER 22

Conducts a new *Macbeth,* directed by Adrian Noble, starring Željko Lučić and Maria Guleghina.

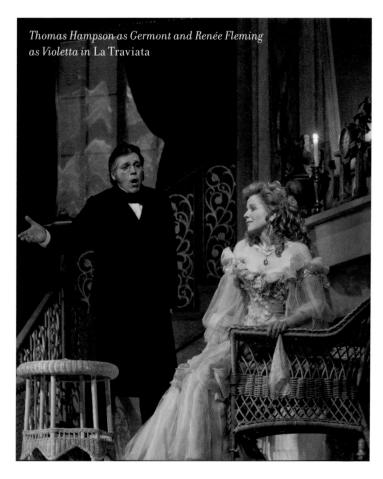

Thomas Hampson as Germont and Renée Fleming as Violetta in La Traviata

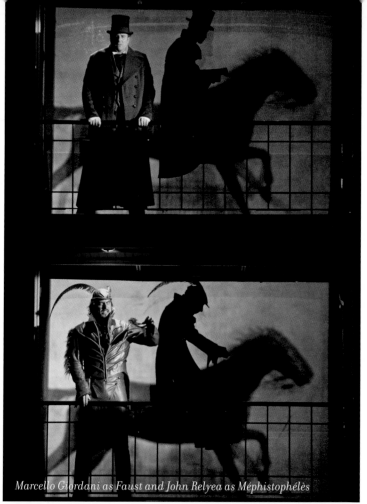

Marcello Giordani as Faust and John Relyea as Méphistophélès

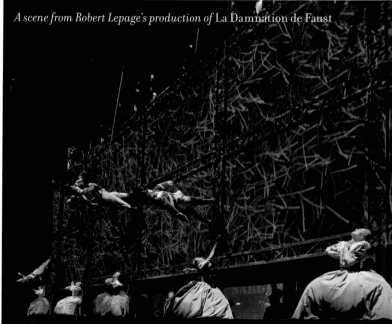

A scene from Robert Lepage's production of La Damnation de Faust

2008

SEPTEMBER 22

As part of the Opening Night Gala starring Renée Fleming, he conducts Act II of *La Traviata* with Ramón Vargas and Thomas Hampson.

NOVEMBER 7

Leads Robert Lepage's new production of Berlioz's *La Damnation de Faust,* starring Susan Graham, Marcello Giordani, and John Relyea, a work he previously performed with the MET Orchestra at Carnegie Hall in 1996.

Susan Graham: At the beginning of my Met career, I was doing small parts—Second Lady in *Die Zauberflöte,* Tebaldo in *Don Carlo*—and they were terrifying because the margin of error is so great. Jimmy took the time to help me and make me feel a part of things. I did one Cherubino in *Le Nozze di Figaro,* filling in for Frederica von Stade. At first I was too nervous to remember much, but when Jimmy was looking at me during "Voi che sapete," I honestly felt as if I could fly. That was when I began to know what happens when you're in the zone with him, that magic carpet ride.

And then came *Der Rosenkavalier.* I had just done my first run of it elsewhere, so it was very fresh in my mind, but when I started to work on it with Jimmy, he showed me something new in virtually every phrase. He has amazing insight into the character, the expression, the artistic approach in phrasing text, how you fit with the clarinet that's accompanying you at that moment. He'd say something like, "What are you, as Octavian, trying to get out of the Marschallin in this moment?" It would shape the musical impulse, or the way I'd go after a certain word. When I finally set foot into that second act, with a sparkly white costume and a shiny rose in my hand, and I heard that sublime music, I sort of lost track of where I was. I looked down at Jimmy, and when he pointed at me to sing, I just hoped I was in the right place at the right time. The look on his face told me that I was, and then the blood returned to my brain. To be on stage in the opera that I love most,

with Jimmy spinning those phrases out for my first time at the Met, was pretty incredible.

Several years later, Octavian figured prominently in another of my greatest experiences with Jimmy. I was singing Idamante in *Idomeneo,* a very tricky role. The first aria right out of the starting block is high-flying and frog-strangling. At the final dress rehearsal, during intermission, Jimmy called my dressing room. Now, he is famous for knowing singers, but it's not just as a breed: he knows the individual, and he knows what buttons to push for each. He could see I was struggling with that aria, and he said, "Okay, what's your favorite role to sing? What role just gives you joy, and

you don't really have to think about it?" I told him that it was Octavian, and he said, "Sing Idamante like it's Octavian." What that did was change my breath and support—and give me confidence. That made all the difference. Jimmy knew that I was somebody who wanted so desperately to do things right that I might not go fully into it, especially the first time around. And he knew that I could feel committed about Octavian. I've drawn on that "sing like it's Octavian" many times since, because it's a metaphor for anything. If you're feeling insecure, act like you're not. Find a way to trick your mind into accomplishing what you can't seem to through more traditional routes. It's brilliant.

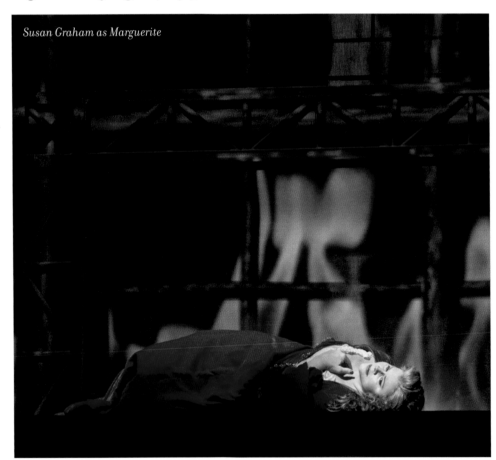

Susan Graham as Marguerite

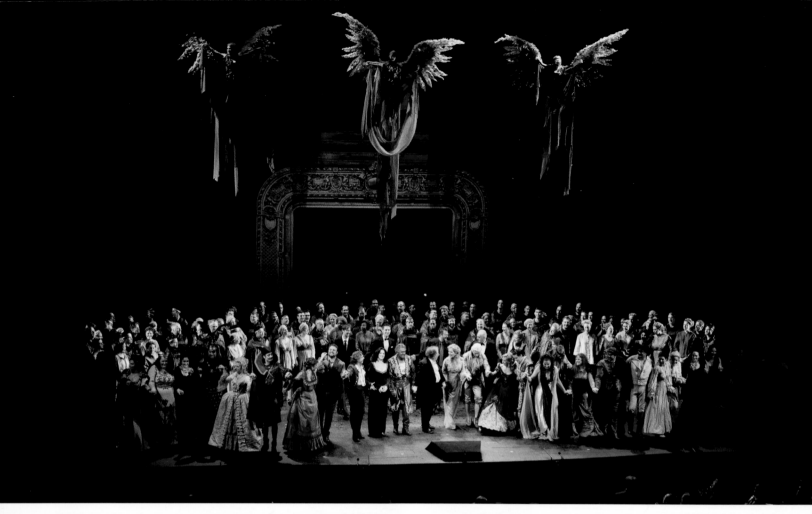

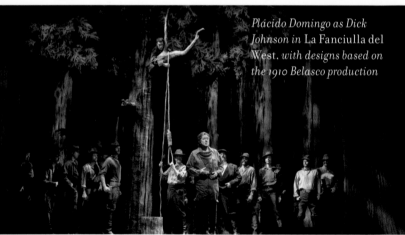

Plácido Domingo as Dick Johnson in La Fanciulla del West. *with designs based on the 1910 Belasco production*

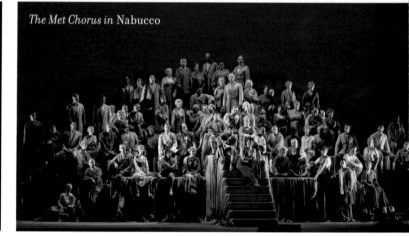

The Met Chorus in Nabucco

2009

Conducts the Met's 125th Anniversary Gala, which recreates scenes from historic Met productions and also pays tribute to Levine's longtime collaborator Plácido Domingo on the occasion of his 40th Met anniversary.

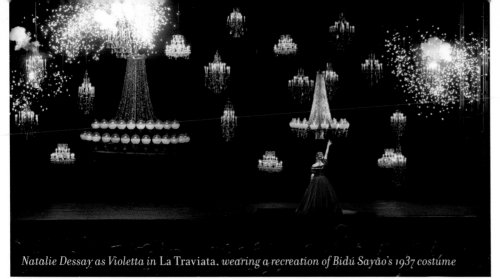

Natalie Dessay as Violetta in La Traviata, *wearing a recreation of Bidú Sayão's 1937 costume*

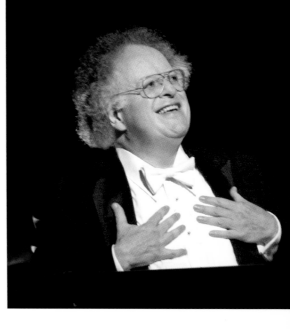

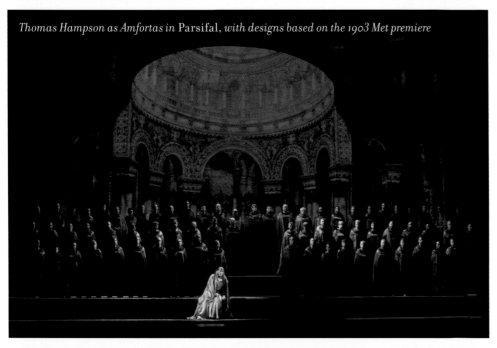

Thomas Hampson as Amfortas in Parsifal, *with designs based on the 1903 Met premiere*

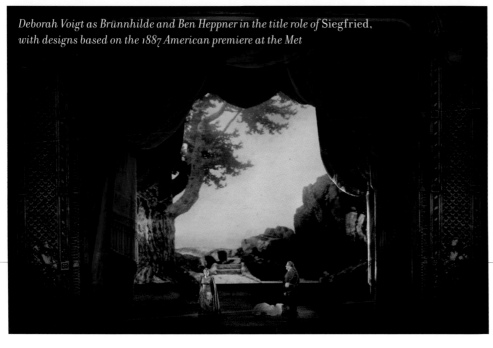

Deborah Voigt as Brünnhilde and Ben Heppner in the title role of Siegfried, *with designs based on the 1887 American premiere at the Met*

Levine with Otto Schenk

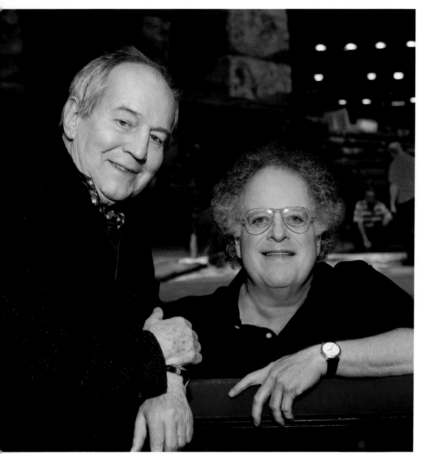

Peter Gelb and Levine present Wotan's spear to James Morris,
who retired the role after 89 performances in the span of 22 years

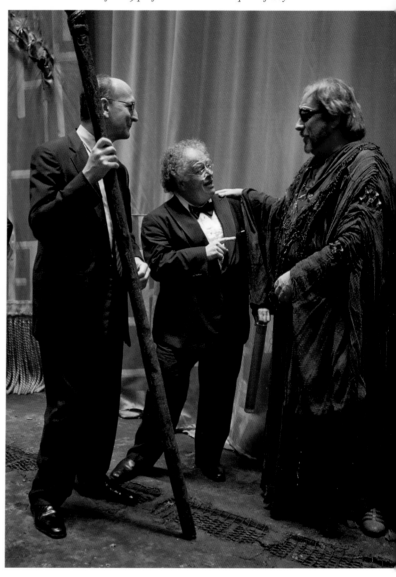

MAY 4–9

Conducts the final cycle of Otto Schenk's
Ring production. It's the 21st complete cycle
of this staging—all of which were conducted
by Levine.

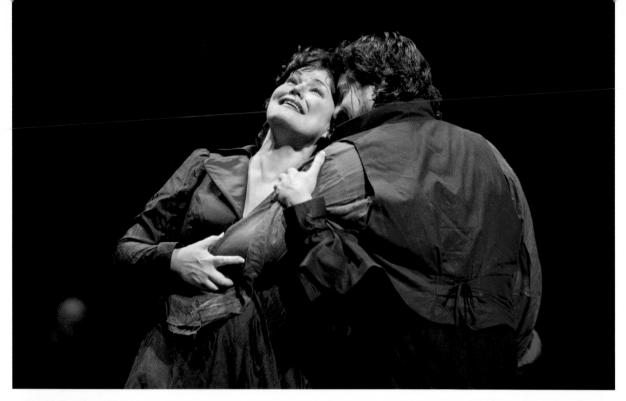

Karita Mattila in the title role of Tosca *and Marcelo Álvarez as Cavaradossi*

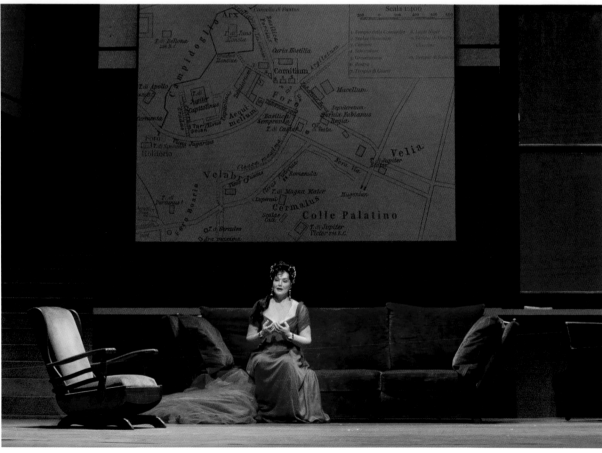

A scene from Luc Bondy's production of Tosca

SEPTEMBER 21

Opens the season with a new *Tosca*, directed by Luc Bondy and starring Karita Mattila, Marcelo Álvarez, and George Gagnidze.

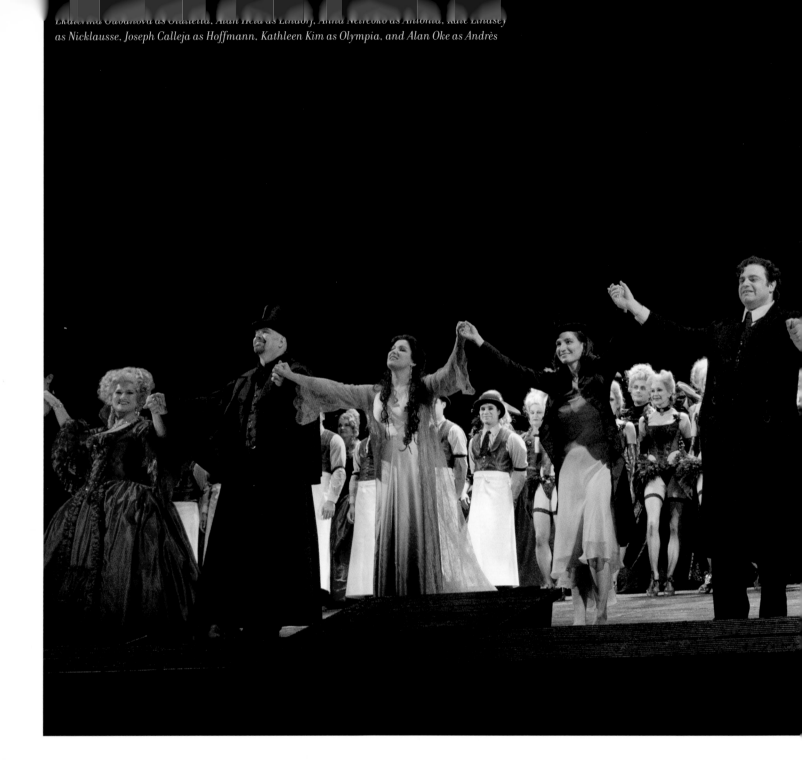

DECEMBER 3

Leads Bartlett Sher's new production of *Les Contes d'Hoffmann,* starring Joseph Calleja, Anna Netrebko, Kate Lindsey, and Alan Held.

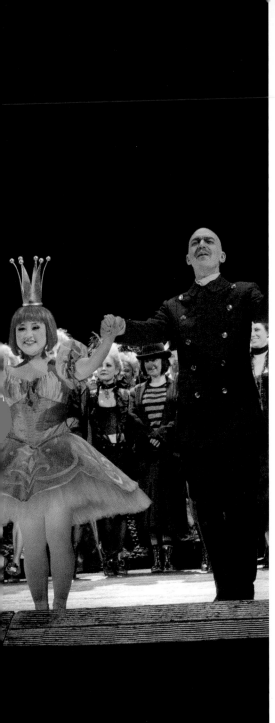

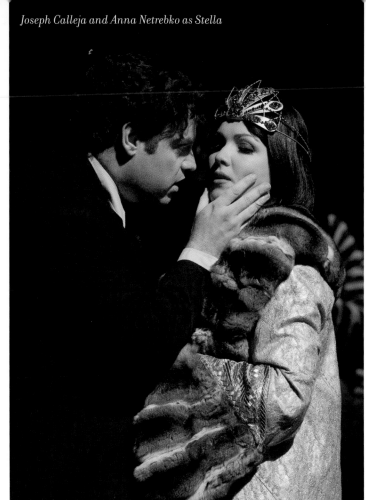

Joseph Calleja and Anna Netrebko as Stella

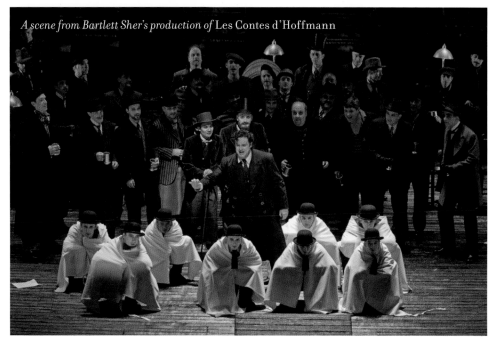

A scene from Bartlett Sher's production of Les Contes d'Hoffmann

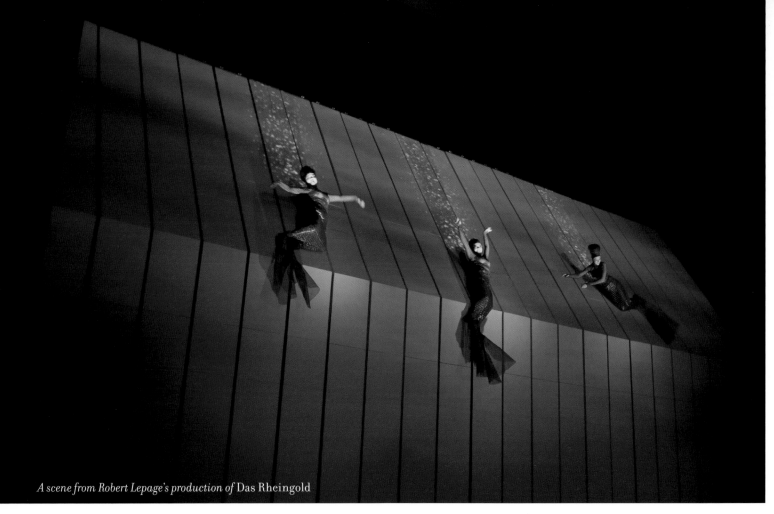

A scene from Robert Lepage's production of Das Rheingold

Robert Lepage: Any director who's offered his first *Ring* cycle is immediately overwhelmed by the sheer size of the adventure, whether it be conceptual or dramaturgical. Of course James Levine certainly knows how big the whole *Ring* is. But he constantly reminds you how simple this intimate family story has to remain.

During the rehearsals of *Das Rheingold,* I felt very privileged to see him work with the singers on the details of Wagner's complex musical score and discovered to my great amazement how great an acting coach he is. He really, truly believes, as I do, that any libretto's subtext can be found in the score. During the first orchestra rehearsal, I noticed how he kept shouting something to the singers above the swell of the orchestra pit. I couldn't understand what he was saying to them, but it certainly seemed to make a big difference on stage. I kept changing seats, getting closer and closer, trying to catch the word he was constantly hammering at them. When I got close enough, I realized he was actually saying: "Text!" So with James Levine, the basic rule seems to be: not only is it important to be heard—it is *fundamental* to be understood.

This certainly came as a pleasant surprise to me, for however absorbed in the music he might seem to be, his main concern is obviously that of a storyteller.

2010

SEPTEMBER 27

Leads his 31st Opening Night, the premiere of a new production of *Das Rheingold,* the first part of a new *Ring* cycle directed by Robert Lepage.

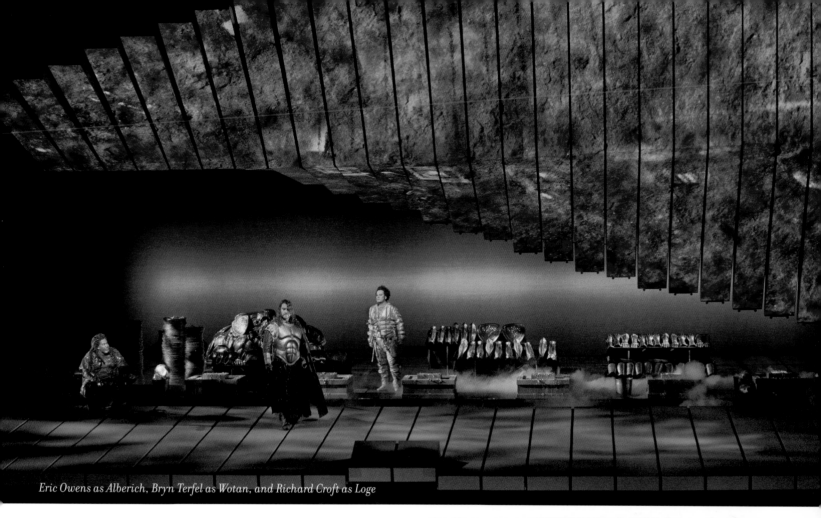

Eric Owens as Alberich, Bryn Terfel as Wotan, and Richard Croft as Loge

JL: After 21 cycles of the old one in 20-odd years, it's time for a new one, for the company and the audience. The Bayreuth Festival used to do new *Ring* productions regular as clockwork. Everything about the way Robert's production looks is completely new—its imagery, its technique. But it is a telling of Wagner's story, not of some other story. It's comprehensible in every detail from front to back, and the imagery is very strong. Also, judging by *Rheingold,* it works for the singers tremendously well. The acoustic makes for a particular kind of sound that flows from the orchestra up to the singers and back out, and yet the singers are clearly related to the scenery. I'm looking forward to the whole thing!

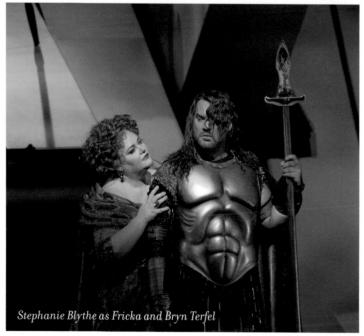

Stephanie Blythe as Fricka and Bryn Terfel

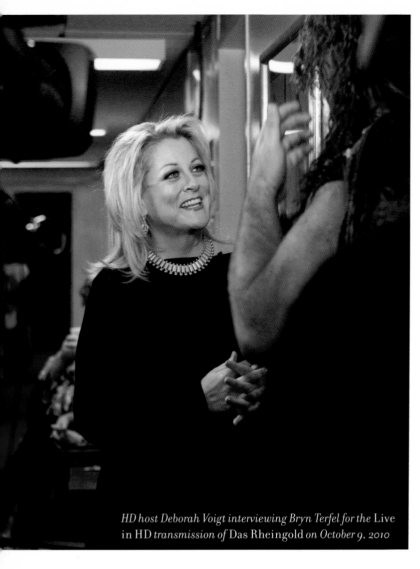

HD host Deborah Voigt interviewing Bryn Terfel for the Live in HD *transmission of* Das Rheingold *on October 9, 2010*

Deborah Voigt: I can't think of another conductor who has influenced me in such a practical sense with my singing. It's all well and good for someone to say, "Well, this doesn't really work," but the gestures in Jimmy's conducting language really speak to singers. I remember that when we did *Ariadne,* I was having trouble with a particular note. It wasn't a high note, a money note, but it just wasn't working well for me. The performance started, we got to that moment, and I looked out in the pit—Jimmy knew, of course, that I was having trouble with it—and he made eye contact with me and went the expanse of the breath with me, including the preparation for it. And I nailed it. Every time I sing Ariadne I think about that moment, and that preparation, and it's never, ever given me trouble again.

My favorite role with him was Sieglinde in *Die Walküre,* one of the roles I feel I was put on the earth to sing. Jimmy takes great joy when he sees joy on the stage. Sometimes he'll be conducting away and he'll just look up and smile at you, and you know that you're on the same wavelength, feeling blessed to be doing this together. But he challenged me with that role, too. Even within the run of performances, we'd get to "O hehrstes Wunder," and I remember thinking, "Omigosh, what's he trying to make me do?" Yet he knew that I could do what he was asking, even when I wouldn't have challenged myself in that way. Having his belief that you can is something very special. I don't know how he knows, except that he loves singers, and he understands our psychology. Singer thinking is a whole other bag, and he really gets that—how fragile we can be and how heroic we can be.

It was hard for me to leave that role behind. The only time I've sung Brünnhilde's Immolation Scene in concert was with Jimmy at Tanglewood. And when that theme, Sieglinde's "O hehrstes Wunder," came up at the end, tears were coming to my eyes. But I feel ready to move on. I ran into Jimmy in the hallway when I was hosting the HD transmission of *Rheingold,* and we just said hi and gave each other a kiss. But after I got home that day, there was a message on my phone: "Hey, it's Jimmy. I just wanted to tell you that you look so good and you look so happy, and I'm just so excited about everything that's coming up, and I just can't wait to get to work on it." It really helped, because it is a bit daunting—understatement—and overwhelming to be the Met's new Brünnhilde in a *Ring* cycle.

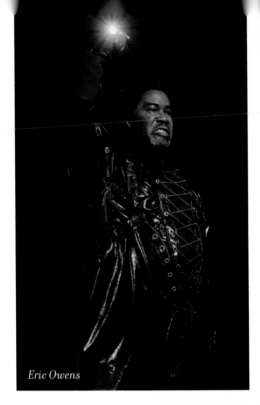

Eric Owens

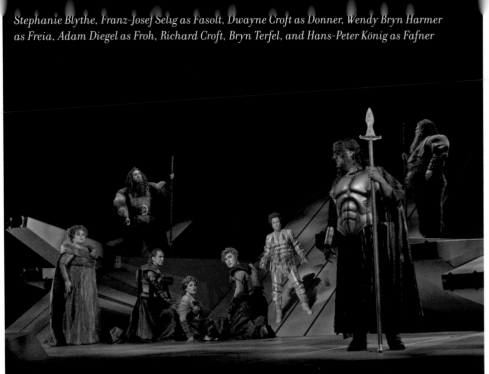

Stephanie Blythe, Franz-Josef Selig as Fasolt, Dwayne Croft as Donner, Wendy Bryn Harmer as Freia, Adam Diegel as Froh, Richard Croft, Bryn Terfel, and Hans-Peter König as Fafner

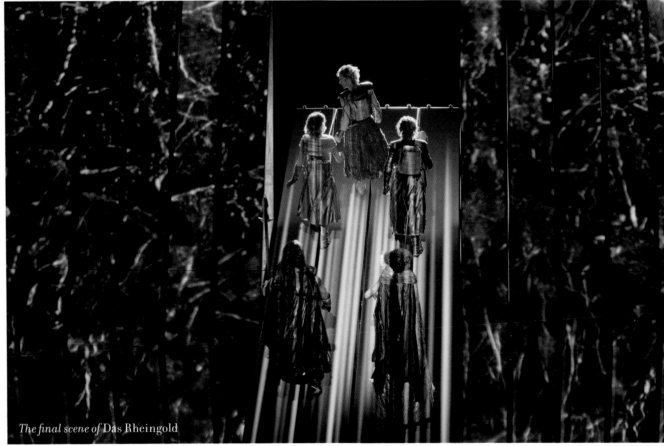

The final scene of Das Rheingold

Mariusz Kwiecien: When I came to America I had this very Eastern European technique, using lots of chest register and not enough head register. Every baritone wants to have this rich, rich voice. But you have it or you don't. And Maestro said, "Your voice is rich enough. Just put it high into your head and give the squillo because the Met will love your voice when you do." I have this advice in my ears now if I ever start to have problems with my singing, and it always works. He is like a doctor for voices. He's heard singers who are better and much more famous than I, and then he's heard how they survived, how they sang this or that role and for how long a time. And he always tells me to wait until the voice shows me where it wants to go, because the voice hates it if you push it—let it sing, let it follow the music.

Maestro always gives me the right energy, the right color of thoughts, for my roles, even if I know something well, like *Don Pasquale*—and it was the first time he conducted it. He always uses poetic words to move my imagination, to change the character of my singing and not only the tempo or volume. When I watch him working with the orchestra, it is the same. He is always poetic, and that's what I love. When somebody says, "Do it faster," or "Do it slower," you then forget it because it doesn't use your imagination. But when he uses his small stories and examples or says, "You have to use the energy like strong wind in between leaves on a tree," then you remember, because you imagine how that sounds.

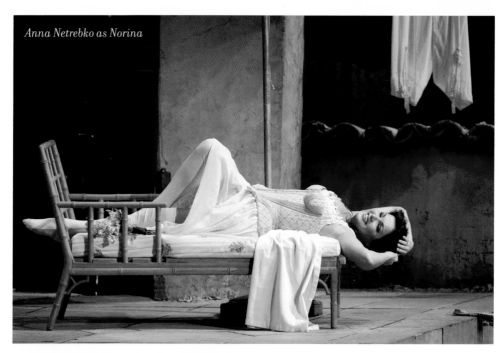

Anna Netrebko as Norina

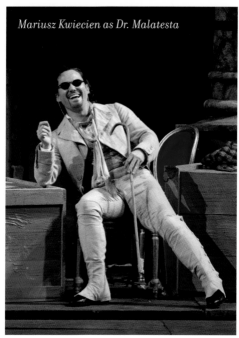

Mariusz Kwiecien as Dr. Malatesta

JL: Is it not a miracle that comedies like *Elisir* and *Pasquale* are still so viable for a contemporary audience if they're well done? I get such a kick out of that. This was a very happy experience because we had John, an American singer, in the title role, and he did a very stylish job. The tenor couldn't be beaten—Matt is a sensational homemade lyric tenor, one of the most beautifully accomplished ones this country has produced. Mariusz did a very good job, with a wonderful mercurial vitality, performance after performance. And Anna, she's a throwback—the genuine article, like the old ones. She's a tremendous talent, with a great respect for the piece and for the work. And her feel for the acting of real characters is so strong, as is her comic timing. She's also wonderful with her colleagues. This whole cast was a pleasure to work with.

OCTOBER 29

Adds Donizetti's *Don Pasquale* to his repertoire, starring John Del Carlo, Anna Netrebko, Matthew Polenzani, and Mariusz Kwiecien.

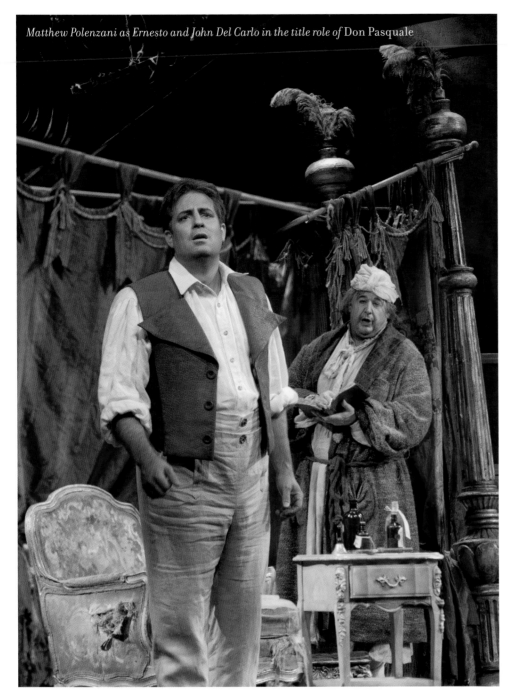
Matthew Polenzani as Ernesto and John Del Carlo in the title role of Don Pasquale

Matthew Polenzani: One of the great things about Jimmy is that if somebody's having a bad night, he tries to help. I'll never forget a performance I was in, when one of the singers was struggling. I have seen conductors in a situation like this pick up the phone and call to find out where the cover is. But Jimmy, in the pit, had a serene, placid, joyful expression on his face, and his whole body was radiating positive energy. He was trying to coax the singer back to himself. And by the next act he sang gorgeously. Hand a big chunk of the credit to Jimmy, who gave him everything he could. He lived and breathed every second with him. You might have thought, by the expression on Jimmy's face, that he was listening to Caruso in his greatest triumph. That made a huge impression on me, and I've told that story to at least three or four young conductors.

Years ago, I did Elliott Carter's fiendishly difficult *In Sleep, in Thunder* with Jimmy and the MET Chamber Ensemble in Weill Hall. At the time, all I could think about was how difficult it was to learn and to sing. But in retrospect, I realize that it wasn't that hard, knowing that Jimmy was standing there with me, and that if I made an error he'd know how to get me back. That's one of the wonderful things about him: he has a way of keeping you calm and excited at the same time.

JL: If I had it to do over again, I'd do it the same, because every move was really organic. I could never have done this in "career moves." People always said to me, "What's next for you?" But I can't think that way; I'm busy thinking about the music, the artists, the ensemble, the improvement of the details... For an American kid, the Met has always been an opera mecca temple. I made a prime life commitment. No one does that out of duress—you do it when it's natural. It would have felt very unnatural to stop it arbitrarily. The honeymoon with the orchestra and chorus never ended. The repertoire and the relationship never stopped growing.

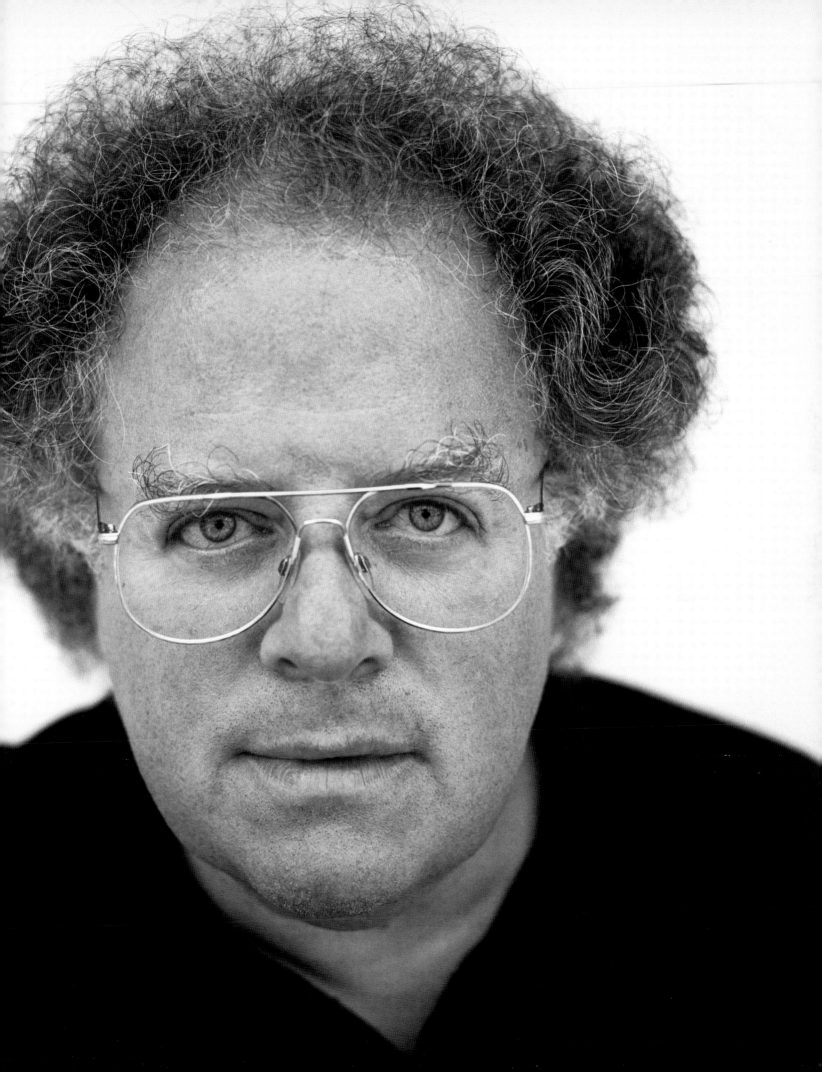

Appendix James Levine at the Metropolitan Opera
Performances

82 *Otello*	33 *Gianni Schicchi*	12 *Oedipus Rex*	
67 *Le Nozze di Figaro*	33 *Suor Angelica*	12 *Le Rossignol*	
67 *Die Walküre*	32 *Luisa Miller*	12 *Le Sacre du Printemps*	
62 *Tannhäuser*	32 *Rise and Fall of the City of Mahagonny*	12 *La Traviata*	
61 *Don Giovanni*	30 *Lulu*	11 *Bluebeard's Castle*	
60 *Don Carlo*	30 *Die Meistersinger von Nürnberg*	11 *Erwartung*	
57 *La Forza del Destino*	30 *I Vespri Siciliani*	11 *Fidelio*	
55 *Falstaff*	28 *Manon Lescaut*	11 *I Lombardi*	
53 *La Bohème*	27 *Götterdämmerung*	10 *Pagliacci*	
53 *Parsifal*	27 *Siegfried*	10 *Salome*	
51 *Così fan tutte*	26 *The Bartered Bride*	9 *La Damnation de Faust*	
49 *Der Rosenkavalier*	26 *Rigoletto*	9 *Orfeo ed Euridice*	
46 *Idomeneo*	26 *Les Troyens*	8 *Cavalleria Rusticana*	
45 *Lohengrin*	25 *Un Ballo in Maschera*	8 *Faust*	
44 *Aida*	24 *Andrea Chénier*	8 *Lucia di Lammermoor*	
44 *Carmen*	23 *Il Trovatore*	7 *Norma*	
44 *Das Rheingold*	21 *Les Contes d'Hoffmann*	6 *Il Barbiere di Siviglia*	
43 *Die Entführung aus dem Serail*	20 *Der Fliegende Holländer*	6 *Benvenuto Cellini*	
43 *Die Zauberflöte*	19 *L'Italiana in Algeri*	6 *L'Elisir d'Amore*	
42 *Porgy and Bess*	18 *Nabucco*	6 *L'Enfant et les Sortilèges*	
41 *Ariadne auf Naxos*	17 *Stiffelio*	6 *Les Mamelles de Tirésias*	
39 *Wozzeck*	16 *Francesca da Rimini*	6 *Parade*	
38 *Pelléas et Mélisande*	15 *Eugene Onegin*	5 *Don Pasquale*	
38 *Tristan und Isolde*	15 *Samson et Dalila*	3 *Madama Butterfly*	
37 *Macbeth*	15 *Turandot*		
37 *Tosca*	13 *The Ghosts of Versailles*		
36 *Elektra*	13 *The Rake's Progress*		
36 *Simon Boccanegra*	12 *La Cenerentola*		
35 *La Clemenza di Tito*	12 *Ernani*		
35 *Il Tabarro*	12 *The Great Gatsby*		
	12 *Moses und Aron*		

Totals include tour and concert performances

Premieres During Levine's Tenure

1976	*Esclarmonde* (Massenet)	1996	*A Midsummer Night's Dream* (Britten)
1977	*Dialogues of the Carmelites* (Poulenc)	1997	*La Cenerentola** (Rossini)
1977	*Lulu** (Berg)	1998	*Capriccio* (R. Strauss)
1978	*Billy Budd* (Britten)	1999	*Moses und Aron** (Schoenberg)
1979	*Rise and Fall of the City of Mahagonny** (Weill)	1999	*Susannah* (Floyd)
1981	*Parade* (Satie)	1999	*The Great Gatsby**† (Harbison)
1981	*Les Mamelles de Tirésias* (Poulenc)	2000	*The Merry Widow* (Lehár)
1981	*L'Enfant et les Sortilèges* (Ravel)	2001	*Doktor Faust* (Busoni)
1981	*Le Sacre du Printemps** (Stravinsky)	2001	*The Gambler* (Prokofiev)
1981	*Oedipus Rex** (Stravinsky)	2002	*War and Peace* (Prokofiev)
1982	*Idomeneo** (Mozart)	2002	*Sly* (Wolf-Ferrari)
1984	*Rinaldo* (Handel)	2002	*Il Pirata* (Bellini)
1984	*La Clemenza di Tito** (Mozart)	2002	*A View from the Bridge* (Bolcom)
1985	*Porgy and Bess** (Gershwin)	2003	*Benvenuto Cellini** (Berlioz)
1986	*Samson* (Handel)	2004	*Rodelinda* (Handel)
1988	*Giulio Cesare* (Handel)	2005	*Cyrano de Bergerac* (Alfano)
1989	*Erwartung** (Schoenberg)	2005	*An American Tragedy*† (Picker)
1991	*Káťa Kabanová* (Janáček)	2006	*Mazeppa* (Tchaikovsky)
1991	*The Ghosts of Versailles**† (Corigliano-Hoffman)	2006	*The First Emperor*† (Dun)
1992	*The Voyage*† (Glass)	2008	*Satyagraha* (Glass)
1993	*Stiffelio** (Verdi)	2008	*Doctor Atomic* (Adams)
1993	*Rusalka* (Dvořák)	2009	*From the House of the Dead* (Janáček)
1993	*I Lombardi** (Verdi)	2010	*Attila* (Verdi)
1994	*Lady Macbeth of Mtsensk* (Shostakovich)	2010	*The Nose* (Shostakovich)
1996	*The Makropulos Case* (Janáček)	2010	*Armida* (Rossini)

* Conducted by James Levine
† World Premiere

Opening Nights

September 17, 1973
Il Trovatore

September 23, 1974
I Vespri Siciliani

September 18, 1978
Tannhäuser

September 24, 1979
Otello

December 10, 1980
Mahler:
Symphony No. 2 in C Minor

September 21, 1981
Norma

September 20, 1982
Der Rosenkavalier

September 26, 1983
Les Troyens

September 24, 1984
Lohengrin

September 22, 1986
Die Walküre

September 21, 1987
Otello

September 26, 1988
Il Trovatore

September 25, 1989
Aida

September 23, 1991
25th Anniversary of Metropolitan
Opera House at Lincoln Center
Rigoletto: Act III
Otello: Act III
Die Fledermaus: Act II

September 21, 1992
Les Contes d'Hoffmann

September 27, 1993
Plácido Domingo and Luciano
Pavarotti's 25th Anniversary
Die Walküre: Act I
Otello: Act I
Il Trovatore: Act III

September 26, 1994
Il Tabarro/Pagliacci

October 2, 1995
Otello

September 30, 1996
Andrea Chénier

September 22, 1997
Carmen

September 28, 1998
Samson et Dalila

September 25, 2000
Don Giovanni

September 24, 2001
A Celebration of Giuseppe Verdi
Un Ballo in Maschera: Act I
Otello: Act III
Rigoletto: Act III

September 23, 2002
Opening Night Gala Performance
Fedora: Act II
Samson et Dalila: Act II
Otello: Act IV

September 20, 2004
Otello

September 19, 2005
Opening Night Gala Performance
Le Nozze di Figaro: Act I
Tosca: Act II
Samson et Dalila: Act III

September 25, 2006
Madama Butterfly

September 24, 2007
Lucia di Lammermoor

September 22, 2008
Opening Night Gala Starring
Renée Fleming
James Levine conducted
La Traviata: Act II

September 21, 2009
Tosca

September 27, 2010
Das Rheingold

Telecasts

April 22, 1972
Metropolitan Opera Gala
Honoring Sir Rudolf Bing

March 15, 1977*
La Bohème
Scotto, Niska, Pavarotti,
Wixell, Plishka

November 7, 1977*
Rigoletto
Cotrubas, Jones, Domingo,
MacNeil, Díaz

April 5, 1978*
Cavalleria Rusticana/Pagliacci
Troyanos, Domingo, Shinall
Stratas, Domingo, Milnes

September 25, 1978*
Otello
Scotto, Kraft, Vickers,
Gibbs, MacNeil

November 21, 1978*
The Bartered Bride
Stratas, Gedda, Vickers, Talvela

January 20, 1979*
Luisa Miller
Scotto, Kraft, Domingo, Milnes,
Giaiotti, Morris

September 24, 1979
Otello
Cruz-Romo, Love, Domingo,
Ciannella, Milnes

November 27, 1979*
Rise and Fall of the City of Mahagonny
Stratas, Varnay, Cassilly, MacNeil

February 16, 1980*
Elektra
Nilsson, Rysanek, Dunn,
Nagy, McIntyre

February 21, 1980*
Don Carlo
Scotto, Troyanos, Moldoveanu,
Milnes, Plishka, Hines

February 24, 1980
Gala of Stars

March 29, 1980*
Manon Lescaut
Scotto, Domingo, Elvira

December 20, 1980*
Lulu
Migenes, Lear, Riegel, Mazura

March 28, 1981
La Traviata
Cotrubas, Domingo, MacNeil

November 14, 1981*
Il Trittico
Scotto, Taillon, Moldoveanu,
MacNeil, Bacquier

December 15, 1981
Rigoletto
Eda-Pierre, Jones, Pavarotti,
Quilico, Berberian

January 16, 1982*
La Bohème
Stratas, Scotto, Carreras,
Stilwell, Morris

February 28, 1982*
In Concert at the Met
Troyanos, Domingo

March 28, 1982*
In Concert at the Met
Price, Horne

October 7, 1982*
Der Rosenkavalier
Te Kanawa, Troyanos, Blegen,
Pavarotti, Hammond-Stroud, Moll

November 6, 1982*
Idomeneo
Cotrubas, Behrens, von Stade,
Pavarotti, Alexander

December 20, 1982*
Tannhäuser
Marton, Troyanos, Cassilly,
Weikl, Macurdy

January 30, 1983*
In Concert at the Met
Domingo, Milnes

March 26, 1983*
Don Carlo
Freni, Bumbry, Domingo, Quilico,
Ghiaurov, Furlanetto

October 8, 1983*
Les Troyens
Troyanos, Norman,
Domingo, Monk

October 22, 1983*
Metropolitan Opera Centennial Gala

December 17, 1983*
Ernani
Mitchell, Pavarotti,
Milnes, Raimondi

March 24, 1984*
La Forza del Destino
Price, Giacomini, Nucci, Giaiotti

April 7, 1984*
Francesca da Rimini
Scotto, Domingo, Lewis, MacNeil

December 29, 1984*
Simon Boccanegra
Tomowa-Sintow, Moldoveanu,
Milnes, Plishka

January 3, 1985
Aida
Price, Cossotto, McCracken,
Estes, Macurdy

December 14, 1985*
Le Nozze di Figaro
Vaness, Battle, von Stade,
Allen, Raimondi

January 10, 1986*
Lohengrin
Marton, Rysanek, Hofmann,
Roar, Macurdy

January 11, 1986*
L'Italiana in Algeri
Horne, Ahlstedt, Monk, Montarsolo

February 28, 1987*
Carmen
Mitchell, Baltsa, Carreras, Ramey

April 4, 1987*
Turandot
Marton, Mitchell, Domingo, Plishka

March 12, 1988*
Ariadne auf Naxos
Norman, Battle, Troyanos, King

June 4, 1988
Celebration Concert
Metropolitan Opera in Japan
Battle, Domingo

September 18, 1988*
In Recital at the Met
Pavarotti

October 15, 1988*
Il Trovatore
Marton, Zajick, Pavarotti,
Milnes, Wells

February 1, 1989
Bluebeard's Castle/Erwartung
Norman, Ramey

April 8, 1989*
Die Walküre
Behrens, Norman, Ludwig,
Lakes, Morris, Moll

October 7, 1989*
Aida
Millo, Zajick, Domingo,
Milnes, Burchuladze

April 5, 1990
Don Giovanni
Vaness, Mattila, Upshaw,
Hadley, Ramey, Furlanetto

April 23, 1990*
Das Rheingold
Ludwig, Jerusalem, Wlaschiha,
Morris, Rootering, Salminen

April 26, 1990*
Siegfried
Behrens, Svendén, Jerusalem,
Zednik, Wlaschiha, Morris

May 5, 1990*
Götterdämmerung
Behrens, Lisowska, Ludwig,
Jerusalem, Raffell, Salminen

January 26, 1991*
Un Ballo in Maschera
Millo, Blackwell, Quivar,
Pavarotti, Nucci

February 9, 1991*
Die Zauberflöte
Battle, Serra, Araiza, Hemm, Moll

September 23, 1991*
*The Silver Anniversary Gala
at Lincoln Center*

November 16, 1991*
L'Elisir d'Amore
Battle, Pavarotti, Pons, Dara

January 10, 1992*
The Ghosts of Versailles
Stratas, Fleming, Horne, Clark,
Quilico, Hagegård

March 28, 1992*
Parsifal
Meier, Jerusalem, Weikl,
Mazura, Moll

October 10, 1992*
Falstaff
Freni, Bonney, Horne,
Lopardo, Plishka, Pola

November 13, 1993*
Stiffelio
Sweet, Domingo, Chernov, Plishka

December 21, 1993
I Lombardi
Flanigan, Pavarotti,
Beccaria, Ramey

January 22, 1994*
Elektra
Behrens, Voigt, Fassbaender,
King, McIntyre

September 26, 1994*
Il Tabarro/Pagliacci
Stratas, Domingo, Pons
Stratas, Pavarotti, Pons

January 26, 1995*
Simon Boccanegra
Te Kanawa, Domingo,
Chernov, Lloyd

October 13, 1995*
Otello
Fleming, Bunnell, Domingo,
R. Croft, Morris

February 27, 1996
Così fan tutte
Vaness, Mentzer, Bartoli,
Hadley, D. Croft, Allen

March 12, 1996
La Forza del Destino
Sweet, Domingo,
Chernov, Scandiuzzi

April 27, 1996*
James Levine 25th Anniversary Gala

October 15, 1996
Andrea Chénier
Guleghina, White, Pavarotti, Pons

March 25, 1997
Carmen
Gheorghiu, Meier,
Domingo, Leiferkus

November 12, 1997
La Cenerentola
Bartoli, Vargas, Alaimo, Corbelli

September 28, 1998*
Samson et Dalila
Borodina, Domingo, Leiferkus

November 11, 1998
Le Nozze di Figaro
Fleming, Bartoli, Mentzer,
D. Croft, Terfel

November 22, 1998
*Luciano Pavarotti
30th Anniversary Gala*

December 18, 1999*
Tristan und Isolde
Eaglen, Dalayman, Heppner,
Ketelsen, Pape

October 14, 2000*
Don Giovanni
Fleming, Kringelborn, Hong,
Groves, Terfel, Furlanetto

October 28, 2000*
Fidelio
Mattila, Welch-Babidge, Heppner,
Polenzani, Struckmann, Pape

April 6, 2001*
Nabucco
Guleghina, White, Jones,
Pons, Ramey

October 6, 2001*
Wozzeck
Dalayman, Clark,
Neumann, Struckmann

December 8, 2001*
Die Meistersinger von Nürnberg
Mattila, Heppner, Polenzani,
Morris, Allen, Pape

April 3, 2003*
Ariadne auf Naxos
Voigt, Dessay, Mentzer, Margison

* Commercial Release

Live in HD

December 30, 2006*
The Magic Flute
Huang, Miklósa, Polenzani,
Gunn, Pape

April 28, 2007
Il Trittico
Guleghina, Frittoli, Mykytenko,
Blythe, Licitra, Pons, Corbelli

January 12, 2008*
Macbeth
Guleghina, Pittas, Lučić, Relyea

February 16, 2008*
Manon Lescaut
Mattila, Giordani, D. Croft

March 22, 2008
Tristan und Isolde
Voigt, DeYoung, Smith,
Schulte, Salminen

September 22, 2008
Opening Night Gala
Starring Renée Fleming
Fleming, Vargas, Hampson

November 22, 2008
La Damnation de Faust
Graham, Giordani, Relyea

January 24, 2009
Orfeo ed Euridice
de Niese, Murphy, Blythe

December 19, 2009
Les Contes d'Hoffmann
Kim, Netrebko, Gubanova,
Lindsey, Calleja, Held

February 6, 2010*
Simon Boccanegra
Pieczonka, Giordani,
Domingo, Morris

October 9, 2010
Das Rheingold
Blythe, R. Croft, Owens,
Terfel, Selig, König

November 13, 2010
Don Pasquale
Netrebko, Polenzani,
Kwiecien, Del Carlo

* Commercial Release

Outdoor Transmissions

SHOWN IN TIMES SQUARE
AND LINCOLN CENTER PLAZA

September 22, 2001*
World Trade Center Relief Benefit

May 11, 2002*
Tosca
Guleghina, Licitra, Morris

September 25, 2006
Madama Butterfly
Gallardo-Domas, Zifchak,
Giordani, D. Croft

September 24, 2007
Lucia di Lammermoor
Dessay, Giordani, Kwiecien, Relyea

September 22, 2008†
Opening Night Gala
Starring Renée Fleming
Fleming, Vargas, Hampson

September 21, 2009
Tosca
Mattila, Álvarez, Gagnidze

September 27, 2010
Das Rheingold
Blythe, R. Croft, Owens,
Terfel, Selig, König

* Lincoln Center Plaza only
† Times Square and
  Fordham University's
  Lincoln Center Campus

Feature Film

February 18, 1983
La Traviata
Stratas, Domingo, MacNeil

Recorded with the Metropolitan
Opera Orchestra and Chorus

Met Discography

1972
*Metropolitan Opera Gala
Honoring Sir Rudolf Bing
Manon Lescaut*: "Tu, tu, amore? Tu?"
Caballé, Domingo
DEUTSCHE GRAMMOPHON

1974
I Vespri Siciliani
Caballé, Gedda, Milnes, Díaz
METROPOLITAN OPERA
HISTORIC BROADCAST

1982
In Concert at The Met
Price, Horne
RCA

La Traviata
Original Motion Picture Soundtrack
Stratas, Domingo, MacNeil
ELEKTRA RECORDS

1985
Parsifal
Rysanek, Vickers, Estes, Mazura, Moll
METROPOLITAN OPERA
HISTORIC BROADCAST

1987
Die Walküre
Behrens, Norman, Ludwig,
Lakes, Morris, Moll
DEUTSCHE GRAMMOPHON

1988
Das Rheingold
Ludwig, Jerusalem, Wlaschiha,
Morris, Moll, Rootering
DEUTSCHE GRAMMOPHON

Siegfried
Behrens, Svendén, Goldberg,
Zednik, Wlaschiha, Morris
DEUTSCHE GRAMMOPHON

Live in Tokyo 1988
Battle, Domingo
DEUTSCHE GRAMMOPHON

1989
Schoenberg
Erwartung & Brettl-Lieder
Norman
PHILIPS

Götterdämmerung
Behrens, Studer, Schwarz,
Goldberg, Weikl, Salminen
DEUTSCHE GRAMMOPHON

L'Elisir d'Amore
Battle, Pavarotti, Nucci, Dara
DEUTSCHE GRAMMOPHON

The Compact *Ring*
Highlights from
Der Ring des Nibelungen
DEUTSCHE GRAMMOPHON

1990
Le Nozze di Figaro
Te Kanawa, Upshaw, von Otter,
Hampson, Furlanetto
DEUTSCHE GRAMMOPHON

Aida
Millo, Zajick, Domingo, Morris, Ramey
SONY

1991
Parsifal
Norman, Domingo, Morris,
Wlaschiha, Moll
DEUTSCHE GRAMMOPHON

Luisa Miller
Millo, Quivar, Domingo, Chernov,
Rootering, Plishka
SONY

Il Trovatore
Millo, Zajick, Domingo,
Chernov, Morris
SONY

Wagner Overtures & Preludes
The Met Orchestra
DEUTSCHE GRAMMOPHON

La Traviata
Studer, Pavarotti, Pons
DEUTSCHE GRAMMOPHON

1992
Don Carlo
Millo, Zajick, Sylvester, Chernov,
Furlanetto, Ramey
SONY

Verdi Ballet Music
The Met Orchestra
SONY

Mussorgsky *Pictures at an Exhibition*
& Stravinsky *Le Sacre du Printemps*
The Met Orchestra
DEUTSCHE GRAMMOPHON

Manon Lescaut
Freni, Pavarotti, D. Croft
DECCA

1993
Mozart Opera Arias
Battle
DEUTSCHE GRAMMOPHON

Rigoletto
Studer, Graves, Pavarotti,
Chernov, Scandiuzzi
DEUTSCHE GRAMMOPHON

Beethoven Symphony No. 3
("Eroica") & Schubert Symphony
No. 8 ("Unfinished")
The Met Orchestra
DEUTSCHE GRAMMOPHON

Berg *Wozzeck* Excerpts, Three
Pieces for Orchestra, *Lulu*-Suite
Fleming
SONY

1994
Idomeneo
Murphy, Vaness, Bartoli,
Domingo, Hampson
DEUTSCHE GRAMMOPHON

Der Fliegende Holländer
Voigt, Heppner, Morris, Rootering
SONY

Opera Arias
Terfel
DEUTSCHE GRAMMOPHON

1995
Wagner Orchestral Music
The Met Orchestra
DEUTSCHE GRAMMOPHON

Strauss *Don Quixote & Tod
und Verklärung*
The Met Orchestra
DEUTSCHE GRAMMOPHON

Maestro of The Met:
James Levine + Friends
Compilation
DEUTSCHE GRAMMOPHON

1996
James Levine's 25th Anniversary
Gala Excerpts
DEUTSCHE GRAMMOPHON

I Lombardi
Anderson, Pavarotti, Leech, Ramey
DECCA

1997
James Levine Anniversary
Collection
Compilation
METROPOLITAN OPERA
HISTORIC BROADCAST

1998
I Want Magic!
American Opera Arias
Fleming
DECCA

2009
Celebrating 125 Years: Historic
Met Performances 1937–2005
METROPOLITAN OPERA

2010
James Levine: Celebrating
40 Years at The Met
Collection
METROPOLITAN OPERA

Orchestral Concerts

Between May 3, 1991 and January 24, 2010, Levine conducted the MET Orchestra in 61 concerts at Carnegie Hall.

May 3, 1991
Berg: Three Pieces for Orchestra, Op. 6
Berlioz: *La Mort de Cléopâtre*
    Norman
Wagner: *Siegfried Idyll*
Wagner: Immolation Scene,
    from *Götterdämmerung*
    Norman
Wagner: Overture to *Rienzi* (Encore)

May 5, 1992
Mahler: Ten songs from
    Des Knaben Wunderhorn
    Hampson
Mussorgsky/Ravel: *Pictures at an Exhibition*
Wagner: Prelude to Act III, from *Die
    Meistersinger von Nürnberg* (Encore)

May 9, 1992
Mozart: Piano Concerto No. 12 in A Major,
    K. 414
    Levine, piano
Mahler: *Das Lied von der Erde*
    Meier, Sylvester

February 28, 1993
Schubert: Symphony No. 8 in B Minor,
    D. 759 ("Unfinished")
Berg: Seven Early Songs
    Meier
Stravinsky: *Le Sacre du Printemps*
Sibelius: *Valse Triste* (Encore)
Dvořák: Slavonic Dance, Op. 72, No. 7
    (Encore)

May 9, 1993
Berg: Three Excerpts from *Wozzeck*
    Fleming
Berg: Violin Concerto
    Perlman, violin
Berg: Symphonic Pieces from *Lulu*
    Fleming
Berg: Three Pieces for Orchestra, Op. 6

March 6, 1994
Bolcom: Fantasia Concertante
    Ouzounian, viola
    Grossman, cello
Mahler: *Rückert-Lieder*
    Horne
Beethoven: Symphony No. 3 in E-flat Major

May 1, 1994
Mozart: "Ch'io mi scordi di te?...Non temer,
    amato bene" K. 505
    Bartoli
    Levine, piano
R. Strauss: *Tod und Verklärung*
Ravel: "Vocalise-étude in the form
    of a Habanera"
Berlioz: "Zaïde"
Mozart: "Deh vieni non tardar"
    from *Le Nozze di Figaro* (Encore)

Rossini: "Nacqui all'affano"
    from *La Cenerentola* (Encore)
    Bartoli
Debussy: *La Mer*
Rossini: "Non più mesta"
    from La Cenerentola (Encore)
    Bartoli

January 22, 1995
R. Strauss: *Le Bourgeois Gentilhomme* Suite
    Gniewek, violin
R. Strauss: Four Songs, Op. 27
R. Strauss: *Four Last Songs*
    M. Price
R. Strauss: *Don Quixote*
    Grossman, cello
    Ouzounian, viola

February 26, 1995
Dvořák: Romance in F Minor for Violin
    and Orchestra, Op. 11
    Gniewek, violin
Schuller: *Of Reminiscences and Reflections*
Mahler: *Das Lied von der Erde*
    Heppner, Hampson

May 7, 1995
Stravinsky: *Firebird* Suite
Liebermann: Concerto for Flute
    and Orchestra, Op. 39
    Galway, flute
Doppler/Galway: Andante and Rondo
    for Two Flutes and Orchestra
    Galway, flute
    Parloff, flute
"Brian Boru March" (Encore)
"The Londonderry Air" (Encore)
Rimsky-Korsakov: "The Flight of the
    Bumble-Bee" from *Tsar Sultan* (Encore)
    Galway, flute
Gershwin: *An American in Paris*
Brahms: Hungarian Dance No. 1 (Encore)

October 15, 1995
Mahler: *Kindertotenlieder*
    Terfel
Mahler: Symphony No. 6 in A Minor

March 10, 1996
Mozart: Symphony No. 38 in D Major
Wagner: *Wesendonck Lieder*
Wagner: "Träume" (Encore)
    Norman
Cage: *Atlas Eclipticalis*
Prokofiev: Symphony No. 5 in B-flat Major

April 21, 1996
Bartók: *The Miraculous Mandarin* Suite,
    Sz. 73
Bartók: Violin Concerto No. 2, Sz. 112
    Chang, violin
Brahms: Symphony No. 1 in C Minor,
    Op. 68

October 20, 1996
Mozart: Piano Concerto No. 24 in C Minor,
    K. 491
    Perahia, piano

Mahler: Symphony No. 4 in G Major
    Murphy
    Gniewek, violin

November 10, 1996
Berlioz: *La Damnation de Faust*, Op. 24
    von Otter, Sabbatini, van Dam, Robbins

December 8, 1996
Verdi: Requiem
    Fleming, Quivar, Pavarotti, Ramey

November 9, 1997
Rossini: Overture to *Semiramide*
Haydn: Sinfonia Concertante in B-flat Major
    Gniewek, violin
    Grossman, cello
    Ferrillo, oboe
    Rogers, bassoon
Gluck: "Oh, del mio dolce ardor"
    from *Paride ed Elena*
Handel: "Lascia la spina" from *Il Trionfo
    del Tempo e del Disinganno*
Haydn: "Al tuo seno fortunato"
    from *L'Anima del Filosofo*
    Bartoli
Mendelssohn: Symphony No. 4 in A Major,
    Op. 90 ("Italian")
Rossini: "Bel raggio lusinghier"
    from *Semiramide* (Encore)
    Bartoli

February 22, 1998
Bach: Fugue (Ricercar) in Six Voices
    from *The Musical Offering*
Tchaikovsky: Violin Concerto in D Major,
    Op. 35
    Vengerov, violin
Ligeti: *Atmosphères*
Berlioz: *Symphonie Fantastique*, Op. 14

May 10, 1998
Brahms: Piano Concerto No. 1 in D Minor,
    Op. 15
Brahms: Hungarian Dances Nos. 1, 3, and 2
    (Encores)
    Kissin, piano
Tan Dun: *Death and Fire*
Ravel: Suite No. 2 from *Daphnis et Chlöe*

November 15, 1998
Mozart: Bassoon Concerto in B-flat Major,
    K. 191
    Rogers, bassoon
Babbitt: Piano Concerto No. 2*
    Taub, piano
Ives: *The Unanswered Question*
Ives: *Central Park in the Dark*
Dvořák: Symphony No. 8 in G Major,
    Op. 88

April 25, 1999
Mozart: Symphony No. 41 in C Major,
    K. 551 ("Jupiter")
Mahler: *Das Lied von der Erde*
    von Otter, Heppner

May 2, 1999
Mozart: Clarinet Concerto in A Major,
    K. 622
    Morales, basset clarinet
Mozart: Piano Concerto No. 20 in D Minor,
    K. 466
    Brendel, piano
Webern: Symphony, Op. 21
Brahms: Symphony No. 2 in D Major,
    Op. 73
Brahms: Hungarian Dance No. 1 (Encore)

November 7, 1999 Matinee
Wagner: Prelude to Act I,
    from *Die Meistersinger von Nürnberg*
Cage: *Atlas Eclipticalis*
Schuller: *Of Reminiscences and Reflections*
Milhaud: *Le Boeuf sur le Toit*, Op. 58
Rachmaninoff: Piano Concerto No. 2
    in C Minor, Op. 18
Rachmaninoff: Prelude in C-sharp Minor
    (Encore)
Rachmaninoff: Prelude in G Minor (Encore)
    Kissin, piano

December 5, 1999
Schoenberg: *Verklärte Nacht*
Messiaen: *Et exspecto resurrectionem
    mortuorum*
Ravel: *Shéhérazade*
    Borodina
Debussy: *Danse Sacrée and Danse Profane*
    Hoffman, harp
Berlioz: *La Mort de Cléopâtre*
    Borodina

May 10, 2000
Verdi: Overture to *La Forza del Destino*
Tchaikovsky: "Polonaise"
    from Eugene Onegin
Smetana: "Polka" from *The Bartered Bride*
R. Strauss: "Dance of the Seven Veils"
    from *Salome*
Mozart: "Giunse alfin...Deh vieni non
    tardar," from *Le Nozze di Figaro*
Stravinsky: "Quietly, night,"
    from *The Rake's Progress*
    McNair
Berg: Symphonic Pieces from *Lulu*
    Welch-Babidge
Wagner: *A Faust Overture*
Wagner: Prelude and Liebestod,
    from *Tristan und Isolde*

May 21, 2000
Bartók: *Bluebeard's* Castle, Sz. 48
    von Otter, Ramey, Krénusz
Bartók's Concerto for Orchestra, Sz. 116
J. Strauss: "Ohne Sorgen" Polka (Encore)
Massenet: "Meditation" from *Thaïs* (Encore)
    Gniewek, violin

December 3, 2000
    Gergiev, conductor
Scriabin: *Prometheus, The Poem of Fire*
    Toradze, piano
Shostakovich: Symphony No. 4 in C minor

March 11, 2001
Mahler: Symphony No. 9

April 29, 2001
Verdi: Requiem
    Fleming, Borodina, Giordani, Pape

May 6, 2001
Schoenberg: *Gurrelieder*
    Voigt, Urmana, Heppner, Polenzani,
    Fink, Haefliger

January 27, 2002
Berg: *Seven Early Songs*
    Fleming
Mahler: Symphony No. 6 in A Minor

May 5, 2002
Haydn: *The Creation*
    Hong, Bostridge, Pape

May 19, 2002
Bolcom: Seventh Symphony:
    A Symphonic Concerto*
Mozart: Symphony No. 41 in C Major,
    K. 551 ("Jupiter")
R. Strauss: Burleske in D Minor
    for Piano and Orchestra
    Thibaudet, piano
Ravel: *Boléro*

October 13, 2002
Nielsen: Concerto for Flute and Orchestra,
    Op. 119
    Parloff, flute
Shen: Legend for Percussion and Orchestra*
    Zuber, percussion
Mahler: Symphony No. 1 in D Major

February 2, 2003
Mozart: Sinfonia Concertante for Violin
    and Viola in E-flat Major, K. 364
    Eanet, violin
    Ouzounian, viola
Brahms: Double Concerto in A Minor
    for Violin and Cello, Op. 102
    Chan, violin
    Figueroa, cello
Rachmaninoff: Piano Concerto No. 3
    in D Minor, Op. 30
Bizet/Volodos: *Carmen* Variations (Encore)
    Volodos, piano

May 10, 2003
Berlioz: Overture to *Benvenuto Cellini,*
    Op. 23
Berlioz: *Roman Carnival* Overture, Op. 9
Berlioz: *La Mort de Cléopâtre*
    Borodina
Berlioz: *Symphonie Fantastique,* Op. 14

May 11, 2003
Berlioz: *Le Corsaire*: Overture
Berlioz: *Harold in Italy*
    Ouzounian, viola
Berlioz: *Symphonie Fantastique*

May 16, 2003
Brahms: *Schicksalslied,* Op. 54
Stravinsky: Symphony of Psalms
Mozart: Mass in C Minor, K. 427
    Murphy, Graham, Polenzani, Relyea

May 18, 2003
Brahms: *Schicksalslied,* Op. 54
Stravinsky: Symphony of Psalms
Mozart: Mass in C Minor, K. 427
    Murphy, Graham, Polenzani, Relyea

October 12, 2003
Berlioz: *Le Corsaire* Overture
Berlioz: *Harold in Italy,* Op. 16
    Ouzounian, viola
Brahms: Piano Concerto No. 2
    in B-flat Major, Op. 83
Mendelssohn: Scherzo in B Minor (Encore)
Chopin: *Valse Brillante,* Op. 34, No. 3
    (Encore)
Brahms: Hungarian Dance No. 1 (Encore)
Brahms: Waltz in A-flat Major, Op. 39,
    No. 15 (Encore)
    Kissin, piano

May 16, 2004
Schoenberg: *Pelleas und Melisande*
Wolf: "Kennst du das Land"
    Borodina
Brahms: Symphony No. 4 in E Minor,
    Op. 98

May 21, 2004
R. Strauss: Concerto for Oboe
    and Small Orchestra
Ravel: *Don Quichotte à Dulcinée*
Mahler: *Lieder eines fahrenden Gesellen*
    Hvorostovsky
Beethoven: Symphony No. 7 in A Major,
    Op. 92

May 23, 2004
Berg: Violin Concerto
Bach: Largo from Sonata in C Major
    (Encore)
    Tetzlaff, violin
Mahler: Symphony No. 9

January 9, 2005
Weber: Overture to *Euryanthe*
Brahms: Violin Concerto in D Major, Op. 77
    Shaham, violin
Varèse: *Amériques*
Gershwin: *An American in Paris*

January 23, 2005
Weber: Overture to *Oberon*
Carter: Variations for Orchestra
Mahler: *Das Lied von der Erde*
    von Otter, Heppner

January 30, 2005 Matinee
Weber: Overture to *Der Freischütz*
Webern: Symphony, Op. 21
Mozart: "Mentre ti lascio," K. 513
Mendelssohn: "Es ist genug," from *Elijah*

Mahler: Three songs from *Rückert-Lieder*
    van Dam
Wuorinen: *Grand Bamboula,*
    for String Orchestra
Dvořák: Symphony No. 8 in G Major,
    Op. 88

January 8, 2006
Tchaikovsky: *Romeo and Juliet*
    Fantasy Overture
Tchaikovsky: "Letter Scene,"
    from *Eugene Onegin*
Berg: Five Orchestral Songs, Op. 4
    ("Altenberg Lieder")
    Fleming
Wagner: Overture and Venusberg Music
    from *Tannhäuser*
R. Strauss: Final Scene from *Capriccio*
    Fleming, Robbins

January 29, 2006
Bartók: Suite from *The Miraculous Mandarin,*
    Sz. 73
Schoenberg: *Erwartung*
    Silja
Stravinsky: *Le Sacre du Printemps*

January 14, 2007
Brahms: Symphony No. 3 in F Major,
    Op. 90
Wuorinen: *Theologoumenon**
Beethoven: Violin Concerto in D Major,
    Op. 61
Bach: Sonata in C, Allegro Assai (Encore)
    Tetzlaff, violin

May 13, 2007
Carter: *Three Illusions*
Mendelssohn: Symphony No. 3 in A Minor,
    Op. 56 ("Scottish")
Carter: *Dialogues* for Piano
    and Chamber Orchestra
    Hodges, piano
Mozart: Symphony No. 41 in C Major,
    K. 551 ("Jupiter")

May 20, 2007
R. Strauss: *Le Bourgeois Gentilhomme* Suite
Schoenberg: "Lied der Waldtaube,"
    from *Gurrelieder*
    DeYoung
Thomas: Overture to *Mignon*
Berlioz: *La Mort de Cléopâtre*
Wagner: "Träume" (Encore)
    DeYoung
Ravel: Suite No. 2 from *Daphnis et Chlöe*

February 17, 2008
Webern: Six Pieces for Orchestra, Op. 6
Mozart: Piano Concerto No. 24 in C Minor,
    K. 491
Beethoven: Bagatelle, Op. 33 (Encore)
    Brendel, piano
Berg: Three Pieces for Orchestra, Op. 6
R. Strauss: Final Scene from *Salome*
    Voigt

May 22, 2008
Carter: Variations for Orchestra
Schumann: Piano Concerto in A Minor,
    Op. 54
    Biss, piano
Tchaikovsky: Symphony No. 4 in F Minor,
    Op. 36

October 5, 2008
Beethoven: *Grosse Fuge* in B-flat Major,
    Op. 133
Messiaen: *Et exspecto resurrectionem
    mortuorum*
Brahms: Violin Concerto in D Major, Op. 77
J. S. Bach: Partita No.3 in E Major,
    Gavotte en rondeau (Encore)
    Tetzlaff, violin

January 25, 2009
Mozart: "Ch'io mi scordi di te?...Non temer,
    amato bene" K. 505
    DiDonato
    Levine, piano
Wuorinen: *Time Regained,*
    a Fantasy for Piano and Orchestra*
    Serkin, piano
Rossini: *La Regata Veneziana*
Rossini: "Non più mesta"
    from *La Cenerentola* (Encore)
    DiDonato
Mendelssohn: Symphony No. 4 in A Major,
    Op. 90 ("Italian")

May 21, 2009
Stravinsky: *Pétrouchka*
Brahms: Piano Concerto No. 1 in D Minor,
    Op.15
    Lang, piano

December 20, 2009
Elgar: *Sea Pictures,* Op. 37
    Blythe
Mahler: Symphony No. 5 in C-sharp Minor

January 24, 2010
Schubert: Symphony No. 8 in B Minor,
    D. 759 ("Unfinished")
R. Strauss: "Das Bächlein" Op. 88, No. 1
R. Strauss: "Ich wollt' ein Sträusslein
    binden" Op. 68, No. 2
R. Strauss: "Allerseelen" Op. 10, No. 8
R. Strauss: "Zueignung" Op. 10, No. 1
R. Strauss: "Morgen" Op. 27, No. 4
R. Strauss: "Ständchen" Op. 17, No. 2
R. Strauss: "Wiegenlied" Op. 41, No. 1
R. Strauss: "Amor" Op. 68, No. 5
R. Strauss: "Grossmächtige Prinzessin"
    from *Ariadne auf Naxos*
R. Strauss: Rondo from "Grossmächtige
    Prinzessin" (Encore)
    Damrau
Beethoven: Symphony No. 5 in C Minor,
    Op. 67

* World Premieres

Chamber Repertoire

Between October 1998 and October 2010, Levine led the MET Chamber Ensemble in 38 concerts at Carnegie Hall's Weill Recital Hall and Zankel Hall.

Andriessen: *Hout* for Tenor Saxophone, Marimba, Guitar and Piano

Babbitt: *All Set* for Jazz Ensemble, *Phenomena* for Soprano and Tape, *The Head of the Bed, Three Theatrical Songs, Two Sonnets*

Bach: Brandenburg Concerti Nos. 1–6, Cantata: *Ich habe genug*

Bartók: *Contrasts* for Clarinet, Violin and Piano

Beethoven: Quintet for Piano and Winds, Septet for Strings and Winds

Berg: Chamber Concerto for Piano and Violin with 13 Wind Instruments, Four Pieces for Clarinet and Piano

Berlioz: Excerpts from *Les Nuits d'été*

Boulez: *Dérive I, Improvisation I sur Mallarmé, Improvisation II sur Mallarmé, Mémoriale (... explosante-fixe ... Originel), sur Incises*

Brahms: *Liebeslieder-Walzer, Neue Liebeslieder,* Serenade No. 2, Two Songs with Viola Obbligato

Cage: *Amores* for Prepared Piano and Percussion, *Living Room Music* for Percussion and Speech Quartet

Carter: *A Mirror on Which to Dwell; Dialogues* for Piano and Chamber Orchestra; *In Sleep, in Thunder; In the Distances of Sleep**; *Luimen;* Sonata for Flute, Oboe, Cello and Harpsichord; *Syringa; Tempo e tempi*

Dallapiccola: *Commiato* for Soprano and Chamber Ensemble; *Piccola musica notturna; Tre poemi* for Soprano and Chamber Orchestra

Debussy: *Chansons de Bilitis, Danse sacrée et danse profane,* Sonata for Cello and Piano

Dutilleux: *Les Citations*: Diptych for Oboe, Harpsichord, Double Bass and Percussion

Feldman: "The Viola in My Life (I)"

Foss: *Time Cycle* (chamber version)

Harbison: *Between Two Worlds; Mottetti di Montale;* Music for Eighteen Winds; *North and South; November 19, 1828*

Kirchner: *Music for Twelve*

Kurtág: *Hommage à R. Sch.*

Ligeti: Chamber Concerto for 13 Instrumentalists, *Ramifications* for 12 Solo Strings

Mendelssohn: Octet for Strings

Messiaen: *Quatuor pour la fin du temps*

Milhaud: *La Création du monde, Le Boeuf sur le toit, Sonatine* for Viola and Cello

Mozart: Divertimento, K. 287; Divertimento, K. 131; Piano Concerto No. 12, K. 414; Quartet for Piano and Strings, K. 478; Quintet for Piano and Winds, K. 452; *Gran Partita,* K. 361; Serenade for Strings, *Eine kleine Nachtmusik,* K. 525; Sonata for Violin and Piano, K. 296; String Quintet, K. 516; Trio for Violin, Cello and Piano, K. 502; Trio for Viola, Clarinet and Piano, K. 498, *Kegelstatt*

Perle: Serenade No. 1 for Viola and Chamber Ensemble

Poulenc: *Le Bal masqué*; Sonata for Clarinet and Piano; Trio for Piano, Oboe and Bassoon

Ravel: *Chansons madécasses, Don Quichotte à Dulcinée, Trois poèmes de Stéphane Mallarmé*

Satie: *Socrate,* symphonic drama in three parts; *Trois mélodies*

Schoenberg: Chamber Symphony for 15 Solo Instruments, Op. 9; Five Orchestral Pieces, Op. 16 (chamber version); Six Little Piano Pieces, Op. 19; *Pierrot lunaire,* Op. 21; Serenade, Op. 24

Schubert: *Auf dem Strom, Der Hirt auf dem Felsen, Quartettsatz,* Octet for Strings and Winds, *Trout* Quintet for Piano and Strings, "Grand Duo" for Piano Four-Hands

Schuller: Grand Concerto for Percussion and Keyboards

Schumann: Fantasy Pieces for Clarinet and Piano; duets for tenor and soprano: *Ich denke dein, In der Nacht, Liebhabers Ständchen, Tanzlied, Unterm Fenster*; Quintet for Piano and Strings; Romances for Oboe and Piano

J. Strauss, Jr.: *Kaiserwalzer* (arr. Schoenberg), *Rosen aus dem Süden* (arr. Schoenberg)

R. Strauss: *Le Bourgeois Gentilhomme* Suite, *Metamorphosen*: Study for 23 Solo Strings

Stravinsky: *Histoire du soldat,* Octet for Wind Instruments, *Ragtime, Renard,* Three Pieces for Clarinet Solo

Varèse: *Density 21.5* for Solo Flute, *Octandre* for Eight Instruments

Verdi: String Quartet

Wagner: *Siegfried Idyll*

Webern: Four Pieces for Violin and Piano, Op. 7; Three Little Pieces for Cello and Piano, Op. 11; Four Songs, Op. 12; Six Songs, Op. 14; Five Canons, Op. 16; Three Traditional Rhymes, Op. 17; Three Songs, Op. 18; Concerto for Nine Instruments, Op. 24

Wolf (orch. Stravinsky): Two Sacred Songs from *Spanisches Liederbuch*

Wuorinen: *New York Notes, Dante Trilogy* (chamber version), *The Great Procession, The River of Light* (chamber version)

Xenakis: *La Déesse Athéna*

* World Premieres

Index

Photo Credits

For the Metropolitan Opera

Ken Howard
63, 82 (*Act II*), 106 (*Act I*), 153 (*Fleming*), 168, 174–175, 184, 187, 188, 189, 190, 191, 193, 194, 196, 197, 198–199, 200, 201, 202 (*Domingo; chorus*), 203, 205, 206–207, 207, 208, 209, 211, 213

Marty Sohl
94, 156 (*scene*), 163 (*Heppner*), 178, 183, 185, 192, 195, 202 (*bows*), 204 (*Schenk and Levine*), 210, 212

Beatriz Schiller
64, 106 (*Act II*)

Robert Caplin
204 (*Gelb, Levine, and Morris*)

For the Metropolitan Opera Archives

Louis Mélançon
16 (*Bing*), 18, 19, 20, 21, 22 (*stage*), 24, 26, 27, 29, 30, 31, 32, 33

James Heffernan
12–13, 34, 35, 36–37, 38, 39, 40, 41, 42, 43, 45 (*Hines, van Dam, and Stratas*), 46–47, 48, 49, 52 (*scene; Milnes and Giacomini*), 53, 56 (*Orth and Moll*), 58–59, 60 (*Rysanek and Nilsson*), 61, 70, 132

Winnie Klotz
52 (*Scotto*), 55, 66–67, 71, 74, 75, 76–77, 78, 79, 80, 81, 82 (*Act III*), 83, 84, 85, 86, 87, 88, 90 (*scene*), 91, 92, 93, 97, 98, 99, 100 (*Levine and Taddei*), 101 (*von Stade*), 102, 103, 104, 105, 107 (*Marton*), 108, 109, 112–113, 113, 114, 115, 117, 118, 119, 128–129, 133, 134, 135, 136, 138, 139, 140, 141, 142, 143, 144, 147, 148, 149, 151, 152, 153 (*Fleming and Domingo; Domingo*), 154, 156 (*Domingo*), 157, 160, 161, 162, 163 (*Voigt and Polaski; Voigt and Heppner*), 164, 165, 166 (*Racette; Álvarez*), 167, 169, 170–171, 179, 180, 181

Hastings-Willinger & Associates
8

Archival material
11, 15, 17, 22 (*program*)

Special Contributors

© Brigitte Lacombe
214–215

Copyright © Beth Bergman
23 (1972), 28 (1973), 45 (*Stratas and Gibbs,* 1977), 50 (1978), 54 (1979), 56 (*scene,* 1979), 57 (1979), 60 (*bows,* 1980), 95 (1984), 99 (1985), 100 (*Raimondi and Battle,* 1985), 101 (*Allen and Vaness,* 1985), 107 (*Zeffirelli and Domingo,* 1987), 116 (1990)

© Henry Grossman
51, 90 (*Domingo, Troyanos, Levine, and Norman*), 146, 155, 158, 159 (*Morris; von Stade; Levine*)

© Steve Sherman
inside front cover, 62, 65, 120, 121, 123, 124, 125, 126–127, 150, 166 (*composers*), 173

© Koichi Miura
cover, 110, 111, 131, 177

© Jörg Reichardt
69

© Evan Schneider
inside back cover, 159

© Christian Steiner
137

From TIME Magazine, 1/17/1983
©1983 Time Inc. Used under license.
89

Courtesy of James Levine
16 (*Levine*), 72–73, 145, 172

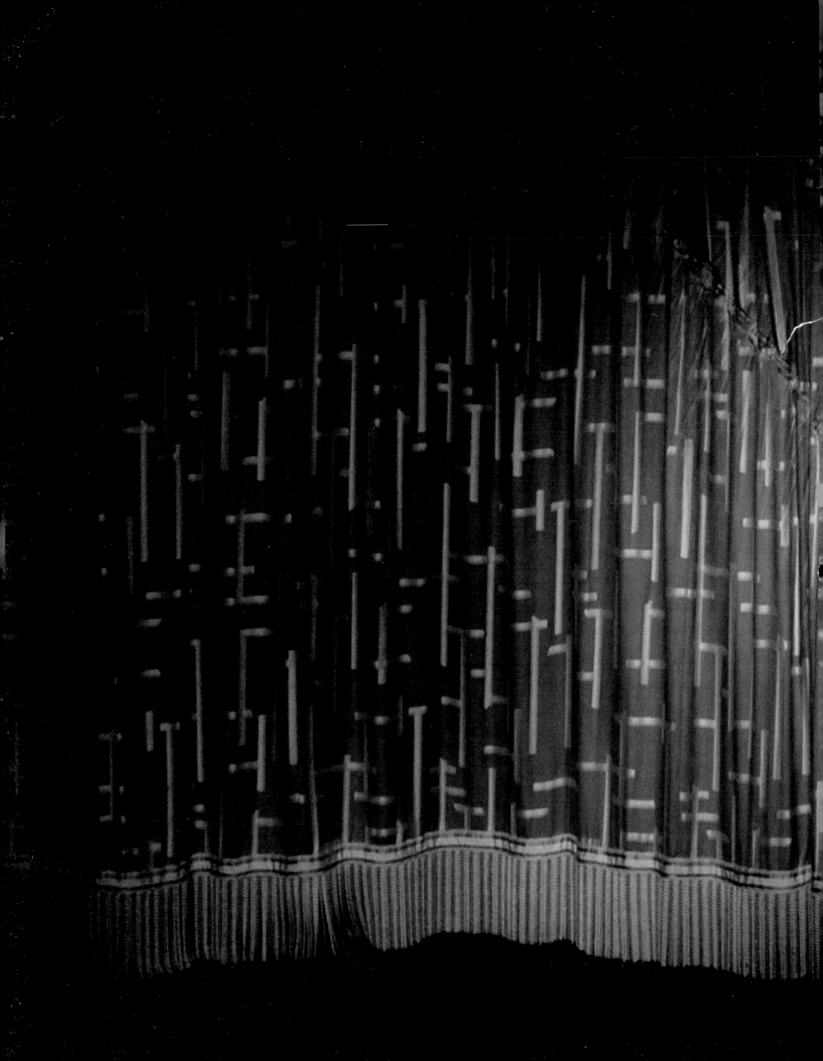